Publications of the

CENTRE FOR REFORMATION AND RENAISSANCE STUDIES

SERIES EDITOR Konrad Eisenbichler

Essays and Studies, 7

Victoria University
in the
University of Toronto

Sins of the Flesh

Responding to Sexual Disease in Early Modern Europe

EDITED BY KEVIN SIENA

Toronto
Centre for Reformation and Renaissance Studies
2005

CRRS Publications
Centre for Reformation and Renaissance Studies
Victoria University in the University of Toronto
Toronto, Ontario M5S 1K7
Canada

Tel: 416/585-4465
Fax: 416/585-4430
Email: crrs.publications@utoronto.ca
www.crrs.ca

Printed in Canada

Library and Archives Canada Cataloguing in Publication

Siena, Kevin Patrick
Sins of the flesh : responding to sexual disease in early modern Europe / by Kevin Siena.

Essays and studies ; 7)
Includes bibliographical references and index.
ISBN 0-7727-2029-0
1. Sexually transmitted diseases—Europe—History—16th century.
2. Sexually transmitted diseases—Europe—History—17th century.
3. Sexually transmitted diseases—treatment—Europe—History—16th century.
4. Sexually transmitted diseases—Treatment—Europe—History—17th century.
5. Sexually transmitted diseases in literature. I. Victoria University Toronto, Ont.).
Centre for Reformation and Renaissance Studies II. Title. III. Series: Essays and studies (Victoria University (Toronto, Ont.). Centre for Reformation and Renaissance Studies) ; 7.

RC201.6.A1S54 2005 306.4'61 C2005-901669-8

The editor and publisher gratefully acknowledge the generous support of the Social Sciences and Humanities Research Council of Canada, The Lupina Foundation through the Comparative Program on Health and Society, and Trent University.

Cover illustration:
Palma il Giovane. "Mars and Venus" (National Library, London)

Cover design: Ian MacKenzie, Paragraphics
Typesetting: Becker Associates

Table of Contents

Introduction

> Some are covered from the head to the knee with a rough scabies dotted with black and hideous lumps, which spares no part of the face (except the eyes), the neck, the chest, or the pubis. They had become so filthy and repugnant that... they hoped to die...Others by contrast, moaned and wept and uttered heartrending cries because of the ulceration of their male organ.[1]46
>
> Joseph Grünpeck, 1503

> For to refraine the filthy lusts of men and women, God hath permitted thys sickness to raigne among them, as a punishment for sinne.[2]46
>
> Surgeon Peter Lowe, 1596

When people wished a pox upon someone in early modern Europe they meant business. Along with plague, the pox (the most common English term for the disease traditionally thought to be syphilis) stood as one of the most evocative and frightening physical disorders of the day. As Grünpeck's quotation illustrates, the disease was portrayed as horribly debilitating and intensely painful. Its victims suffered; they all too often died. As Lowe's claim indicates, the pox was also almost universally depicted as a sign of moral depravity. Of course in early modern Europe all diseases were interpreted in providential terms; outward signs of illness stood for internal moral failure.[3] Yet the link between disease and sin was forged nowhere stronger than in the pox. Its sufferers, disfigured by the ulcers, baldness, and collapsed noses characteristic of infection, bore not just symptoms, but symbols. Wishing a pox on one's enemies meant wishing that they be struck with a condition that might render them the victims of more than just physical torture, but possibly also moral condemnation, ridicule, and social scorn.

---

[1]Cit. in Quétel, *History of Syphilis,* p. 19

[2]Lowe, *Easie, Certaine, and Perfect Method,* cap. 2.

[3]For useful discussions of providential interpretations of illness that address the pox in particular see Cunningham and Grell, *Four Horsemen of the Apocalypse*, chap. 5 and Arrizabalaga, Henderson and French, *The Great Pox,* 38–55. For a thoughtful microhistory that explores the multiple readings of bodily signs in the period (in a case the author suggests was syphilis) see Ruggiero, 'Strange Death of Margarita Marcellini.'

The pox was a particularly potent image because it represented deviance on so many levels. Its symptoms were abhorrent: nasty, stinking, and putrid. In the binary tandem of purity and impurity,[4] it stood for filth. And it was more. It was ugly in a world that valued beauty, tainted in a world that valued purity, and sinful in a world that valued probity. It seemed almost entirely void of any positive associations. The essays that follow hope to show that the pox represented one of early modern Europe's most significant cultural markers. Playwrights dramatized it. Satirists mocked with it. Doctors theorized about it. Quacks profited from it. Moralists lectured about it. Patients lamented it. And virtually everyone feared it. This collection takes as a point of departure that the rise of the pox needs to be registered as a more significant development in the course of early modern European history than has largely been allowed

The history of the disease remains unsettled. Indeed, from the moment it stepped onto the European stage in the 1490s it became the cause of wildly imaginative interpretations. Of course this idea – that the disease entered Europe in the 1490s – has itself generated 500 years of controversy that continues to this day.[5] I will address that issue in a moment, but there is little dispute that the *idea* of a new disease, which was given a new name, or to be precise a set of new names, did arise in Europe in the closing decade of the fifteenth century. The most famous incident related to the onset of the pox was an ill-fated and oft-discussed siege of Naples by the army of King Charles VIII of France in 1494–95.[6] For early modern commentators and modern historians alike this siege became ground zero in the history of this disease. The pox first demonstrated its fury by ravaging the bodies of the invading French army forced to retreat, defeated not in the battlefield but in the bordellos, or so the story goes. This tale served a peculiar function in early venereal disease treatises. It offered the narrative structure of a good story whose moral remained open-ended. Indeed writers spun the tale in a variety of ways, illustrating just how hard the European imagination would work to interpret this disease. Over time the defeat of the French became a form of germ warfare, a construction of the disease recently noted elsewhere in Renaissance literature.[7] Some claimed that the Italians spiked the French army's wine casks with the blood of lepers; others portrayed

[4]The classic expression of these categories is Douglas, *Purity and Danger.*

[5]For an overview of the debate see Quétel, *History of Syphilis,* pp. 33–49.

[6]Quétel, *History of Syphilis,* pp. 9–11; Cunningham and Grell, p. 249; Rosebury, *Microbes and Morals*, p. 25; Lowe, *An Easie, Certaine and Perfect Method*, cap. 2; Clowes, *A Brief and Necessary Treatise*, p. 149.

[7]Qualtiere and Slights, 'Contagion and Blame,' pp. 19–20.

Jews as the nefarious agents responsible for this concoction.[8] Still others saw the bodies of Italian prostitutes as the vehicle of infection. The Italians allegedly set infected women upon their besiegers, casting prostitutes out of the city who, like Trojan horses in reverse, carried death hidden within them. Two centuries later commentators would still trumpet that 'these courtizans so sauced the French that in a short time this Venereal *Lues* raged through the camp.'[9] The broad range of interpretations of this lone event begins to hint at the anxiety that surrounded the new disease.

Anna Foa was right to say that Europeans found ways to deal with this anxiety without breaking into outright panic. One way they did this was to use traditional intellectual and iconographic tools to represent the disease. In several ways, Europeans recycled essentially medieval ideas (most notably those derived from leprosy) as they scrambled to interpret the new scourge that seemed to appear out of nowhere. These efforts certainly helped to present the pox in less mysterious terms and mitigated its terror, as Foa cogently argues.[10] Nonetheless, there remained a truly frantic element to early responses to the disease, captured particularly well in the words of a young Albrecht Dürer who in 1506 exclaimed 'Pray to God for me that I may be saved, especially from the French Disease, because I know nothing of which I am so much afraid, nearly every man has it, and it eats up many people so that they die.'[11] The pox instilled this kind of fear as much for its horrible symptoms as for the unsettling implications it held for a changing and unpredictable world in which a new disease could strike out of nowhere.

An historiography has emerged specific to the history of sexually transmitted disease. Like many topics in medical history, it fell first to doctors themselves to conduct this inquiry. Early twentieth-century studies on the history of the pox tended to appear not in history journals but in medical journals, like the *British Journal on Venereal Disease*.[12] Identifying famous historical figures that may have had the pox was one recurring

---

[8]Foa, 'New and the Old,' pp. 39–40.

[9]Maynwaring, *History and Mystery of the Venereal Lues,* pp. 15–16; Harvey, *Little Venus Unmasked*, p. 4

[10]Foa, 'New and the Old,' pp. 38–42; It is notable that J. S. Cummings does use the term 'paranoia' to describe the initial reactions to the disease, 'Pox and Paranoia in Renaissance Europe.'

[11]Cit. in Timken-Zinkann, 'Some Aspects of Epidemics,' pp. 358–359.

[12]Examples include Cumston, 'Syphilis in the 15th and 16th centuries,' and Moore, 'Joseph Grünpeck and his Neat Treatise.' This is not to overshadow the important work done by such foundational medical historians as Karl Sudhoff, whose compilation of early printed treatises was invaluable to the field. See *The Earliest Printed Literature on Syphilis*.

theme that abounded in early histories, an interest that shows no sign of abating.[13] However, work on sexual disease intensified especially in the 1980s and 1990s. In part this was a logical extension of a number of academic pursuits. Scholarship on the history of sexuality blossomed in the wake of Foucault's work and the parallel explosion of research on gender and the body.[14] Simultaneously, scholars from a range of disciplines moved into the history of medicine, applying elements of what was then being called the 'new cultural history' to health and disease. The work of cultural anthropologists, especially Mary Douglas' work on pollution, began to influence historians' explorations of illness,[15] while representations of pathology stirred literary critics and art historians inspired by Susan Sontag's work on disease as metaphor and Sander Gilman's work on illness and iconography.[16] Scholarship on sex and scholarship on medicine could not be kept long apart; the early modern period was well served by the likes of Thomas Laqueur and Roy Porter to name just two who bridged the fields.[17] The pox itself thus became quickly poised as a point of convergence where a range of important lines of scholarship met. It is indicative that an article on early modern syphilis can be found in the inaugural volume of the *Journal of the History of Sexuality* in 1990.[18] Literary critics especially have been at the forefront of recent work on early modern sexual disease. For example, exploration of images of the pox in early modern English literature has produced important contributions by Greg

---

[13]J. D. Rolleston, 'Venereal Disease in Literature,' p. 180; Rosebury, pp. 146–164. It should be noted that this is just one aspect of Rosebury's important book, which indeed predates the rise in interest sparked by the HIV pandemic. The most recent such exploration is Hayden, *Pox: Genius, Madness, and the Mysteries of Syphilis*.

[14]The undoubted influence of Foucault's *History of Sexuality* in turning significant attention to the topic should not, of course, obscure important work on sex in history that preceded it. Here the prolific career of Vern Bullough is illustrative. For a discussion of the culture and climate in which early historians of sexuality worked see Bullough, 'Sex in History: A Redux,' pp. 3–11.

[15]Douglas, *Purity and Danger*. An example of Douglas' influence on medical history in this period is R.I. Moore's discussion of leprosy in *The Formation of a Persecuting Society*, pp. 45–65 and 100–123.

[16]Sontag, *Illness as Metaphor* and *AIDS and its Metaphors*, Gilman, *Disease and Representation*.

[17]Laqueur, *Making Sex*; Roy Porter's prolific output makes rehearsing his catalogue impossible here. Two of his earlier contributions linking the history of sex and the history of medicine were 'Spreading Carnal Knowledge or Selling Dirt Cheap ?' and 'The Secrets of Generation Display'd.' More substantial later work included Porter and Hall, *The Facts of Life*.

[18]Boehrer, 'Early Modern Syphilis,'

Bentley, Johannes Fabricius, Raymond Anselment, and Margaret Healy all since 1989.[19]

However, the increased attention to the history of STDs sparked in the 1980s can hardly be attributed to mere shifting trends of scholarship. It is often useful to remember that we are all destined to become primary sources. It will be immediately apparent to those who reflect on this scholarship that it came in the wake of the first wave of the HIV pandemic. As the 1980s wore on, not even Ronald Reagan's infamous refusal to say the word 'AIDS' could keep the topic out of public debate. As scientists worked to identify and treat the new disease, scholars in the humanities sought to help understand it by setting it in context. It was French historian Claude Quétel who offered the most comprehensive history of sexually transmitted disease that explored the early modern period. Originally published in French in 1986, Quétel's *Le mal de Naples: histoire du syphilis* traced the history of the famed French Pox from the late fifteenth century to the late twentieth century, drawing explicit comparisons between the history of syphilis and the early history of HIV/AIDS. In a similar vein, Richard Davenport-Hines wove together a history of sexual disease with a history of homosexuality to launch a spirited polemic against intolerance in 1990.[20] In early modern syphilis scholars had a topic with profound contemporary resonance: a sexually transmitted infection that seemed to appear out of nowhere, which initially lacked any proven treatment, and which frequently killed its victims. In terms of emphasis, Quétel's book can itself represent the general weighting of the research that would ensue on the topic; while the early modern period received some good coverage,[21] the lion's share of attention has fallen on the nineteenth and twentieth centuries, leaving a great deal of work still to do on earlier centuries.[22]

---

[19]Bentley, *Shakespeare and the New Disease;* Fabricius, *Syphilis in Shakespeare's England*; Anselment, *Realms of Apollo* pp. 131–171; Margaret Healy, *Fictions of Disease*, chaps. 4 and 5.

[20]Davenport-Hines, *Sex, Death and Punishment.* For his treatment of syphilis see especially pp. 16–54.

[21]Roughly two thirds of Quétel's book addresses the period after 1800.

[22]Important monographs on the modern period that emerged in this wave of scholarship include Brandt, *No Magic Bullet* and Cassell, *Secret Plague.* More recent contributions on VD in the modern age include Spongberg, *Feminizing Venereal Disease;* Davidson, *Dangerous Liaisons;* Davidson and Hall (eds.) *Sex, Sin and Suffering*; J.D. Oriel, *Scars of Venus*; and Baldwin, *Contagion and the State,* pp. 355–523. On VD and Empire see Levine, *Prostitution, Race and Politics.* The eighteenth century has been well served by a collection similar to this one, Merians (ed.) *The Secret Malady.*

Until recently most of this research has focused on 'syphilis.' This is hardly surprising. Prior to HIV/AIDS syphilis was the most deadly and fearsome form of sexual infection. However, an important revisionist history has stressed that it is inappropriate to focus early modern studies on the history of 'syphilis.' Jon Arrizabalaga, Roger French and John Henderson's influential *The Great Pox: The French Disease in Renaissance Europe* (1997) made several important contributions, including the call for clearer terminology.[23] The term 'syphilis' does emerge in the Renaissance. Specifically, it was the title character in Girolamo Fracastoro's 1530 epic poem about the onset of the new disease.[24] However, the term did not stick; early modern commentators almost never used the word. Instead, in the vernacular they employed terms like 'the French Disease,' 'the foul disease,' 'the venereal disease,' or 'the pox,' while in Latin they wrote of *morbus gallicus* or *lues venerea*. The call for modern scholars to employ terms that contemporaries used is more than a matter of linguistic perfectionism. It is an attempt to avoid the pitfalls of an historical methodology called retrospective diagnosis, the practice of applying modern diagnostic categories to previous periods of history. Scholars propose that there are two core problems with such an approach. First, it demands translating between linguistic and conceptual worlds separated by several centuries and, secondly, it suffers from a kind of essentialism, privileging our own categories as supposedly fixed and stable.[25]

Renaissance commentators had their own disease concept – *the* venereal disease – a single ailment that included a range of conditions that we would now separate. Thus patients suffering from what we term syphilis and what we term gonorrhea received the same diagnosis, as did a wide range of patients likely suffering from other genito-urinary or skin conditions that we would diagnose entirely differently. It is thus impossible to assume that what they termed the pox was what we term syphilis in all (or even a majority of) cases. Presuming that all sixteenth-century 'venereal' patients were syphilitics is almost certainly a flawed assumption, obscuring rather than clarifying early modern medical realities.

The case of 'syphilis' versus the 'French Disease' has become one of the prime examples used to demonstrate the issues that attend retrospective diagnosis as an historical method.[26] However, that does not mean that

---

23 Arrizabalaga, Henderson and French, *The Great Pox*, pp. 1–19.

24 Fracastoro, *Syphilis, Sive Morbo Gallico*.

25 Harley, 'Rhetoric and the Social Construction of Sickness,' p. 419

26 For example, Mary Lindemann uses this case to explain the concept in her useful survey, *Medicine and Society*, p. 22

everyone has abandoned the study of syphilis in the early modern world. Some commentators have responded that this approach is too limiting, preventing scholars from exploring longer continuities of disease-history.[27] Others simply explore different questions. For example, paleopathologists continue to investigate one of the great historico-scientific questions of all time – did syphilis come from the New World – and are less interested in discursive intricacies. Their primary focus is a bacterium, *Treponema pallidum*, and whether or not it can be found in pre-Columbian bones in Europe.[28]

None of the articles in this volume take up that interesting question. It is simply not one that literary critics or historians are likely to be able to answer. While early modern descriptions of symptoms, whether textual or graphic, present rich material for humanities scholars to decode, they are far too vague by themselves to settle the legendary debate on 'the Columbian Exchange.'[29] Were the patients whom Peter Lowe described as suffering from 'apostumes,' 'running of the reins,' 'ulcers,' and 'pustles' syphilitic?[30] Many feel that it is impossible to know.

This begins to suggest that reading this disease is a complex process. Jonathan Gil Harris suggests that we need a multitude of readings to unpack early modern representations of the pox. Even more than Arrizabalaga, Henderson and French, who demanded that we contextualize the disease by employing terms that contemporaries used, Harris demands that we always remember that syphilis should not be reified to assume an objective place prior to the text, but rather is produced and constantly reproduced *by* the text. Indeed, it is a text, or in Harris' terms a 'pathotext.' For Harris both the identification ('syphilis') and its chronology ('early modern') have to be themselves read as multi-faceted textual products, produced over time, and laden with layer upon layer of meaning. Harris suggests using the notion of the palimpsest to describe the disease; just like the writing slate which, though it could be wiped clean, still left remnants behind, the pox carried with it artefacts of meaning inherited from previous discourses

---

27Healy, p. 252, n 6; for an excellent example of a history that makes the bacterium *Trepenoma pallidum* its primary historical actor (while still acknowledging that diseases can be socially constructed) see Sheldon Watts' chapter on syphilis in *Epidemics and History*, pp. 122–166.

28For a sample of recent research on the question see *L'Origine de la Syphilis en Europe*, eds. Dutour, et. al. One of the most recent studies suggests that the disease was already in Europe prior to 1493. Mays, Crane-Kramer and Bayliss, 'Two Probable Cases of Treponemal Disease of Medieval Date from England.'

29This phrase was coined by Crosby, *Columbian Exchange*.

30Lowe, *An Easie, Certaine and Perfect Method,* chap. 5.

stretching back centuries. To steal a phrase from Clifford Geertz, the pox demands very thick description indeed.[31]

Harris explores how this necessitates at least three different types of readings – medical, metaphoric, and historicist – which all yield different insights. On the surface this is hardly surprising, but Harris presses to take the revisionist stance one-step further. Shifting from 'syphilis' to 'pox' in the name of using a term that contemporaries employed is, for Harris, essentially an historicist reading. However, it is merely historicist and it obscures the fundamental textuality of the disease as well as the anachronistic alternative analyses (metaphoric and medical) that uncover unique elements crucial to reading the disease. Most challengingly he declares that he actually prefers 'syphilis' to the historicist 'pox.' This is not because he argues for thinking in terms of a fixed biological entity that entered Europe after 1492 – far from it. He prefers the term because it immediately announces and constantly recalls the multi-layered and textual nature of pathology.

Harris analyzes a play called *The Three Ladies of London* to demonstrate his approach. He displays the great influence of the disease in this period by exploring a play in which the pox played no overt role. No character is sexually infected and no character offers a monologue on the disease. Rather, it lurks beneath the play's surface, demonstrating how Harris' call for multiple diachronic readings is particularly apt. On the one hand, the presence of dermatological markers on certain characters invites a medical reading in which we might compare characters' blemishes to syphilitic symptoms. However, these blemishes also call for a metaphoric reading. Harris explores how the spot was employed as a marker indicating not real, physical sickness, but invisible spiritual flaws. The spot was a metaphor for sin. This usage merely continued a centuries-old tradition of employing blemishes as metaphors for deeper, invisible flaws of the soul.

However, a third, historicist analysis brings a uniquely early modern reading, an economic one. The pox also became an entity that moved about, crossing national and other boundaries. In so doing it became a commodity. Harris situates the disease within the enormous global trade that emerged after 1492 and proposes that the growth of trade dramatically affected understandings of the disease. There emerged a profound economic awareness of the pox as it was imported and exported, like so many spices and silks in the age of nascent globalization. Indeed, English physician Gideon Harvey would later use just that term, commodity, to

---

[31] Geertz, *Interpretation of Cultures*, pp. 3–30. I do not mean to imply that Harris applies the methodology that Geertz describes here. Harris offers a critique of Geertz in *Foreign Bodies*, pp. 4–5.

describe the pox's threat to England. '[T]o prevent the importation of the like commodities for the future,' he claimed, 'part of the Custom house must be converted into Lazarettos to search all Foreigners before they set foot on shore.'[32] Whereas many of the metaphoric uses to which the pox was put harkened back to older notions of pathology, this economic understanding was new.[33]

Classic texts in the Hippocratic Canon such as *Airs Waters and Places* had long established a connection between illness and location. Now the post-1492 commodified pox threatened to transform the traditional connection between pathology and place.[34] Rather than fixed in a specific climate disease now roamed freely, in part thanks to developing scientific understandings of contagion, which Harris has explored elsewhere.[35] Like its close cousin plague, the pox would not be corralled. It took to the roads and high seas, becoming cargo and currency in a new age in which diseases could be traded like bitter fruits between peoples, nations, and continents.

This would have a major impact on understandings and representations of this disease. As has been often noted, one of the most prevalent responses to the new disease was projection; country after country took turns laying blame, usually by naming it after a rival.[36] Over time the pox would represent many things, but it was perhaps in discussions of nation that it performed its most elaborate and significant symbolic work. Because the body was a primary metaphor for nation, the urge to preserve a clean national body and the anxiety of possible infection from without gave sixteenth and seventeenth-century commentators a powerful discourse to help formulate early notions of national identity.[37] Metaphors of clean and

---

32Harvey, *Great Venus Unmask'd,* p. 98.

33Harris develops this idea further through extensive readings of the pathological and the economic in English Renaissance drama in *Sick Economies,* on syphilis see especially pp. 29–51.

34For an overview see Wear, *Knowledge and Practice,* pp. 184–190.

35Harris emphasizes the rise of Paracelsian chemistry that began to present disease more as a result of foreign entities invading the body than as the traditional Galenic imbalance of humours. *Foreign Bodies*, pp. 20–26; Arrizabalaga, Henderson and French stress the role played by the pox in forcing a revision of medical theories on contagion, *The Great Pox,* pp. 234–251; See also Nutton, 'The Seeds of Disease,' pp. 1–34.

36Quétel, *History of Syphilis* pp. 10, 16; Foa, 'New and the Old,' p. 26;

37One of the founding expressions of this idea was Hale, *The Body Politic.* See Scholz, *Body Narratives* for a useful review of discussions on the reciprocal relation between individual and political bodies, pp. 1–12. Particularly pertinent to this volume is her analysis of the import of gendered presentations of purity and somatic metaphors of nation, pp. 81–105; Harris stresses that in the context of England the Reformation marked a key turning point in corporeal metaphors, shifting attention from the Catholic

dirty, sick and healthy, stood at the forefront of this project. Writers never tired of medical metaphors, discussing how nations needed to be purged, cleansed, or healed.[38] Just as nations could be plagued, so too could they be poxed.

This dynamic went far beyond merely naming the disease after one's enemies. Several contributors seek to explore in greater detail the processes by which the pox became linked to the foreign. It is not surprising that we see (imagined) foreign sexual habits openly criticized. For example, warnings about the lechery of Jews or the wanton nature of New World natives were not uncommon.[39] However, seemingly innocuous aspects of foreign cultures could also be vilified through association with sexual disease. Roze Hentschell demonstrates how for the English the 'French Disease' was very much that, a pathologizing of all things French. In some ways the French Disease was not the pox, but French-ness itself, which was seen as no less threatening, no less invasive. English authors warned that adopting French fashions was tantamount to being infected. Significantly, there was convenient slippage between speaking about French clothing and the French Disease. Authors moved effortlessly between the two forging powerful metaphoric links. To dress like the French was to be like the French, and to be like the French was to be diseased. Critics presented the same qualities of luxury and lechery that compelled English men and women to adorn themselves with French fashions as the primary motives that also drove them towards the pox. Hentschell demonstrates how it is frequently impossible to disentangle anxiety about the pox from uneasiness that surrounded the foreign.

Clothing was just one aspect of this phenomenon in action. Language was another. Here the model of sexual disease as dangerous commodity that both Harris and Hentschell suggest was vital. Anxieties about foreign language share many of the same characteristics as anxieties about imported cloth. Diane Cady shows how English writers constructed foreign language not just pathologically, as a disease, but sexually pathological, as a venereal disease. Foreign tongues were frequently depicted as feminine, producing a drive to present English as a masculine language by trumpeting its (manly)

---

body of Europe to the national body politic, as well as arguing for the continued importance of political body metaphors despite shifting medical paradigms. See pp. 30–34 and 141–146.

[38]Harris, *Foreign Bodies,* p. 3.

[39]Quétel, *History of Syphilis,* pp. 33–37, Foa, 'New and the Old,' pp. 31–33, 37; Siena, 'Pollution, Promiscuity and the Pox,' pp. 569–571; On other links between the disease and New World natives see Eamon, 'Cannibalism and Contagion' pp. 1–31 and Horowitz, 'The New World and the Changing Face of Europe' pp. 1181–1201.

Teutonic roots. Foreign languages thus became feminized invaders that wormed their way in, corrupting the English tongue in a mess of gender confusion and linguistic transvestism. Here foreign words themselves became a disease threatening to pollute, and a feminine disease at that. Moreover, writers singled out women as particularly prone to promoting this linguistic pollution at home, being especially drawn to foreign words seen as frivolous ornaments for their speech akin to cosmetics for their face or French fashions for their body.

Again we witness significant slippage. Cady shows how many of the same characteristics that allegedly rendered women prone to wanton sexuality simultaneously made them prone to verbal promiscuity, generating a kind of linguistic anxiety that went hand in hand with men's sexual anxiety.[40] Wanton women would spread pollution one way or another, whether through their mouths as language or through their bodies as pox. Here there are important parallels between depictions of linguistic pollution and theories of sexual pollution. A dominant medical explanation for the pox was as a poison generated by the mixture of different men's seed in the wombs of promiscuous women.[41] Paralleling this, words from different languages mixed in women's mouths just as seeds of different men might mix in their wombs. Either, contemporaries held, was a hazardous mixture. However, as Cady shows in her analyses of plays like *Jack Drum's Entertainment* and *Englishmen for my Money,* the stories of linguistic and sexual pollution did not just mirror one another; they frequently intersected. The politics of Cady's reading are also vital, for they demonstrate that the gendered presentations of language as sexual disease functioned on two levels. Portrayals of foreign language as sexual disease helped to galvanize the nation, while portrayals of women's speech as threatening to that nation underscored gender oppression.

Given the anxiety that surrounded the disease and the clear moral issues that it raised, it is worth considering the influence of the pox on Europe's moral climate. Some have suggested that we can point to the rise of the pox as a factor influencing the increased asceticism of the sixteenth century. As Robert Jütte put it, some historians have found the coincidence of the advent of the pox and the rise of what many term puritanism 'conspicuous.'[42]

---

[40]The work on masculinity and adultery is important here. Breitenberg, 'Anxious Masculinity,' pp. 377–398; Turner, *Fashioning Adultery*, pp. 83–105; Foyster, *Manhood in Early Modern England*, pp. 103–146; Gowing, *Domestic Dangers*, chap. 6.

[41]Schleiner, 'Infection and Cure through Women,' pp. 505–506; Siena, 'Pollution, Promiscuity and the Pox,' pp. 562–566.

[42]Jütte, 'Syphilis and Confinement,' p. 100.

To borrow a phrase from Theodore Rosebury, there may be a connection between 'microbes and morals.'[43] Such connections will be more convincing to those who believe that a new micro-organism entered Europe in the 1490s. However, even if we accept that as the case, a clear verdict remains difficult and caution is prescribed to avoid monocausal explanations for complex historical developments. An example is sociologist Stanislav Andreski's thesis, imaginative though it may be, that the onset of syphilis explains both puritanism and the witch hunts.[44]

Andreski's conclusions have proven too sweeping for many; however, his underlying premise – that the disease sent cultural shockwaves through Europe – remains a useful insight. The presence of a deadly disease linked to sex must have confirmed the beliefs of those who saw the world in providential terms and who viewed disease as one of the clearest ways that God communicated his displeasure. After the rise of the pox the internal logic of providential thought could only have strengthened the connection between sex and sin.[45] What other message could people have taken once the wrath of God so clearly targeted sexuality ? The increasingly puritanical attitudes of the sixteenth and early seventeenth centuries are undoubtedly part of the larger drift toward moral purification in the age of the religious wars. And clearly the Reformation context is crucial here. However, historians might do well to consider the role of the pox itself in contributing to the atmosphere in which calls for moral purification intensified. Moreover, the new disease likely ensured that sex took a central role in the eyes of reformers, alongside alehouses, gambling and popular religion. All that being said, it bears reminding that the connection between the pox and moral policing campaigns was somewhat more complex than it first appears.

The policing of sodomy helps demonstrate the point. Authorities in Renaissance Lucca developed a unique regulating agency, the *Offizio sopra l'Onestà*, or Office of Decency, specifically charged to police sodomy. Mary Hewlett shows that the Lucchese *Onestà* long predates the outbreak of the pox. Thus, sodomy was already considered a threat worthy of policing well before *mal francese* entered the equation. The advent of the pox seemed merely to provide authorities with a number of vital new tools to enhance

---

[43]Rosebury, *Microbes and Morals;* however, Rosebury's scepticism of the American origin leads him to question this connection, p. 196*;* Fabricius, pp. 16–20, 32; Allen, pp. 45–48; Bullough and Bullough, *Women and Prostitution,* pp. 146–156.

[44]Andreski *Syphilis, Puritanism, and Witch Hunts*. Anthropologist Eric Ross recently advanced ostensibly the same claims, though without acknowledging Andreski's research. 'Syphilis, Misogyny and Witchcraft in 16th-Century Europe.'

[45]Davenport-Hines, *Sex, Death and Punishment*, pp. 32–33.

their policing efforts. Links were soon formed between sodomy and sexual infection that were so close as to blur the line between the two. Authorities began to use diagnosis of the pox as cause to investigate sodomy. In other words, medical diagnosis began to provide legal cause to investigate criminal (sexual) behaviour. More than just providing possible leads, the city forced medical personnel and institutions to participate in investigations and prosecutions. The city required doctors to provide the *Onestà* with details of infected patients (who would then be investigated) and sent its own agents into Lucca's pox hospitals to interrogate patients in its hunt for sodomites. These steps helped to medicalize sodomy itself. Medical authorities essentially began to diagnose sodomy, as physicians, surgeons and midwives all interpreted bodily signs to offer medical 'proof' of anal sex, further harnessing medical knowledge to the cause of moral policing. Finally, the significant numbers of foreigners and new immigrants arrested and tried by the *Onestà* enhances the arguments of Harris, Hentshell, and Cady, even further by showing in yet another context how apprehension about sex and disease manifested itself in attempts to police the boundaries that separated the internal from the external.

Policing efforts to the north in Venice also involved forms of incarceration. Laura McGough's study of female reformatories explores the dynamic links between myths about the pox, emerging scientific theories of contagion, and institutional efforts to quarantine women. Not just any women, McGough shows how authorities specifically targeted beautiful women in the name of public health. McGough explores the histories of the *Convertite* and the *Zitelle*, two institutions that grew directly out of the city's pox hospitals. These penitentiaries sought to enclose women identified as a public health threat. Cultural apprehension about the unsettling power of female beauty made attractive women seem especially dangerous to Venetian authorities. Initially the *Convertite* cloistered women after they had been treated in the hospital, making the reformatory an extended arm of the city's larger response to the pox. However, the connection between policing and the pox is again complicated. While the *Convertite* incarcerated women who had contracted disease, the later *Zitelle* quarantined young women *before* they were ever infected. Administrators expressly targeted beautiful young girls for institutional quarantine, ostensibly to protect them, but really to protect Venice *from* them. The threat that these women might one day spread infection seems to have been justification enough. McGough draws links between these institutions, myths about the advent of the pox that blamed beautiful prostitutes, and medical theories of contagion to show that Venice quarantined beauty in the name of public health.

But just what was the connection between sex and this disease? This was one of the many questions that early scientists struggled to answer. Jon

Arrizabalaga explores university medicine and the response to the French Disease during its first decade in Europe. He demonstrates that there was no uniform response to the pox on the part of Europe's medical elite. The medico-scientific response was instead a kind of intellectual scramble.[46] There was significant confusion about the role played by sex in spreading the disease. The important medical historian Owsei Temkin suggested that it took several decades before doctors linked the pox to sex.[47] However, Arrizabalaga demonstrates that a close reading of the earliest medical treatises does not fully support that claim. Some of the very earliest doctors did link the disease to sex. The trouble was that not everyone made the connection. Moreover, those who did disagreed on what the nature of that connection was. Copulation and contagion were linked, but how ?

That question was not easily resolved because the open, fluid, and multi-faceted nature of Latin Galenism allowed for a wide range of explanations. A key issue all doctors had to address was why the disease seemed to strike the genitals. Some physicians indeed pointed to sexual intercourse as the primary means of transmission through contagion. However, others suggested that the disease was linked to an astrological event in the constellation of Scorpio (which ruled the genitals) and this explained the connection between the pox and the sex organs. Still others played down the connection with sexuality altogether. The connection between sex and illness was further complicated because sex was not just viewed as a means of getting sick in this period; it was also an important way to stay healthy. Sex played a vital role in maintaining the all-important humoural balance within the Galenic medical economy and it performed vital functions within theories of the six non-naturals, (air, food and drink, sleep, movement and rest, retention and evacuation, and the emotions). Sustaining a healthy sex life was one way to ward off or recover from illness. Therefore, the connections between sex and the French Disease, although forged from a very early date, did not immediately result in doctors' advice to abstain from sex. In fact, some physicians actually advised infected patients to continue having sex in order to recover their health. However, once physicians linked the disease to sex we find them moving quickly to condemn prostitutes, indicating that the policing efforts described by McGough were informed by medical science from a very early date.

One of the most important of these earliest theorists was the astrologer Joseph Grünpeck, one of the most frequently cited early authorities on the

---

[46]On these debates see Arrizabalaga, Henderson and French, *The Great Pox,* pp. 56–87, and Quétel, *History of Syphilis,* pp. 19–22, 25–29.

[47]Temkin, 'On the History of "Morality and Syphilis",' pp. 472–474.

disease. Indeed, his words open this book. Darin Hayton would suggest that this is likely what Grünpeck would have wanted. New dilemmas cry out for new solutions. Once the pox struck, the young unknown astrologer aggressively offered himself as an intellectual leader, explaining the theoretical underpinnings of this mysterious new disease. For Grünpeck, the answer lay in sophisticated (though to our eye clearly problematic) astrology. By generating an astrological explanation for the disease Grünpeck tried to establish himself as a scientific thinker of great weight.

However, Hayton demonstrates that Grünpeck's real agenda was political, namely, his own career advancement. Grünpeck's highly creative astrology, which seemed to bend and twist to try to square the timing of the rise of the pox with an elaborate scheme of celestial occurrences, is trumped only by his even more affected attempts at impressing Emperor Maximilian I in pursuit of a position at court. Maximilian expressed significant anxiety about the French Disease and Grünpeck jumped at the chance to make a name for himself by weaving the emperor's concerns into his medico-astrological treatises on the pox. It is hard not to view Grünpeck as an opportunist, for the advent of a new disease presented a tremendous opportunity to advance himself as a saviour in the face of a crisis. The strategy worked. Grünpeck won his position at court. However, he could hardly have predicted when he first wrote against the French Disease that he, too, would find himself infected. Grünpeck's tone changed dramatically as his perspective shifted from confident aspiring courtier to suffering diseased victim, something Domenico Zanrè highlights in a different context.

Zanrè explores several Cinquecento Tuscan satirists and analyzes the multiple ways they put the pox to rhetorical use. On the one hand we get a glimpse of how the pox functioned in contemporary satire. Sexual infection was perfect ammunition for the satirist. Not only was the disease morally charged, Margaret Healy has stressed that it was exciting literary material and its 'box-office appeal' may help explain the predominance of representations of the pox on the early modern stage.[48] Italian writers were no less apt than their English counterparts to put this symbolic tool to work. Zanrè demonstrates how one Tuscan writer utilized burlesque to express contemporary dissatisfaction with literary conventions. Again we see what a flexible metaphoric instrument sexual infection was. Unsurprisingly the pox was a common topic in such satire, and Zanrè shows how it was used not just to advance literary criticism but also to demonize particular groups, most

---

[48]Healy, *Fictions of Disease,* pp. 152–153.

notably prostitutes, demonstrating that the *literati* could join the ranks – alongside Arrizabalaga's medical scientists and McGough's municipal bureaucrats – of those who condemned these women.

However, ribald satire did not always dominate, even among bawdy satirists. Within the writings of a single author, Zanrè detects vastly different presentations of the *mal francese*. While this might result from an author's different political aims at varying points in his career (as evidenced by Grünpeck), it could also be a product of one's personal encounter with the pox (as also evidenced by Grünpeck!). Zanrè compares earlier and later works by Agnolo Firenzuola that reveal a dramatic change of tone. Writing at age 26, the youthful and optimistic Firenzuola recounted his adventure with the pox, which he believed he had conquered. Seven years later it became clear to him that the disease was not so easily shrugged off and that his confidence in renaissance medicine may have been overstated, as was sadly so often the case. Older, wiser, and now fearing death, he offers a much more sober piece of interior self-reflection. Zanrè's reading points us in a useful direction, for we too rarely hear the voices of patients. For all that has been done on the history of the pox, the history of doctors has outstretched the history of patients. Yet the patient-experience is a crucial component of the story that scholars must engage more directly.[49] We need much more work on how people who believed themselves to be infected not only understood their disease but strategized to deal with it.

One way of thinking about patients is to consider what options health care providers made available to them (although, of course, this continues to emphasize health care providers, rather than health care recipients.) Class played a significant role in determining one's medical options. Patients of means had no dearth of medical practitioners to choose from. The poor, however, frequently had to rely on charity when they fell ill. The poxed poor presented a conundrum for early modern charities. As debates heated up in the sixteenth century about the deserving and non-deserving poor early modern hospitals had to grapple with whether or not a pauper infected with the pox constituted a worthy object of charity. It was not a question easily solved. However, my own study of London's royal hospitals demonstrates that those in charge of these institutions never considered the 'foul' beyond the pale of charity. A breakdown of the patient population shows that, far from shunning the poxed as some of scholars have suggested, London's royal hospitals made treating them one of their most important services. Yet, the above-mentioned tension never dissipated. 'Foul' became

[49]On the call for patient-centred histories of medicine see the work of Roy Porter: 'The Patient's View,' pp.175–198; and Porter (ed.) *Patients and Practitioners*.

its own category. Policies unique to the foul wards – including public whipping – reveal a great deal about prevailing attitudes towards those struck with this disease.

The force of the response to the pox can also be felt in the marketplace. The fear that the pox inspired was not just a product of the disease's supposed newness, nor its connection with sexuality, though these obviously had a major impact. The breadth and force of the responses to the pox that this book seeks to chart also stemmed from the mundane fact that it was simply everywhere. The prevalence of 'venereal' patients in hospitals is just one piece of evidence suggesting that a significant portion of the population came to be diagnosed with this disease, regardless of what pathogen they may or may not have harboured.

It is not surprising then that the market responded vigorously to meet such widespread demand.[50] Evidence from England shows that healers of all stripes scrambled to offer treatment. The medical of division of labour, which was supposed to see different forms of healing restricted to particular kinds of healers – physicians, surgeons, apothecaries – was in practice difficult to enforce and compromised at the best of times. When it came to the pox with so much market share at stake, monopolies were ignored as all manner of practitioners flooded the market peddling their 'cures.' In London, we have seen that quacks had great success playing to patients' concerns for privacy, promising discreet treatment and trying to undercut traditional healers with a range of new marketing techniques aimed at luring poxed patients. These included promises of secret backdoor entrances, inconspicuous therapies, and even female assistants to cater to shy women.[51]

Yet David Gentilcore shows that this may have varied significantly in different contexts. His research on Italian charlatans shows that they occasionally participated in the sale of patent medicines to venereal patients. However, unlike English empirics, Italian charlatans traded in the French Disease surprisingly rarely. This seems the result of Italian medical regulation. In the regulated Italian medical market *ciarlatani* felt themselves to be under the scrutiny of medical authorities charged with governing medical practice. Italy's medical marketplace had little trouble providing lots of available care for Italians with the French Disease. Gentilcore's exploration of the records of Italian medical authorities demonstrates the

---

[50]The classic case for the model of the medical marketplace was advanced by Cook in *Decline of the Old Medical Regime,* pp. 28–69.

[51]Siena, 'The "Foul Disease" and Privacy;' Porter, *Health for Sale,* pp. 142 and 151–155.

richness and varied character of the medical scene in early modern Italy. His analysis of almost 1,600 charlatans' licenses allows for our closest look yet at these unique practitioners' activities. However, the evidence on *ciarlatani* depicts a scene in which it was the traditional healers, physicians and surgeons, who provided the bulk of treatment for venereal disease. *Ciarlatani* who strayed beyond the limits set by their licenses and offered forms of care restricted to more elite practitioners often faced disciplinary action. Thus the Italian medical marketplace may not have been quite the wild-west show of unbound entrepreneurship that the English scene is often depicted as having been.

The differences in the pictures emerging from the English and Italian medical scenes may result from the nature of sources or the nature of local medical regulation,[52] but a cultural component may also be at work. At least one study has compared Italian and English medical responses to the French Disease and has suggested that the latter were much more prone to moralize about the pox. While Italian doctors openly discussed ways to prevent infection (while still having sex) their English counterparts frequently issued moral warnings about God's wrath, refusing to provide information on prophylaxis lest they become the facilitators to sin.[53] This may indicate a more restricted, puritanical view of the disease in England than in Italy. The practice of publicly whipping venereal patients, something not apparent in the Italian pox hospitals that have been studied, may offer another piece of evidence for this view. It may be – and this is speculative – that a particularly harsh view of infection in England made patients there more receptive to the promises of privacy that English quacks were all too ready to make. In other words, differences in demand (to continue with the market model) may account for this seeming difference in supply when it came to treatment for the pox in different parts of Europe. Whatever the case, the differences between the Italian and English contexts offer an opportunity to make an important point about the state of early modern STD studies. The majority of work – including most contributions in this volume – has comprised isolated case studies. Comparative work involving multiple contexts marks one of our most pressing needs.

The contributions below have been organized into sections on medical, literary, and institutional responses. However, I resisted organizing this introduction according to these themes or discussing the articles in order of their appearance to make the point that these divisions are porous.

---

[52]On English medical regulation see Cook, *Decline of the Old Medical Regime* and *Trials of an Ordinary Doctor*; and Pelling, *Medical Conflicts in Early Modern London*.

[53]Schleiner, 'Moral Attitudes Towards Syphilis and its Prevention,' pp. 389–410.

Connections and cross fertilizations abound in the essays that follow. There are many ways in which the articles below speak across the synthetic sections into which they have been arranged. Readers are invited to navigate their own journey through these pages looking for the themes outlined here as well as those of their own discovery. Organization aside, we hope that these articles can together demonstrate the richness and importance of the subject and, most of all, inspire further research on sex and disease in the early modern era. Hardly a definitive statement, this volume is offered as an invitation. It seeks to demonstrate where some research on the topic is heading and invite others along for the ride. The pox had a major impact on the early modern world that has not yet been fully acknowledged. Margaret Pelling was undoubtedly correct when she recently suggested that 'venereal disease remains seriously underestimated as a force for social change' in this period.[54] We hope that the essays that follow can play a small part in remedying that situation, but we acknowledge that we still have a long way to go.

Trent University
Peterborough, Canada

Acknowledgements
I gratefully acknowledge the generous support provided by the Social Sciences and Humanities Research Council of Canada, The Lupina Foundation through the Comparative Program on Health and Society, and Trent University. A few people also deserve special thanks: Chris Metcalfe, Margret Hovanec, Peter Warrian, Stuart Heath and especially Konrad Eisenbichler.

CITED WORKS

Allen, Peter Lewis, *The Wages of Sin: Sex and Disease, Past and Present.* Chicago: University of Chicago Press, 2000.

Andreski, Stanislav. *Syphilis, Puritanism, and Witch Hunts: Historical Explanations in the Light of Medicine and Psychoanalysis with a Forecast about AIDS.* New York: St. Martin's Press, 1989.

Anselment, Raymond. *Realms of Apollo: Literature and Healing in Seventeenth-Century England.* Newark: University of Delaware Press, 1995.

Arrizabalaga, Jon, John Henderson, and Roger French. *The Great Pox: The French Disease in Renaissance Europe.* New Haven: Yale University Press, 1997.

Baldwin, Peter. *Contagion and the State in Europe, 1830–1930.* Cambridge: Cambridge University Press, 1999.

---

[54]Pelling, *Common Lot*, p. 28. See also her spirited call for greater integration of the disease into general histories of the period, *Medical Conflicts*, pp. 340–341.

Beier, A.L. *Masterless Men: The Vagrancy Problem in England 1560–1640*. London: Methuen, 1985.

Bentley, Greg. *Shakespeare and the New Disease: The Dramatic Function of Syphilis in 'Troilus and Cressida,' 'Measure for Measure,' 'Timon of Athens.'* New York: Peter Lang, 1989.

Boehrer, Bruce T. 'Early Modern Syphilis' *Journal of the History of Sexuality*, 1 (1990): 197–214.

Brandt, Allan M. *No Magic Bullet: A Social History of Venereal Disease in the United States Since 1880*. New York: Oxford University Press, 1985.

Breitenberg, Mark. 'Anxious Masculinity: Sexual Jealousy in Early Modern England' *Feminist Studies*, 19:2 (1993): 377–398.

Bullough, Vern and Bonnie Bullough, *Women and Prostitution: A Social History*. New York: Prometheus, 1987.

Bullough, Vern, 'Sex in History: A Redux' pp. 3–22 in *Desire and Discipline: Sex and Sexuality in the Premodern West*, eds. Jacqueline Murray and Konrad Eisenbichler. Toronto: University of Toronto Press, 1996.

Carmichael, Ann. *Plague and the Poor in Renaissance Florence*. Cambridge: Cambridge University Press, 1986.

Cassell, Jay, *Secret Plague: Venereal Disease in Canada since 1830*. Toronto: University of Toronto Press, 1987.

Clowes, William. *A Brief and Necessary Treatise, Touching on the Cure of the Disease now called Lues Venerea*. London: Edm. Bollifant, 1596.

Cook Harold, *The Decline of the Old Medical Regime in Late Stuart London*. Ithaca: Cornell University Press, 1986.

Cook, Harold, *Trials of an Ordinary Doctor: Joannes Groenvelt in Seventeenth-Century London*. Baltimore: The Johns Hopkins University Press, 1994.

Crosby, Alfred. *The Columbian Exchange: Biological and Cultural Consequences of 1492*. Westport, CT: Greenwood, 1972.

Cummins, J. S. 'Pox and Paranoia in Renaissance Europe' *History Today*, 38 (1988): 28–35.

Cumston, Charles. 'Syphilis in the 15th and 16th Centuries, Especially at Paris' *British Journal of Dermatology*, 35 (1923): 331–334.

Cunningham, Andrew and Ole Peter Grell. *The Four Horsemen of the Apocalypse: Religion, War, Famine and Death in Reformation Europe*. Cambridge: Cambridge University Press, 2000.

Davenport-Hines, Richard. *Sex, Death and Punishment: Attitudes to Sex and Sexuality in Britain Since the Renaissance*. London: Collins, 1990.

Davidson, Roger. *Dangerous Liaisons: A Social History of Venereal Disease in Twentieth Century Scotland*. Amsterdam: Rodopi, 2000.

Davis, Natalie Zemon. 'Poor Relief, Humanism and Heresy' pp. 17–64 in her *Society and Culture in Early Modern France*. Stanford, CA: Stanford University Press, 1975.

Douglas, Mary. *Purity and Danger: An Analysis of the Concepts of Pollution and Taboo* London: Routledge and Kegan Paul, 1966.

Eamon, William. 'Cannibalism and Contagion: Framing Syphilis in Counter-Reformation Italy' *Early Science and Medicine*, 3:1 (1998): 1–31.

Fabricius, Johannes. *Syphilis in Shakespeare's England.* London: Jessica Kingsley, 1995.

Foa Anna. 'The New and the Old: The Spread of Syphilis (1494–1530)' pp. 26–45 in *Sex and Gender in Historical Perspective,* eds. Edward Muir and Guido Ruggiero. Baltimore: The Johns Hopkins University Press, 1990.

Foyster, Elizabeth A. *Manhood in Early Modern England: Honour, Sex and Marriage.* London: Longman, 1999.

Geertz, Clifford. *The Interpretation of Cultures.* New York: Basic Books, 1973.

Gilman, Sander. *Disease and Representation: Images of Illness from Madness to AIDS.* Ithaca, NY: Cornell University Press, 1988.

Gowing, Laura. *Domestic Dangers: Women, Words, and Sex in Early Modern London.* Oxford: Clarendon Press, 1996.

Hale, David George. *The Body Politic: a Political Metaphor in Renaissance English Literature.* The Hague: Mouton, 1971.

Harley, David. 'Rhetoric and the Social Construction of Sickness and Healing' *Social History of Medicine,* 12:3 (1999): 407–435.

Harris, Jonathan Gil. *Foreign Bodies and the Body Politic: Discourses of Social Pathology in Early Modern England.* Cambridge: Cambridge University Press, 1996.

Harris, Jonathan Gil. *Sick Economies: Drama, Mercantilism, and Disease in Shakespeare's England.* Philadelphia: University of Pennsylvania Press, 2004.

Harvey, Gideon. *Great Venus Unmasked: Or a More Exact Discovery of the Venereal Evil, or French Disease.* 2nd ed. London: B. G. for Nath Brook, 1672.

Harvey, Gideon. *Little Venus Unmasked: Or a Perfect Discovery of the French Pox.* London: James Partridge, 1685.

Hayden, Deborah. *Pox: Genius, Madness, and the Mysteries of Syphilis.* New York: Basic Books, 2003.

Healy, Margaret. *Fictions of Disease in Early Modern England.* New York: Palgrave, 2001.

Horowitz, Elliot. 'The New World and the Changing Face of Europe' *Sixteenth Century Journal,* 28:4 (1997): 1181–1201.

Jütte, Robert. *Poverty and Deviance in Early Modern Europe.* Cambridge: Cambridge University Press, 1994.

Jütte, Robert. 'Syphilis and Confinement: Hospitals in Early Modern Germany' pp. 97–115 in *Institutions of Confinement: Hospitals, Asylums, and Prisons in Western Europe and North America, 1500–1950,* eds. Norbert Finzsch and Robert Jutte. Cambridge: Cambridge University Press, 1996.

Laqueur, Thomas. *Making Sex: The Body and Gender from the Greeks to Freud.* Cambridge, MA: Harvard University Press, 1990.

Lindemann, Mary. *Medicine and Society in Early Modern Europe.* Cambridge: Cambridge University Press, 1999.

Levine, Philippa. *Prostitution, Race and Politics: Policing Venereal Disease in the British Empire.* London: Routledge, 2003.

L'Origine de la Syphilis en Europe, avant ou après 1493? eds. Olivier Dutour, György Palfi, Jacques Berato, and Jean-Pierre Brun. Paris: Centre Archeologique du Var ; Errance, 1994.

Lowe, Peter. *An Easie, Certaine, and Perfect Method, to Cure and Prevent the Spanish Sicknes.* London: James Roberts, 1596.

Mays, Simon, Gillian Crane-Kramer and Alex Bayliss, 'Two Probable Cases of Treponemal Disease of Medieval Date from England' *American Journal of Physical Anthropology,* 120 (2003): 120–133.

Maynwaring, Everad. *The History and Mystery of the Venereal Lues.* London: J.M., 1673.

Moore, Merril, 'Joseph Grünpeck and his Neat Treatise' *British Journal of Venereal Disease,* 11 (1935): 1–27.

Moore, R.I. *The Formation of a Persecuting Society: Power and Deviance in Western Europe, 950–1250.* Oxford: Oxford University Press, 1990.

Nutton, Vivian 'The Seeds of Disease: An Explanation of Contagion and Infection from the Greeks to the Renaissance' *Medical History,* 27 (1983): 1–34.

Oriel, J. D. *The Scars of Venus: A History of Venereology.* London: Springer-Verlag, 1994.

Patients and Practitioners: Lay Perceptions of Medicine in Pre-industrial Society ed. Roy Porter. Cambridge: Cambridge University Press, 1985.

Pelling, Margaret. *The Common Lot: Sickness, Medical Occupations and the Urban Poor in Early Modern England.* London: Longman, 1998.

Pelling, Margaret. *Medical Conflicts in Early Modern London: Patronage, Physicians, and Irregular Practitioners 1550–1640.* Oxford: Oxford University Press, 2003.

Porter, Roy. 'Spreading Carnal Knowledge or Selling Dirt Cheap? Nicholas Venette's *Tableau de l'amour conjugal in eighteenth-century England' Journal of European Studies,* 14 (1984): 233–255.

Porter, Roy. '"The Secrets of Generation Display'd": Aristotle's Master-piece in Eighteenth-Century England' *Eighteenth-Century Life,* 9:3 (1985): 1–21.

Porter, Roy. 'The Patient's View: Doing Medical History from Below' *Theory and Society,* 14 (1985): 175–198.

Porter, Roy. *Health For Sale: Quackery in England 1660–1850.* Manchester: Manchester University Press, 1989.

Porter, Roy and Hall, Lesley. *The Facts of Life: The Creation of Sexual Knowledge in Britain 1650–1950.* New Haven: Yale University Press, 1995.

Pullan, Brian. *Rich and Poor in Renaissance Venice* Cambridge MA: Harvard University Press, 1971.

Qualtiere, Louis F. and William W. E. Slights. 'Contagion and Blame in Early Modern England: The Case of the French Pox' *Literature and Medicine,* 22:1 (2003): 1–23.

Quétel, Claude. *The History of Syphilis,* trans. Judith Braddock and Brian Pike, Baltimore: The Johns Hopkins University Press, 1990.

Rolleston, J. D. 'Venereal Disease in Literature' *British Journal of Venereal Disease,* 10 (1934): 175–182.

Rosebury, Theodore. *Microbes and Morals: The Strange Story of Venereal Disease.* New York: Viking Press, 1971.

Ross, Eric B. 'Syphilis, Misogyny and Witchcraft in 16th-Century Europe' *Current Anthropology* 36:2 (1995): 333–337.

Ruggiero, Guido. 'The Strange Death of Margarita Marcellini: *Male,* Signs, and the Everyday World of Pre-modern Medicine' *American Historical Review,* 106:4 (2001): 1141–1158.

Schleiner, Winfried. 'Infection and Cure through Women: Renaissance Constructions of Syphilis' *Journal of Medieval and Renaissance Studies,* 24:3 (1994): 499–517.

Schleiner, Winfried. 'Moral Attitudes Towards Syphilis and its Prevention in the Renaissance' *Bulletin of the History of Medicine,* 68 (1994): 389–410.

Scholz, Susanne. *Body Narratives: Writing the Nation and Fashioning the Subject in Early Modern England.* New York: St. Martin's Press, 2000.

Sex, Sin and Suffering: Venereal Disease and European Society Since 1870. eds. Roger Davidson, and Lesley Hall. London: Routledge, 2001.

Siena, Kevin P. 'Pollution, Promiscuity, and the Pox: English Venereology and the Early Modern Discourse on Social and Sexual Danger' *Journal of the History of Sexuality,* 8:4 (1998): 553–574.

Siena, Kevin P. 'The "Foul Disease" and Privacy: The Effects of Venereal Disease and Patient Demand on the Medical Marketplace in Early Modern London' *Bulletin of the History of Medicine,* 75:2 (2001):199–224.

Slack, Paul. *The Impact of Plague in Tudor and Stuart England.* London: Routledge, 1985.

Sontag, Susan. *Illness as Metaphor.* New York: Straus and Giroux, 1978.

Sontag, Susan. *AIDS and its Metaphors.* New York: Straus and Giroux, 1989.

Spongberg, Mary. *Feminizing Venereal Disease: The Body of the Prostitute in the Nineteenth-Century.* London: Macmillan, 1997.

Temkin, Owsei. 'On the History of "Morality and Syphilis"' pp. 472–484 in his *The Double Face of Janus and Other Essays in the History of Medicine.* Baltimore: The Johns Hopkins University Press, 1977.

The Earliest Printed Literature on Syphilis, Being Ten Tractates from the Years 1495–1498, ed. Karl Sudhoff. Florence: R. Lier, 1925.

The Secret Malady: Venereal Disease in Eighteenth-Century Britain and France ed. Linda E. Merians. Lexington, KY: University of Kentucky Press, 1996.

Timken-Zinkann, R. F. 'Some Aspects of Epidemics and German Art about 1500' *Medical History,* 8:4 (1969): 355–362.

Turner, David M. *Fashioning Adultery: Gender, Sex and Civility in England, 1640–1740.* Cambridge: Cambridge University Press, 2002.

Watts, Sheldon. *Epidemics and History: Disease, Power and Imperialism.* New Haven: Yale University Press, 1997.

Wear, Andrew. *Knowledge and Practice in English Medicine, 1550–1680.* Cambridge: Cambridge University Press, 2001.

Scientific and Medical Responses

Medical Responses to the 'French Disease' in Europe at the turn of the Sixteenth Century[1]

Jon Arrizabalaga

To Roger French, (1938–2002) *in memoriam*

The 'French Disease' (*morbus gallicus*) is the most popular name for an apparently new condition that quickly spread throughout Europe in the 1490s. It was perceived as a loathsome and incurable disease consisting of severe aches in the bones and of sores usually beginning in the genitals, but eventually covering the whole body. Like plague and other infectious diseases, it damaged all social strata and ravaged the most humble people, but its wide diffusion among courts and urban patriciate – along with the quantity and expressiveness of surviving historical sources referring to these elites – has promoted an image of the 'French Disease' as a condition typical of the privileged social strata.

Latin Galenism, the medical system then dominant among university practitioners who covered the health demands of social elites, was characterized by plural, open, and equivocal views about disease causality. This meant that physicians initially related the French Disease to a range of various kinds of causes (divine punishment, corrupt air, harmful star constellations, and bad life regime, among others), which could be at work either collectively or separately. It did not, however, prevent some of the

---

[1]This article has been partly worked out in the framework of the project BHA2002-00512 of the Dirección General de Investigación, Spanish Ministry of Science and Technology. Previous versions of it were presented as papers to the *IV Jornadas de Historia de la Medicina y de la Ciencia* (Madrid, Universidad Complutense, September 1995) and to the *International Conference 'Comparative Perspectives on the History of Sexually Transmitted Diseases'* (London, University of London, April 1996); and published as the chapter 'Causalidad, especificidad y prevención del "mal francés" en la medicina universitaria del tránsito entre los siglos XV y XVI' pp. 141–157 in *De la responsabilidad individual a la culpabilización de la víctima. El papel del paciente en la prevención de la enfermedad*, L. Montiel and I. Porras, eds. Aranjuez: Doce Calles, 1997.

earliest university practitioners who coped with the disease from acknowledging that a specific external cause transmissible through contagion by contact – sexual, above all – could also be involved in the spread of this disease. In the works of these earliest practitioners we can detect a rather consistent shift from a pattern of disease prevention, which was then peculiar to the reactions against plague and pestilences, to a new one tending to focus upon coitus. The attention to contagion and coitus also demonstrates that we should rethink the suggestion that the French Disease was not considered venereal until after 1520.[2] A great deal of the earliest medical writers linked the disease to sex in a number of ways.

This paper has two major aims. On the one hand, it is intended to track these new views on disease causality by exploring a number of the earliest medical works on the French Disease.[3] On the other hand, it aims to examine the extent to which these new views determined the prevention measures proposed by the earliest writers on this disease.

The thirteen works from 1496 to 1502 I will examine do not exhaust the extant earliest medical literature on the French Disease, but can be seen as representative. They were written by twelve doctors, most of whom developed their careers in Italy. Five works relate to a courtly disputation on the identity and causes of the new disease held in Ferrara between late March and early April 1497 under the patronage of the local lords, the dukes of Este. They are those written by the three known contenders at the dispute, the medical professors at the university of Ferrara Nicolò Leoniceno (1428–1524) and Sebastiano dall'Aquila (*c.*1440–*c.*1510), and the Estense court physician Corradino Gilino (*fl.*1468–1499),[4] and two provoked by Leoniceno's work, namely its rebuttal by the Bolognese medical professor Natale Montesauro (*fl.* 1484–1501), and the counter-replication to the latter by Antonio Scanaroli (*c.* 1450–1517), a former pupil of Leoniceno practicing in Modena.[5] Three more treatises arose from the papal court of Alexander VI Borgia. They were written by two of his physicians, both of them Spaniards from Valencia who long resided in Rome, namely Gaspar

---

2Temkin, 'On the History of "Morality and Syphilis",' especially pp. 472–474.

3For more information on this topic, see Arrizabalaga, Henderson, and French, *The Great Pox*.

4Leoniceno, *Libellus de epidemia quam vulgo morbum gallicum vocant*; Dall'Aquila, *Interpretatio et cura morbi gallici* (written in 1497), fols. 184^{r}–202^{v}; Gilino, *De morbo quem gallicum nuncupant*. For a facsimile edition of Leoniceno's and Gilino's works see pp. 117–182 and 251–260, respectively, in *The Earliest Printed Literature on Syphilis*.

5Montesauro, *De dispositionibus quas vulgares mal franzoso appellant*; Scanaroli, *Disputatio utilis de morbo gallico*. For a facsimile edition of these works see pp. 279–312 and 313–346, respectively, in *The Earliest Printed Literature on Syphilis*.

Torrella (*c.*1452–*c.*1520) and Pere Pintor (*c.*1423/4–1503).[6] A third Valencian, Joan Almenar (*fl.*1502), was the author of another similar work which was first published in Venice in 1502 and appears to have been strongly influenced by Italian university circles.[7] The three remaining works belong to authors from the Germanic area, namely Konrad Schellig (*fl.* 1496), physician of the elector of the Palatinate and medical professor at Heidelberg university; Johann Widmann (1440–1524), physician of the earl of Württemberg and professor in Tübingen; and Bartholomäus Steber (d. 1506), professor in Vienna. Schellig and Widmann completed parts of their educations in Northern Italian medical faculties – both of them in Padua, and Widmann also in Pavia and Ferrara.[8]

Causes of the French Disease

Latin Galenist practitioners assumed that disease was essentially the result of a humoural imbalance provoked by a concatenation of external and internal, remote and proximate causes operating according to an open and plural pattern, within a framework of permanent interrelations between macro and microcosmos. According to the Christian ontology – unquestioned in Europe until well into the eighteenth century and also shared by Islam and Judaism, the other two major monotheist religions in the Mediterranean area – God's will was the first cause of disease, as it was of all things in His Creation. Yet, Christian natural philosophers' construction of a natural order autonomously ruled by natural laws, save exceptional circumstances (i.e., miracles), meant that theologians kept an intellectual and professional monopoly on the *Primum Movens*. For their part physicians, charged with the task of attending bodily health and bodily disease, were in charge of the secondary causes that determined the state of their patient's health or sickness.

Within this causal system, one single cause could provoke multiple diseases and one single disease could be due to multiple causes. Patients

---

6 Torrella, *Tractatus cum consiliis contra pudendagram seu morbum gallicum. De morbo gallico cum aliis*, and *Dialogus de dolore cum tractatu de ulceribus in pudendagra evenire solitis*; Pintor, *De morbo foedo et occulto his temporibus affligente*. For a facsimile edition of Torrella's earliest work see pp. 182–232 in *The Earliest Printed Literature on Syphilis*.

7 Almenar, *Libellus ad evitandum et expellendum morbum gallicum ut nunquam revertatur*.

8 Schellig, *In pustulas malas morbum quem malum de Francia vulgus appellat*; Widmann, *Tractatus de pustulis et morbo qui vulgato nomine mal de franzos appellatur*; Steber, *A malafranczos morbo gallorum preservatio ac cura*. For a facsimile edition of these three works see pp. 1–22, 233–250 (and 347–352), and 261–278, respectively, in *The Earliest Printed Literature on Syphilis*.

could suffer from 'composite' diseases, that is, diseases resulting from a mixture of two or more 'simple' ones. The 'morbid matter' that was the immediate cause of disease could freely move within a sick body, and this often caused a disease to change its seat during its course. Furthermore, such matter could eventually change in its substance or properties and cause one disease to 'metamorphose' into another.

a. Theurgical causes

The initial perplexity of university practitioners towards the nature and causes of the French Disease contributed to emphasize the open, plural, and equivocal character of the causal views of Latin Galenism. In one way or another, almost all practitioners referred to God as its First Cause. Yet, most focused on 'secondary causes' – those usually subjected to concern by university physicians – while only some of them gave a central role to the First Cause. In both cases, the alleged barrier between the disease-views of university physicians and lay people was much more permeable than traditionally assumed for medieval and Renaissance Europe. This intercommunication was particularly manifest with regard to views on the theurgical causes of the French Disease.

University practitioners like Johann Widmann, Nicolò Leoniceno, Natale Montesauro, or Antonio Scanaroli emphasized their professional interest as physicians for the immediate causes and declared their incompetence to discuss theurgical causes, which were allegedly a topic of theologians' exclusive concern.[9] Others, like Gaspar Torrella, merely echoed the voice of third persons (*alii dicunt*) who claimed that this disease was due to God's punishment.[10] In both cases, the theurgical causes played no role at all in the battery of preventive or therapeutic measures except for occasional standard pious invocations to the Greatest Healer.

A third group of practitioners attached the new disease directly to a divine origin, although not even this was entirely determinant upon their preventive or therapeutic advice. Following the Aristotelian pattern of causality, Joan Almenar stated that knowledge of material, formal, and efficient causes was the competence of the 'bodily physician' (*medicus corporalis*), while that of the final cause belonged to the 'spiritual physician' (*medicus spiritualis*). According to the latter, diseases and other calamities

---

[9]Widmann, *Tractatus de pustulis et morbo qui vulgato nomine mal de franzos appellatur*, fols. 1^{r}–1^{v}; Leoniceno, *Libellus de epidemia quam vulgo morbum gallicum vocant*, sign. c8^{v}–d1^{r}; Montesauro, *De dispositionibus quas vulgares mal franzoso appellant*, fols. 4^{v}–5^{r}; Scanaroli, *Disputatio utilis de morbo gallico*, sign. a2^{v}.

[10]Torrella, *Tractatus cum consiliis contra pudendagram*, sign. a3^{v}.

befell humans as a punishment for their sins; some diseases were specifically related to mortal sins – quotidian fever to pride, podagra to laziness, and leprosy to lust. Since the French Disease was akin to leprosy, Almenar claimed, it should be related to lust. Thus, those wishing to preserve themselves from it or to recover their health should avoid lust.[11] Yet, this did not prevent Almenar from dedicating two complete chapters to medical remedies for treatment and safe prevention of the disease.[12]

Finally, the Ferrarese court physician Corradino Gilino claimed that the outbreak of the French Disease resulted from the apocalyptic punishment that God sent upon the Italian people for their many and grave sins. This peculiar view, which did not prevent Gilino from writing an otherwise standard medical treatise on this disease, was strongly influenced by the apocalyptic atmosphere pervading late fifteenth-century Italy and very influential at the Estense court of Ferrara, which the prophetic activism of the Dominican friar Girolamo Savonarola fuelled from Florence.[13] Gilino's theurgical views fit into a widespread pattern of collective disease in the Old Testament, namely that of the countless and terrible plagues that scourged the Israelites or their enemies. Alternatively, the identification of the French Disease with that of the Biblical patriarch Job was also influential in late fifteenth-century northern Italy among lay people, including medical circles like that of the Estense court. This new identity was by no means surprising since both diseases were perceived as unknown, inexplicable, incurable, and afflicting victims who appeared deformed and loathsome. The dilemma of whether Job's disease and other troubles were divine punishment for sin or undeserved calamities sent upon innocents to prove the sincerity of faith was at work in the contemporary perceptions of the French Disease.[14]

b. Natural Causes: Epidemic Versus Contagion?

All of this did not prevent most early medical writers on the French Disease from concentrating most of their attention on the natural causes of this disease, particularly those 'inferior' or 'proximate' ones. A major discussion revolved around whether it was an epidemic scourge or merely a contagious disease. Latin Galenist physicians assumed that every epidemic disease was also contagious, but the opposite was not true. On the other hand,

[11] Almenar, *Libellus ad evitandum et expellendum morbum gallicum*, sign. A4^{r}–A4^{v}, D1^{v}.

[12] Almenar, *Libellus ad evitandum et expellendum morbum gallicum*, sign. B3^{v}–D1^{v} (treatment), D1^{v}–D2^{v} (prevention).

[13] Gilino, *De morbo quem gallicum nuncupant*, fol. 1^{v}.

[14] Arrizabalaga, Henderson, and French, *The Great Pox*, pp. 44–45, 52–55.

while epidemics were allegedly provoked by universal causes, *contagia* did not require the concurrence of this kind of causes for their outbreak and spread.

Thus, a number of writers understood the French Disease as provoked by a causal chain similar to that typical of the late medieval pestilences: that is, from the 'First Cause' (divine punishment) to that unleashing the epidemic (a corruption of the air) through one or more astral causes (usually, ominous planetary conjunctions). Yet, each medical writer emphasized different links in this chain. Some underlined the role of celestial influences, in consonance with the flourishing of astrological medical views in contemporary Europe.[15] This was the case of Gilino and Almenar,[16] who showed themselves well aware of the theurgical cause, as well as of Konrad Schellig and Bartholomäus Steber, neither of whom discussed theurgy explicitly.[17] Others, like the German Widmann and the Italians Leoniceno, Montesauro and Scanaroli, claimed that, as physicians, they should limit themselves to study the proximate natural causes beginning with the air corruption and leave to theologians and astrologers the discussions of superior causes.[18] Let us take Leoniceno's views as an example. To him the French Disease should be reckoned within the chapter of 'epidemics' – in the Hippocratic meaning of this term, i.e., collective diseases wandering from one place to another. It derived from a warm and humid 'intemperance' of the air, frequently but not exclusively in the summer. He claimed that the French Disease had broken out in Italy during the 1496 summer after an excessive humidity had lasted for over a year and he identified it with Hippocrates' description in *Epidemics*, book 3. This disease was only one of the multiple effects of this peculiar qualitative change of the air, which he considered to be the 'mother of every putrefaction,' in keeping

---

[15]North, 'Celestial Influence – The Major Premise of Astrology,' pp. 45–100; Grant, 'Medieval and Renaissance Scholastic Conceptions of the Influence of the Celestial Region on the Terrestrial,' pp. 1–23; and French, 'Astrology in Medical Practice,' pp. 30–59.

[16]Gilino, *De morbo quem gallicum nuncupant*, fol. [1^r]; Almenar, *Libellus ad evitandum et expellendum morbum gallicum*, sign. A3^v–A4^r.

[17]Schellig, *In pustulas malas morbum quem malum de Francia vulgus appellat*, sign. a2^v; Steber, *A malafranczos morbo gallorum preservatio ac cura*, sign. 5^v–6^r. Schellig was not explicit as to the role of the theurgic cause on the French Disease, but Jacob Wimpheling was in the letter preceding the former's work. At its beginning Wimpheling stated: 'iusta Dei severitas sive propter horrendam et olim inauditam blasphemiam sive propter spurcissimum (quod invaluit) adulterium aut cetera peccata, per syderum fluxus aliasque causas morbum quendam quem nostra tempestate insubres in patriam suam Gallos invexisse lamentantur...' (sign. a1^v).

[18]See note 8, above.

with Aristotelian natural philosophy. To Leoniceno the French Pox was a generic disease which could manifest itself under several species according to the nature of the pathological humour(s) involved in each case.[19]

A third group including Sebastiano dall'Aquila, Pere Pintor and Almenar himself claimed that the French Disease was sometimes an epidemic scourge, sometimes merely a contagious disease. To Dall'Aquila, who identified it with Galen's *elephantiasis*, the French Disease could spread through an 'air infection' or, more often, through 'what physicians call contagion,' particularly that linked to touch. Dall'Aquila underlined three forms of contagion through touch, namely coitus, assiduous sleeping, and nursing. At a secondary level, Dall'Aquila admitted, in agreement with Leoniceno, that 'some air infection' caused by moist weather had contributed to the outbreak of the French Disease, but he denied any role to the immoderate heat that Leoniceno believed had also been involved.[20]

Pintor, on the other hand, qualified the French Disease as a 'dreadful and hidden' (*foedus et occultus*) epidemic disease. He identified it with a third and obscure species of the *variola* kind of disease called *aluhumata* that had been previously described by Avicenna and Rhazes.[21] Like the alleged two other *variola* species, it resulted from a 'corruptive' boiling (as opposite to 'perfective' boiling) of the blood. This blood could originate from the remains of menstrual blood which, according to Galenic assumptions, fed the foetus during pregnancy. These remains could stay for one's whole life after birth or, less often, generate from the consumption of harmful foods and other regime disorders. The kind of blood involved in the French Disease was melancholic, which contemporaries believed could hardly boil. Thus, the risk of suffering from the French Disease was higher in individuals with a melancholy complexion.[22]

Such infected menstrual blood could remain dormant for long periods or even for one's whole life. But at any stage it could also become the material cause of the French Disease as a result of certain 'external causes,' particularly the 'pestilential, corrupted air.'[23] This required enough additional heat to cause this peculiar boiling. Such heat could come from lengthy exposure to the sun, an overly hot and moist spring, or the shaking of the blood itself when nature tried to expel it from the body.[24] Beyond

---

19Leoniceno, *Libellus de epidemia quam vulgo morbum gallicum vocant*, sign. d1ᵛ–d3ʳ.

20Dall'Aquila, *Interpretatio et cura morbi gallici*, fols. 196ʳ⁻ᵛ.

21Pintor, *De morbo foedo et occulto his temporibus affligente*, sign. aᵛ, a1ᵛ, a7ᵛ, d7ᵛ, f3ᵛ–f4ʳ.

22Pintor, *De morbo foedo et occulto his temporibus affligente*, sign. a4ʳ, a6ᵛ, a7ʳ, b2ʳ, c7ʳ–dʳ.

23Pintor, *De morbo foedo et occulto his temporibus affligente*, sign. a4ʳ–a5ʳ.

24Pintor, *De morbo foedo et occulto his temporibus affligente*, sign. a6ᵛ–a7ᵛ.

these external causes, Pintor also judged that there was 'a certain hidden influence or property' arising from some peculiar star constellations lasting from 1483 – the alleged year for the beginning of the epidemic – to 1500 – the date for its end according to his prognosis. As a way of noticeable proof (*sensuale iuditium*) of these astral influences, Pintor argued that prisoners, enclosed monks and nuns, and those living in marshy areas where thick air hung, had not suffered from the French Disease.[25] Yet, Pintor admitted that sometimes the *aluhumata* could also be provoked by a merely inferior cause.[26]

Pintor admitted that the French Disease was always contagious. So sufferers could infect the air of a room, as well as those people accompanying, conversing, eating, or sleeping with them. In passing from one house to another, this 'harmful air' could easily spread over all the city and infect many other people. People's risk of infection grew in proportion to the proximity and length of their contact with a sufferer. Thus, Pintor underlined, the French Disease was extremely contagious when a man has copulated with a woman suffering from it, particularly if he lived with her. Pintor claimed that men were much more receptive to sexual contagion than women and explained this through reasons identical to those used by Torrella in 1497, to which I will refer below.[27]

The Valencian Almenar claimed that the French Disease was a 'harmful epidemic condition' which could even infect through a 'pure influence or corruption of air,' although it worked more often by contagion in the context of social intercourse (*conversatio*). Almenar piously asserted that the clergy (*religiosi*) caught the disease by means of breathing corrupted air, while contagion was the mode of infection for children and adults, the former through being kissed or suckled, the latter through coitus.[28] Yet, Almenar admitted that some individuals could manage to avoid catching the French Disease, despite being inclined to melancholic diseases, following an inadequate life regime, or of having sex with infected people. To explain this surprising feature he argued that their bodies had greater thickness or some peculiar 'individual property' that protected them against the 'impressions' of this disease.[29]

Finally, the views held by the papal physician Gaspar Torrella expressively illustrate the case of those who claimed that the French Disease was

---

25 Pintor, *De morbo foedo et occulto his temporibus affligente*, sign. d^r–d^v.

26 Pintor, *De morbo foedo et occulto his temporibus affligente*, sign. a7^r–b2^r, b6^r, b7^r.

27 Pintor, *De morbo foedo et occulto his temporibus affligente*, sign. d^r–d^v.

28 Almenar, *Libellus ad evitandum et expellendum morbum gallicum*, sign. B1^r.

29 Almenar, *Libellus ad evitandum et expellendum morbum gallicum*, sign. D3^r.

not epidemic, but merely a contagious disease. After having quickly revised the theurgical and astral causes (the latter of which he openly disqualified in his work of 1500), he stated that this disease was usually transmitted through contagion by individual contact, although it could be also developed as a result of an inadequate life regime. While the disease might occasionally be transmitted when someone came into contact with the infectious 'halo' which supposedly surrounded the ill, contagion was predominantly through sexual contact.[30]

In 1497 Torrella intended to prove his professional competence in the face of the French Disease with five medical reports (*consilia*). Three of them illustrated his views on its contagion, although only one of them (the first *consilium*) appears to be a case of direct sexual transmission, allegedly through the corrupt vapours from the uterus entering pores in the member of his patient 'Nicholas the Young' – a pseudonym for Caesar Borgia according to Sudhoff's suggestion.[31] In his male-centred account Torrella asserted that men suffered more from the French Disease than women because on the one hand men had a hotter complexion and on the other the uterus encouraged the corruption of vapours within infected women. It was of first importance, therefore, that men should avoid infected women. However, the reverse was not true according to Torrella. Since the uterus was cold, dry, and dense, it did not suffer damage very easily and it was only after repeated sexual contact with infected men that women became infected.[32] The fourth *consilium* might have been a case of non-sexual contagion, given that it concerns a mature man who caught the pox by sleeping in the same bed as his infected brother.[33] As for the last case (the third *consilium*), Torrella simply speaks of a 30-year old Lombard man who was infected through 'contagion.'[34]

There were also other (albeit less usual) ways to transmit the French Disease according Torrella. The paradigm of this alternative view revolved around an inappropriate life regime in the 'six non-naturals' (*sex res non naturales*) that could equally cause the pox. This was particularly the case in people whose complexions inclined towards the humoural *dyscrasia*, which supposedly unleashed this disease. Torrella warned consistently that those are liable to the French Disease who indulge in anger or melancholy, who 'make use of salted, sharp, and bitter foods or drink ...; who do not

---

30 Torrella, *Tractatus cum consiliis contra pudendagram*, sign. a4^{v}–b1^{r}.

31 *The Earliest Printed Literature on Syphilis*, p. xxxiii.

32 Torrella, *Tractatus cum consiliis contra pudendagram*, sign. c4^{v}–d1^{r} (*consilium* I).

33 Torrella, *Tractatus cum consiliis contra pudendagram*, sign. e1^{r} (*consilium* III).

34 Torrella, *Tractatus cum consiliis contra pudendagram*, sign. e2^{r} (*consilium* IV).

take baths as they used to do; who do not change their clothes; who do not take exercise or massage; who take meals or medicines that bring matter to the skin; who drink sharp and old wines or those sweet and heated too long.'[35] He illustrated this alternative mode of infection by providing three examples of what could happen to *any* individual in absence of his advice. The first was the case of a Catalan university-trained physician who got the disease as a result of having consumed the wrong food and drink during a sea voyage.[36] The second case also involved a sea-voyager who exposed himself excessively to the sun and fell into 'some other inappropriate regime' during the course of his trip.[37] The final case was that of a priest with dyscrased complexion and liver.[38]

Why Does the French Disease Begin in the Genitals?

There was thus a wide plurality of views on the French Disease and causation, which demonstrates the extreme openness of Latin Galenism. The multiple variables required to determine causation assured that the cause-effect relationship was highly indeterminant and hardly resolved in the first decade that followed 1494. This should warn us against hastily applying our own conceptual framework onto theirs. Sexual transmission was clearly one topic in the debate, but it was far from alone. Indeed, the breadth of the dissimilar responses to a central question – why does the disease usually begin in the genitals? – offers a splendid topic to display this.

For some, especially those who, like Almenar and Pintor, directly addressed superior causes, astrology played an important role in linking the disease to the sex organs. Some contemporary university practitioners explained that the French Disease located itself in different parts of the body as a result of the influence of peculiar celestial phenomena, such as planetary conjunctions or oppositions, zodiac projections, and lunar eclipses. The assumption that the zodiac sign of *Scorpio* was projected upon the anatomy and diseases of the genitals was explicit or implicitly at work in the Valencian Almenar and Pintor, among others.[39] Almenar believed that the French Disease tended to begin in the genitals because there was a 'conformity' between these parts and the quality of the new disease

35 Torrella, *Tractatus cum consiliis contra pudendagram*, sign. b1r.

36 Torrella, *Tractatus cum consiliis contra pudendagram*, sign. b1r (*consilium* II).

37 Torrella, *Tractatus cum consiliis contra pudendagram*, sign. d2v (*consilium* II).

38 Torrella, *Tractatus cum consiliis contra pudendagram*, sign. e3r (*consilium* V).

39 Sudhoff, *Graphische und typographische Erstlinge der Syphilisliteratur aus den Jahren 1495 und 1496*, pp. 6–7, plates III–IV.

resulting from the entrance of Saturn in the sign of Aries and other corresponding celestial dispositions that he did not specify.[40] On the other hand, Pintor assigned the signs of the French Disease to melancholic parts (with no care to their chronology) because of the identity of the planets involved in the conjunctions that he associated with the disease's outbreak and spread. Simply put, he located symptoms in the genitals based on the assumption that the conjunction of 1483 – which allegedly marked the disease's beginning – happened under the sign of *Scorpio*.[41] Curiously enough, not all writers who assigned an important role to astrology in their causal views resorted to similar kinds of interpretations when trying to explain the initial genital manifestations of the French Disease. Steber, for instance, explained this feature from the anatomical peculiarities of these parts,[42] while Gilino attributed it to the peculiar tropism of the disease matter as a result of its qualities.[43]

For those like Leoniceno, Montesauro, Scanaroli, and Torrella, all of whom had left the consideration of superior causes to theologians and astrologers, the initial genital location of the French Disease resulted from more 'immediate' causes. Consistent with his causal views and relying on Galen's authority, Leoniceno argued that the disease frequently first appeared in the genitals because these parts were more exposed to putrefaction due to their primary qualities (their natural heat and humidity), to the extent that even the slightest changes in the air could affect them.[44] Dall'Aquila endorsed this idea,[45] but Almenar radically rejected it arguing that, if this were the case, every disease would begin in the genitals.[46] By contrast, Montesauro claimed that the pox first struck the genitals only when it had been transmitted 'by contagion during coitus.' In other cases the disease began in the head, much like the Avicennan *asaphati* with which he identified it. He explained this differential feature by arguing – always according to Avicenna's authority – that genitals became infected during coitus more than other bodily parts, for 'they are protected from air, tend

---

40 Almenar, *Libellus ad evitandum et expellendum morbum gallicum*, sign. D2^{v}.

41 Pintor, *De morbo foedo et occulto his temporibus affligente*, sign. b^{r}.

42 Steber, *A malafranczos morbo gallorum preservatio ac cura*, sign. 5^{v}.

43 By echoing Galen's and Avicenna's authority as to 'cancer,' Gilino stated that as thicker and hotter the morbific matter was (as it was the case of the French Disease), as more often and quickly it tended to go to the sparse and soft members like the pudenda (i.e., 'testicles, vulva, penis and anus'). See Gilino, *De morbo quem gallicum nuncupant*, fols. 2^{v}–3^{r}.

44 Leoniceno, *Libellus de epidemia quam vulgo morbum gallicum vocant*, sign. d2^{r}.

45 Dall'Aquila, *Interpretatio et cura morbi gallici*, fols. 196^{v}–197^{r}.

46 Almenar, *Libellus ad evitandum et expellendum morbum gallicum*, sign. D2^{v}.

towards heat and humidity,' and are placed close to the ways of evacuation for 'superfluous humours.'[47]

Scanaroli shared the ideas of his master Leoniceno whose authority he intended to defend from Montesauro's attack. Thus, he claimed that the French Disease first appeared in parts other than genitals in just two or three per cent of cases. He counterattacked that it was (allegedly) well known that the disease began in the genitals even in 'many virgin children as well as old people who had never tried to copulate.'[48] So the disease was linked to the sexual organs, but not necessarily linked to sexual intercourse. To reinforce these claims, Scanaroli had no qualms about relying on Torrella's authority, despite the clear differences in their interpretations of this question. Indeed, in 1497 Caesar Borgia's doctor had asserted that the genitals, in particular the male penis, were most usually the initial site of the French Disease whether it was caught through contagion – as in the case of the young man in *consilium* I who got the French Disease after having an affair with an infected woman – or through a bad life regime – like the patient in *consilium* II who got sick as a result of an excessive sun irradiation.[49] Indeed, in his new work of 1500 – two years after Scanaroli's – Torrella continued to situate the most common beginning of the disease in the genitals. Now, however, he compared the French Disease with *scabies* so that he gave to this feature an explanation entirely based on the idea of infection. Although 'the genitals become infected first, and then the remaining members,' the infection always began from the member that first came into contact with the disease sores, for 'all that touches the putrid, decays immediately.' Thus, the French Disease could also be spread contagiously to an infant from the breasts, mouth, or face of a wet nurse and, conversely, to another nurse from the mouth or face of the infected infant on the assumption that 'wet nurses often kiss infants.'[50]

---

[47]Montesauro, *De dispositionibus quas vulgares mal franzoso appellant*, fol. 3^{v}; Avicenna, *Liber Canonis Medicine*, lib. III, fen XX, trat. ii, cap. xx: 'Cum ulcera accidunt in istis locis, sunt mala ambulativa quoniam membra ista sunt secundum formam ad quorum partes festinat putrefactio, quoniam sunt protecta ab aere, et declivia ad caliditatem et humiditatem, et approximant meatibus superfluitatum et assimilantur quodammodo ulceribus viscerum et oris. Et eorum deteriora sunt illa que fiunt in lacerto qui est in radice virge, et in ano; et illud immo quoniam indigent exsiccatione forti, et sensus eorum cum hoc est vehemens. Et fortasse necessarium est abscindere virgam ipsam, quum super ipsam putrefiunt ulcera, et perambulant' (Venice, Luca Antonio Junta, 1527, fol. 285^{r}).

[48]Scanaroli, *Disputatio utilis de morbo gallico*, sign. a4^{v}–a5^{r}.

[49]Torrella, *Tractatus cum consiliis contra pudendagram*, sign. c4^{v}, d2^{v}.

[50]Torrella, *Dialogus de dolore cum tractatu de ulceribus in pudendagra evenire solitis*, sign. a6^{v}.

Although all writers linked the genitals to the disease within their discussions of symptoms, they gave a wide range of explanations for this connection. For some, the clear genital manifestations of the French Disease pointed to a link with sexual intercourse. However, the issue remained unresolved and some of the earliest writers remained hesitant to conclude that the French Disease was primarily sexually transmitted. The open, equivocal, and varied belief system that was Latin Galenism allowed for a multiplicity of explanatory reactions to the new disease and left the question of the sexual nature of the new disease quite unsettled.

Preventive Measures

If causality and prevention might be considered two sides of a coin, a close relationship between the causal views of and the preventive measures against the French Disease held by university practitioners at the turn of the sixteenth century should hardly surprise us. But, here again, some discrepancies can be detected among these writers concerning not only their explanations for why the disease struck, but also what patients should do about it.

Invocations to God seeking protection against the French Disease were commonplace for most authors. However, the emphasis fluctuated in relation to their views on the role of the theurgical cause. Indeed, those like Pintor and Almenar who stressed superior causes explicitly claimed that this was the starting point for any medical intervention whether preventive or therapeutic. By contrast, others, like Schellig and Torrella, for whom superior causality played a less central role, restricted themselves merely to introducing a prayer somewhere in their works, preferably at their beginning and/or end.

Otherwise, the core preventive measures involved the prescription of a regimen appropriate to the patient's complexion in order to maintain an appropriate humoural balance. This regime, which relied on adequate use of the 'six non-naturals' (*sex res non naturales*) – prescribing those beneficial and proscribing those harmful – was usually reinforced by phlebotomy and pharmacy. Unsurprisingly, physicians to whom the French Disease was an 'epidemic' emphasized preventive measures concerning the first 'non-natural' (i.e., air and environment). Apart from this detail, the proposed remaining preventive measures were generally traditional. However, their views on the regulation of coitus are very relevant in calibrating the extent to which they constructed the French Disease as venereal at the turn of the sixteenth century.

It is well known that Latin Galenists placed coitus among the 'non-naturals.' However, there were discrepancies among medical writers about where to put it within that schema. Some relied on Ali Abbas's *Pantegni* and

Avicenna's *Canon* and placed coitus within the fifth *necessary* 'non-natural' (inanition and repletion). Others, basing their claims on Joannitius' *Isagoge,* asserted that sexual intercourse was merely one of the unnecessary 'non-naturals' which – like baths – were linked to the third 'non-natural' (exercise and rest) and helped the evacuating action of exercise. Still further, Arnau de Vilanova gave to coitus an independent status as a part of the so-called secondary non-naturals and argued that it was linked at once to three separate non-naturals, namely the third (exercise and rest), the fifth (inanition and repletion), and the sixth (accidents of the soul). For, firstly, coitus was a way to evacuate a product of the third digestion, i.e., the semen produced by both the male testicles and the female ovaries; secondly, it was closely connected to a man's emotional life; and thirdly, its implementation implied bodily agitation and physical movement.[51] Thus, sex played a central role in the six non-naturals, but that role was far from clear.

Latin Galenist practitioners were closely dependent on Arabic medical sources and in their male-centred *regimina sanitatis* they not only agreed that sex was necessary for keeping oneself healthy, but also claimed that a healthy life was impossible without the frequent practice of coitus. In fact, their unanimously positive view of coitus led university practitioners to recommend it as an actual therapeutic remedy for certain diseases, including the French Disease.[52] The evacuating action promoted by coitus, on the one hand, dried and cooled the body and reduced the natural faculties (*virtutes*), while on the other hand, it prevented the natural heat from being extinguished by humoural repletion. Coitus was also supposed to bring general benefits such as body relief, male's delight, comfort, and confidence, as well as local effects such as relief of the head and senses, ejection of spermatic vapours congregated in the brain and heart, relief of pain in kidneys full of superfluities, and the elimination of matter from the apostemes placed at the groins and testicles. Physicians recommended that patients copulate at the end of the gastric and hepatic digestions and the middle of the third digestion, provided that the superfluities from the first and second digestions had been eliminated and that the body was temperate. According to these assumptions, the therapeutic benefits of copulating were greatest in the morning, after having slept, although some extended the timetable from midnight to daybreak and others also recommended it at sunset.[53]

---

[51]Niebyl, 'The non-naturals,' pp. 488–490; Gil-Sotres, with Paniagua and García-Ballester, 'Introducción,' pp. 629–630, 761–762.

[52]For the case of coitus and plague, see Cohn, Jr., *The Black Death Transformed*, p. 242.

[53]Gil-Sotres with Paniagua and García-Ballester, 'Introducción,' pp. 763–766.

Coitus was prescribed for the young and proscribed for the elderly. Physicians advised strong and stout, sanguine complexioned, reddish and hairy men that they could copulate more assiduously; choleric and melancholic, dry complexioned, very thin and convalescent men should instead practice it less often. Coitus should be avoided whenever vital faculties were weak, for instance, in those of very hot or cold complexions, the starving, those who had eaten or drunk excessively, over-worked or exercised, who had taken baths, were suffering from emotional shocks, or had evacuated (e.g. by blood-letting, purging, vomiting, sweating). Medical authorities believed that sex implied the consumption of the *humidum radicale*, the wasting of the natural heat and wearing of the natural faculties. Thus all the therapeutic benefits of moderate coitus could turn harmful if practiced too frequently or for too long. If the body was heated with an unnatural heat, the main bodily members (brain, heart, liver, lungs and stomach, among others) were damaged; harmful and stinking humours invaded the body and were given off through skin, above all at the genitals, damaging the sight, joints, and nerves, drying the complexion, and bringing premature ageing. Therefore, physicians drastically proscribed excessive coitus, particularly when the air was corrupted.[54]

All the university practitioners here studied (except for Leoniceno and Scanaroli) considered the regulation of coitus among measures useful for the prevention of the French Disease. They all agreed that its immoderate practice should always be counter-indicated, while its moderate practice might be permissible to some people. Only Dall'Aquila warned every man, whether ill or healthy, against copulating at all.[55] Schellig strongly advised against 'excessive and violent' coitus, claiming that it generated stink in the body, mouth, and gums, and increased itch and *scabies* by pushing out corrupted matter and stimulating the outlet for hot and putrid vapours to the skin surface.[56]

Among the men who could enjoy moderate coitus without major risk, Schellig, Widmann and Montesauro listed those accustomed to the pleasures of Venus, young or early mature men, healthy, well-nourished, idle, and married.[57] Gilino added that the well-complexioned, the young, and

---

54Gil-Sotres with Paniagua and García-Ballester, 'Introducción,' pp. 766–767; Schellig himself recalled these rules before referring to those concerning the French Disease. See Schellig, *In pustulas malas morbum quem malum de Francia vulgus appellat*, sign. b1^{r}.

55Dall'Aquila, *Interpretatio et cura morbi gallici*, fols. 197^{r}, 200^{r}.

56Schellig, *In pustulas malas morbum quem malum de Francia vulgus appellat*, sign. b1^{r}.

57Schellig, *In pustulas malas morbum quem malum de Francia vulgus appellat*, sign. b1^{r-v}; Widmann, *Tractatus de pustulis et morbo qui vulgato nomine mal de franzos appellatur*, fols. 3^{v}–4^{r}; Montesauro, *De dispositionibus quas vulgares mal franzoso appellant*, fol. 8^{r}.

those accustomed to coitus could practice it even when they were ill.[58] Furthermore, Montesauro warned those accustomed to regular sex not to stop it altogether, for their retained sperm could turn into poison and rot the complexion of the principal members.[59] Finally, Schellig advised that intrinsic causes – i.e., those applying only to healthy and married men –, and not merely extrinsic ones, had to incite these individuals' nature to coitus; and that they might practice it preferably after the first and second digestions, that is at dawn, taking care to rest and sleep later.[60] So, for some early writers maintaining an active sex life, even if regulated, formed a core component of their therapeutic regimen for the French Disease. Instead of advising patients to cease having sex once infected, many doctors prescribed it.

However, other writers, such as Gilino, Almenar, Dall'Aquila, Torrella and Widmann were somewhat more cautious and emphasized the risk of catching the French Disease by contagion (especially during coitus.) For this reason, the Ferrarese court doctor Gilino advised men not to enjoy social gatherings attended by infected men or women, and especially to avoid sex with them. Indeed, he claimed to have witnessed 'the greatest torments [of] those infected by this way.'[61] To Almenar gatherings that promoted excessive social 'intercourse' with people infected with the French Disease or with those generating harmful humours (melancholic, above all) also posed a risk. However, sex with an infected woman carried the highest risk of all.[62] Indeed, Dall'Aquila recommended that healthy individuals – as well as sufferers from the French Disease – should avoid sexual intercourse entirely. He particularly urged them not to engage in it with those known to be infected with the disease. He argued that the over-heating of the womb resulting from the motion of copulation added more humidity to an already extremely humid organ. This humidity, he concluded, quickly became corrupt, and its 'corrupted vapours' rapidly rose from the womb and penetrated through the pores open on the penis.[63] Torrella similarly urged men to avoid sex with infected women because men, he argued, contracted the French Disease by contagion much more readily than women. He must have held strongly the conviction that men caught the disease easily while women resisted it, for it seems to have influenced his

---

58 Gilino, *De morbo quem gallicum nuncupant*, fol. 4^{r}.

59 Montesauro, *De dispositionibus quas vulgares mal franzoso appellant*, fol. 8^{r}.

60 Schellig, *In pustulas malas morbum quem malum de Francia vulgus appellat*, sign. b1^{r-v}.

61 Gilino, *De morbo quem gallicum nuncupant*, fol. 3^{r}.

62 Almenar, *Libellus ad evitandum et expellendum morbum gallicum*, sign. D2^{r}–D2^{v}.

63 Dall'Aquila, *Interpretatio et cura morbi gallici*, fols. 197^{r}, 200^{r}.

therapeutic advice to male patients. He recommended that one of his patients, who allegedly got the disease as a result of a bad regime, avoid coitus as long as possible. However, if the patient found he could not refrain, Torrella advised him to have sex only after his digestion was concluded and, more interestingly, that he should seek out a non-infected woman for his partner.[64] The therapeutic benefit of coitus to his male patient seems here to outweigh the risk of contagion to the woman. Finally, Widmann confined himself to warn men against having sex with 'women covered with sores,' healthy women who had recently copulated with 'men covered with sores,' or prostitutes.[65]

In the face of any damage (*nocumentum*) to the male member after coitus, Almenar recommended his patients to wash their genitals with a compound specific to this aim and then, to apply an abstersive powder. As a general precautionary measure Almenar also advised men and women to clean their genitals thoroughly after sex with a 'clean linen shirt or cloth' – never with the clothes of infected women for they were also infected – and later to wash these parts with hot water or white wine.[66]

In 1500, two years before this prophylactic advice by Almenar, prostitutes eventually became the target of the earliest measures for collective prevention against the French Disease ever proposed by any medical practitioner. It was Torrella who postulated them. In order to eradicate the disease from the world he suggested that prostitutes who suffered from this disease should be identified and confined. Although Torrella complained that no authority (pope, emperor, king, prince or lord) had paid attention to his proposals, he assured readers that the pox could be entirely eradicated if city authorities would empower matrons, with the support of secular officials, to examine prostitutes and commit those found infected to a special institution with its own doctor until they could recover their health.[67] Given the long existing legal tradition in medieval Europe of repressive measures against prostitution, it may be worth remarking that Torrella's measures appear to have been intended for strictly sanitary purposes however much they targeted a historically conspicuous scapegoat for social anxieties.

---

64 Torrella, *Tractatus cum consiliis contra pudendagram*, sign. c4^{v}–d1^{r}, d3^{r}.

65 Widmann, *Tractatus de pustulis et morbo qui vulgato nomine mal de franzos appellatur*, fol. 4^{r}.

66 Almenar, *Libellus ad evitandum et expellendum morbum gallicum*, sign. D2^{r}–D2^{v}.

67 Torrella, *Tractatus cum consiliis contra pudendagram*, sign. c4^{v}–d1^{r}; Torrella, *Dialogus de dolore cum tractatu de ulceribus in pudendagra evenire solitis*, sign. d4^{v}, e6^{v}.

TOWARDS A CONCLUSION

Vivian Nutton has proved that the notion of contagion was not foreign either to Galen or to Renaissance university medicine, and that Fracastoro's merit consisted not in the alleged originality of his theory, but in his ability at systematizing the ideas on contagion contained in Galenic texts and reformulating them in the framework of sixteenth-century Galenism.[68] Thus, a certain conception of causal specificity tied to the notion of contagion was already present in university medical tradition from at least the mid fourteenth century. Put plainly, debates on whether some infectious diseases were the result not merely of a humoural imbalance but of a specific external cause can already be detected in some medical works on the occasion of the Black Death of 1348.

To illustrate the issue, let us take the views by Gentile da Foligno, professor in the medical faculty of Perugia when plague fell on that Italian city and the reply by his colleague at the University of Naples, Giovanni della Penna (*fl.*1344–1387).[69] In the *Consilium contra pestilentiam* written by Gentile in mid June 1348, just before his death, ironically as a result of plague, he claimed that the substantial air corruption of which plague consisted, became apparent through 'perceptible corruptions' (*corruptiones sensibiles*) which could enter human bodies in contact with this air through two main ways; first via the air inhaled, and second via the air absorbed through the pores of the skin. While some bodies could resist the attack of this corruption, others could not (these individual differences, which were interpreted through the Galenic theory of the constitution, unanimously recognized among late-medieval university physicians).[70] When the 'perceptible corruptions' entered a susceptible body, a 'poisonous matter' was generated near the heart and the lungs. This matter did not act by means of its qualities, but through its poisonous-ness – that is, through

---

[68]Girolamo Fracastoro was merely an exponent of this new tendency. Most of his supposed achievements were actually a historical artefact created by the bacteriologists of the 'heroic era.' They actually took him as the beginning of a genealogy they constructed to legitimate their role in late nineteenth- and early twentieth-century medicine. See Nutton, 'The Seeds of Disease' and 'The Reception of Fracastoro's Theory of Contagion'; and Cunningham, 'Transforming Plague: the Laboratory and the Identity of Infectious Disease.'

[69]Arrizabalaga, 'Facing the Black Death,' pp. 259–264.

[70]To these individual peculiarities which made some bodies resistant to the corruption and others liable to suffer damage Gentile dedicated five different *dubia* (nos. 5, 6, 10, 11, 12) plus one more (no. 9) to show 'why men die from the pestilence while oxen and other beasts do not.' See Gentile da Foligno, *Consilium contra pestilentiam*, sign. c1^{v}–c2^{v}, c3^{r}–c4^{r}.

its specific property of being poisonous (*per proprietatem venenositatis*). Through the theory of the multiplication of species Gentile explained how this 'poisonous matter,' even in small amounts, could spread into and eventually infect the entire body.[71] He stressed the power of self-multiplication of this 'poison' which, when in contact with the 'humidities of our body,' acted in the same way as other poisons, turning whatever it touched into its likeness so that it spread by continuity throughout the body. When the poison reached and touched the heart, it turned it into poison, so that the vital spirit lying in the heart yielded to the poisonous form and abandoned it, leaving the heart and the body without movement – that is, dead.[72] Gentile explained how the 'poisonous vapours' shed by an infected body communicated themselves to others through the breath or the skin. As a result, the 'pestilence' spread rapidly by means of contagion (*per contagionem*), passing from person to person and from place to place.[73] At this point Gentile echoed two significant Galenic paragraphs taken from *De differentiis febrium*: the first referred to 'certain seeds of the pestilence' which were thrown from the pestilent body to the surrounding air through the two above-mentioned routes; the second talked about the 'remains of warmth' present in the air long after the 'pestilence' had gone that infected like a 'ferment' in a bread oven.[74] Far from being accepted at the time, Gentile's ideas implying a vague notion of causal specificity were ignored by most contemporary university practitioners and even denied by some. Giovanni della Penna, for instance, claimed that the 'pestilence' affected only those individuals whose choleric matter had become overly heated and corrupted so that it was their personal constitution that eventually made it possible for the 'pestilence' to take root in their 'choleric matter.'[75]

While it was not immediately accepted, the influence of the notion that a sort of specific poisonous matter transmissible through contagion by contact (or otherwise) might be involved in the spread of plague and other pestilences steadily grew among European university medical practitioners during the two hundred years after the Black Death of 1348. Thus, they

---

71On the theory of the 'multiplication of species,' see Crombie, *Robert Grosseteste and the Origins of Experimental Science*, pp. 86, 109–110, 112, 114–115, 117–118, 137–138, 140, 144–149, *passim*; Lindberg, *Theories of Vision from Al-Kindi to Kepler*, pp. 19, 98, 113–116, 223, 254–255, *passim*; and also the bibliography quoted by both of them.

72Gentile da Foligno, *Consilium contra pestilentiam*, sign. c4^{r}–c4^{v}.

73Gentile da Foligno, *Consilium contra pestilentiam*, sign. a2^{r}.

74Gentile da Foligno, *Consilium contra pestilentiam*, sign. a3^{v}: 'Inquit [Galenus] enim [?] circundantem nos aerem inferri quedam pestilentie semina'; and sign. a3^{r}: 'Manent enim reliquie caliditatis, ut in clibano, que velut fermentum inficiunt, ...'.

75Giovanni della Penna, *Consilium in magna pestilentia*, pp. 341–342.

gradually accepted that individuals could get ill from epidemic diseases, not just because of corrupted air disrupting the humoural balance of those leading a bad life regime, but also as a consequence of the direct action on their bodies by external poisonous matter.

The French Disease significantly contributed to the spreading of this idea. When the disease broke out in the 1490s, it was associated with various kinds of causes – external and internal, remote and proximate – which theoretically could be at work either collectively or independently. None of this, however, prevented physicians from relating this 'new' condition – from the very beginning, and increasingly as time went on – to contact with the poisonous matter specific to it. Whether applied to the plague, to the French pox, or to other 'contagious' diseases – among which Fracastoro distinguished *variolae*, *morbilli*, sweating fever, *puncticulae*, *phthisis*, *rabies*, *elephantia*, *lepra* and *scabies* – the idea that individuals got ill *only* from an infectious disease when they entered into contact with its peculiar poisonous matter won many supporters among European university medical practitioners from the mid sixteenth century onwards. Individual contagion became to them a *necessary* condition for the outbreak and spread of infectious disease, however much it also continued to require the concurrence of other causes peculiar to the Galenist causal system. Thus, infectious diseases were perceived more and more as natural species that were born, grew, got old, and died, and which were gradually framed according to 'ontological' parameters instead of the 'physiological' ones traditional to Galenism.

As I have intended to show in this study, the earliest medical writers on the French Disease admitted several modes of contagion by contact, but all of them agreed that coitus was the easiest and most frequent way to contract this condition. Consistently, they also show a path of disease prevention measures that was gradually changing from a pattern peculiar to the reactions against plague and pestilences to a new one tending to focus upon coitus. This necessarily implied a shift between two patterns of blaming disease victims, namely from the traditional response against epidemics which related disease with collective and generic faults, to a new one tending to individualize responsibilities insofar as individual behaviour became perceived as the main determinant of health and disease. Although the identification of the French Disease with the disease of Job in late fifteenth-century northern Italy might point in this direction, it was only from the sixteenth century onward that these new perceptions became clear and openly influential on European university medicine. On that score, the sixteenth-century movements for religious Reformation played a major role in the Protestant as in the Catholic side of Europe.

While it did not take three decades to forge a link between the French Disease and sexuality, as is sometimes thought, there was no consensus on the issue. The ways in which university doctors linked the disease to sex frequently stemmed from their underlying views on the nature of the disease itself, whether it was an epidemic or a contagious distemper, and whether they addressed superior causes or merely immediate causes. Moreover, they also failed to find consensus on the role of sex within a healthy life regimen relative to the six non-naturals. These various strains of early thinking on the French Disease resulted in a revealing range of preventative and therapeutic advice found in early medical writings. The recognition of contagion by contact spurred some writers to warn explicitly against having sex with people known, or in some cases suspected, of being infected. But assumptions about the importance of maintaining an active sex life led others to advise patients with the French Disease to continue having (moderate) sex. Such advice tended to be phrased specifically for male patients. Moreover, assumptions that male physiology was more vulnerable to infection, while women's bodies were infected with greater difficultly, led some physicians to advise infected men to seek out non-infected women for sex as part of their therapeutic regimen of recovery. Doctors clearly linked the disease to sex from the earliest date, but the conclusions they drew from that connection led to a range of conflicting and questionable medical advice.

Among the earliest university practitioners who dealt with the French Disease, Torrella was the one who went furthest in developing new views as to both the causality and the prevention of this condition. In 1497 he argued that the French Disease was usually contracted through contagion by contact (mostly venereal) and, less frequently, as a result of a bad regime, the concurrence of a universal cause such as general air corruption being required for the disease spreading in none of these alternative ways. Yet, three years later (1500), he openly claimed the French Disease to be a contagious disease like *scabies*, its corrupted matter, even just a small amount, multiplied itself and was attracted by bodily members which were eventually turned into its nature and corrupted. Finally, when the digestive *virtus* of liver and veins failed and generated bad blood, the matter multiplied everywhere and the disease affected the entire body.[76] Therefore, little wonder that he emphasized in 1497 the need to avoid coitus with people infected by the French Disease. By 1500 he was the only one proposing a rigorous sanitary control of prostitutes as the best way not only to avoid disease spread but also to eradicate it entirely.

---

[76]Torrella, *Dialogus de dolore cum tractatu de ulceribus in pudendagra evenire solitis*, sign. a6^{v}–a7^{r}.

Cited Works

Almenar, Joan, *Libellus ad evitandum et expellendum morbum gallicum ut nunquam revertatur.* Venice: Bernardinus Venetus de Vitalibus, 1502.

Arrizabalaga, Jon. 'Facing the Black Death: Perceptions and Reactions of University Medical Practitioners' pp. 237–288 in *Practical Medicine from Salerno to the Black Death*, eds. Luis García-Ballester, Roger French, Jon Arrizabalaga, and Andrew Cunningham. Cambridge: Cambridge University Press, 1994.

Arrizabalaga, Jon, John Henderson, and Roger French. *The Great Pox: The French Disease in Early Modern Europe.* New Haven: Yale University Press, 1997.

Avicenna, *Liber Canonis Medicine.* Venice: Lucio Antonio Junta, 1527.

Cohn Jr., S.K. *The Black Death Transformed: Disease and Culture in Early Renaissance Europe.* London: Arnold, 2002.

Crombie, A.C. *Robert Grosseteste and the Origins of Experimental Science, 1100–1700.* Oxford: Clarendon Press, 1953.

Cunningham, Andrew. 'Transforming Plague: The Laboratory and the Identity of Infectious Disease' pp. 209–244 in *The Laboratory Revolution in Medicine*, eds. Andrew Cunningham and Perry Williams. Cambridge: Cambridge University Press, 1992.

Dall'Aquila, Sebastiano. *Interpretatio et cura morbi gallici*, fols. 184^r–202^v in Gatinaria, Marco *et al.*, *De curis egritudinum particularium noni Almansoris practica uberrima* ... Pavia: Jacob de Burgofranco, 1509.

French, Roger. 'Astrology in Medical Practice' pp. 30–59 in *Practical Medicine from Salerno to the Black Death*, eds. Luis García-Ballester, Roger French, Jon Arrizabalaga, and Andrew Cunningham. Cambridge: Cambridge University Press, 1994.

Gentile da Foligno. *Consilium contra pestilentiam.* Colle di Val d'Elsa: n.p., *c.*1479.

Gilino, Corradino. *De morbo quem Gallicum nuncupant.* Ferrara: Laurentius de Rubeis, 1497/1498.

Giovanni della Penna. 'Consilium in magna pestilentia' pp. 341–348 in 'Pestschriften aus den ersten 150 Jahren nach der Epidemie des "Schwartzen Todes", 1348.' *Archiv für Geschichte der Medizin,* 5 (1911–1912), ed. Karl Sudhoff.

Gil-Sotres, P. with Juan A. Paniagua and Luis García-Ballester. 'Introducción' pp. 471–861 in *Arnaldi de Villanova Opera Medica Omnia. X.1. Regimen sanitatis ad regem Aragonum.* Barcelona: Universitat de Barcelona-Fundació Noguera, 1996.

Grant, J.E. 'Medieval and Renaissance Scholastic Conceptions of the Influence of the Celestial Region on the Terrestrial' *Journal of Medieval and Renaissance Studies,* 17 (1987): 1–23.

Leoniceno, Nicolò. *Libellus de epidemia quam vulgo morbum gallicum vocant.* Venice: Aldo Manucio, 1497.

Lindberg, D.C. *Theories of Vision from Al-Kindi to Kepler.* Chicago and London: University of Chicago Press, 1976.

Montesauro, Natale. *De dispositionibus quas vulgares mal franzoso appellant.* Bologna: Giustiniano de Ruberia, 1497/8.

Niebyl, P.H. 'The Non-naturals' *Bulletin of the History of Medicine,* 45:5 (1971): 486–492.

North, J.D.. 'Celestial Influence – The Major Premise of Astrology' pp. 45–100 in *'Astrologi allucinati': Stars and the End of the World in Luther's Time*, ed. Paola Zambelli. Berlin and New York: Walter de Gruyter, 1986.

Nutton, Vivian. 'The Seeds of Disease: An Explanation of Contagion and Infection from the Greeks to the Renaissance' *Medical History*, 27 (1983): 1–34.

Nutton, Vivian. 'The Reception of Fracastoro's Theory of Contagion: The Seed that Fell Among Thorns' *Osiris*, 2nd. Series, 6 (1990): 196–234.

Pintor, Pere. *De morbo foedo et occulto his temporibus affligente*. Rome: Eucharius Silber, 1500.

Scanaroli, Antonio. *Disputatio utilis de morbo gallico et opinionis Nicolai Leoniceni confirmatio contra adversarium eandem opinionem oppugnantem*. Bologna: Benedictus Hectoris, 1498.

Schellig, Konrad. *In pustulas malas morbum quem malum de Francia vulgus appellat que sunt de genere formicarum salubre consilium*. Heidelberg: Friedrich Misch, 1496.

Steber, Bartholomäus. *A malafranczos morbo gallorum preservatio ac cura*. Vienna: Johannes Winterburg, 1498.

Sudhoff, Karl. *Graphische und typographische Erstlinge der Syphilisliteratur aus den Jahren 1495 und 1496*. Munich: C. Kuhn, 1912.

Sudhoff, Karl. 'Introduction' pp. IX–XLV in *The Earliest Printed Literature on Syphilis, Being Ten Tractates from the Years 1495–1498*, ed. Sudhoff. Florence: R. Lier, 1925.

Temkin, Owsei. 'On the History of "Morality and Syphilis" ' pp. 472–484 in his *The Double Face of Janus and Other Essays in the History of Medicine*. Baltimore: Johns Hopkins University Press, 1977.

The Earliest Printed Literature on Syphilis, Being Ten Tractates from the Years 1495–1498, ed. Karl Sudhoff. Florence: R. Lier, 1925.

Torrella, Gaspar. *Tractatus cum consiliis contra pudendagram seu morbum gallicum*, Rome: Pietro della Torre, 1497.

Torrella, Gaspar. *De morbo gallico cum aliis*, 2nd ed. Rome: J. Besicken, *c.*1498.

Torrella, Gaspar. *Dialogus de dolore cum tractatu de ulceribus in pudendagra evenire solitis*. Rome: Johannes Besicken & Martinus de Amsterdam, 1500.

Widmann, Johann. *Tractatus de pustulis et morbo qui vulgato nomine mal de franzos appellatur*. Rome: Stephan Plannck / Strasbourg: Johannes Grüninger, 1497.

Charlatans, the Regulated Marketplace and the Treatment of Venereal Disease in Italy

David Gentilcore

On the 1st of March 1581 a syphilitic, Francesco Maria Marconi, appeared before the tribunal of the College of Physicians in Mantua with a denunciation to make. Marconi recounted how that winter he had been very sick, aggravated by headache. One day while in the square he spotted 'a large handbill' (*un grande ephitafio*) fixed to the column in front of the 'Emperor' apothecary's shop. He had a friend read it out to him. The handbill was advertising the services of someone who offered to treat every sort of disease, including pains caused by the *morbo gallico*. Marconi, accompanied by his friend, went to the (as yet unnamed) practitioner's rented room in town. He told him of his disease. The practitioner offered to treat Marconi for the price of three gold *scudi*, a significant sum. 'And I, who was prepared to pay that sum and more to get better, put my hand to my purse,' Marconi later told the tribunal, and gave the practitioner a *ducatone* by way of down payment. Marconi went again the next day and was given a pill to swallow. The day after that he was given three paper pouches of powder to take on three separate occasions. The practitioner then let blood from Marconi's left hand, gave him three syrups, and then let blood from his left foot. The latter bloodletting 'harmed me a great deal,' Marconi recalled. Then a cupping glass was applied to his chest and his 'ulcer' (meaning one of his sores). Then he was given an electuary three times. 'All of this treatment lasted some twenty-eight to thirty days,' Marconi said. He 'felt all afflicted and dead as a result of those remedies.' He decided not to continue with the practitioner's services, especially since the latter 'still wanted to go inside and ruin me completely' (*voleva ancor andar dentro et rovinarmi al tutto*). Marconi concluded his denunciation with the affirmation that he was quite certain that if he had not left the practitioner he would be dead.

The most important point was never stated: that Marconi wanted his money back. But this must have been understood. Moreover, Marconi did not tell the tribunal anything about his present condition, nor was he asked to. This vagueness regarding the nature of the medicines used, as well as the chronology of the treatment, is a not unusual characteristic of first-hand accounts of illness episodes in early modern Italy. The tribunal even had specifically to ask Marconi the name of the practitioner, for, rather unusually in the case of a denunciation, Marconi did not mention it. He was 'Mastro Giuseppe dell'Isola, and he is old and goes around practising just the same,' Marconi answered. He was then asked to name other sufferers treated by dell'Isola, and Marconi named a ducal steward, a bow-maker, and the present *vicario* (although I could not make out of what). The names might have helped build a case against dell'Isola; but evidently there was nothing against him and the case was dropped. Dell'Isola had not irrevocably harmed Marconi and, once it was discovered that he was a licensed medical practitioner – as the title *mastro* suggests – there was perhaps no reason to proceed against him.[1] At the most, dell'Isola could be accused of not keeping to his end of the bargain to cure Marconi; but then Marconi had not allowed the treatment to run its full course. It is not clear from the denunciation just how long this would have been, so perhaps there had never been any healing contract as such, written or verbal, between the sufferer and the practitioner. In a typical healing contract the practitioner promised to cure the sufferer while the sufferer promised to pay the practitioner an agreed sum. Healing contracts usually identified the nature of the illness, the duration of the treatment, and the cost of the medicines.[2] No money was due, however, if the patient did not get better; and it was up to the patient to determine this. For instance, in a 1566-67 case adjudicated by the Milanese College of Physicians, a barber was accused by a syphilitic of having promised to cure his three gummas (that is, tumours of syphilitic origin) in exchange for payment of sixteen *scudi*. Although the treatment was undertaken and the money paid, the sufferer's condition did not improve. The sufferer-cum-plaintiff wanted his money back.[3] As these surviving denunciations suggest, the practice of

---

[1]ASMa, *Sanitaria*, 1, 'Costituto contro un medico che medicava abusivamente da ciarlatano che avea attaccato un 'grande epitafio' che diceva offizio di medicare ogni sorte di male e in ispecie del morbo gallico, ecc.a.' The title given to the accusation by a later archivist identifies the accused as a doctor (*medico*) – a fact which I have not been able to confirm – 'who practised illicitly as a charlatan.' What was *illicit* about the dell'Isola's activities, whatever sort of practitioner he was, was his mixing of branches of the medical arts which the authorities sought to keep separate: physic (his prescribing and administering of remedies and the framing of diagnoses), surgery (his bloodletting and cupping) and charlatanry (the open advertising of his services).

[2]Pomata, *Contracting a Cure*, pp. 25-55, 140-171.

[3]ASMi, *Studi*, 127, E.

medicine in early modern Italy was policed – if that is not too strong a word – from above. If medicine was a marketplace, it was a regulated one. However imperfect, ineffective, and prone to negotiation this policing and regulation may have been, it did represent an ongoing attempt by the medical elites to keep the 'healing arts' within the bounds they considered appropriate. There were considerations of both a moral and a corporative nature at play, so that not everything can be reduced to the matter of 'competition'. In other words, we are not dealing with the unfettered marketplace so favoured as a model by scholars of early modern England. How the response of therapeutic practices in general, and those of 'charlatans' in particular, was shaped by this regulation is the subject of this essay.

To begin with, it is too often asserted (or assumed) that 'charlatans' treated venereal disease and sold remedies for it.[4] Because of the shame attached to the disease no recognized practitioner would want to treat it and sufferers could get treatment only in secret and by disreputable practitioners. This, it has been argued, left the way wide open for 'quack doctors' of all kinds, resulting in a fringe monopoly. There are three things wrong with this series of assumptions, at least when applied to early modern Italy, and they have to do with notions of shame, the sources of treatment available, and the quack label itself.

The first point is that, despite the way venereal disease was often linked with sin by moralizers, sufferers – at least male ones – were not always and everywhere overcome with shame. Indications to the contrary abound, of course. As unimpeachable an authority as a Neapolitan protophysician, Antonio Santorelli, wrote of the need to tolerate and license 'empirics' since 'many victims would go to them who, because of shame, would not dare go to a doctor or surgeon.'[5] In Giambattista Morgagni's clinical consultations the names of the sufferers are sometimes crossed out – especially if they were nobles – to protect their identity (although this may have been done by the disciple of Morgagni's who preserved the letters for posterity).[6] Yet other accounts suggest that sufferers sought treatment quite openly. When, in 1527, Johannes Senff (Sinapius) undertook what was known as the 'guaiac cure,' it was under the care of an eminent Heidelberg physician. Having rented an apartment in which to create the self-enclosed sauna-like atmosphere necessary for the treatment, Senff hung up a few pictures and invited over some friends for a sort of

[4]Quétel, *History of Syphilis*, p. 87; Porter, *Health for Sale*, p. 149-156; Cunningham and Grell, *Four Horsemen of the Apocalypse*, p. 263.

[5]Santorelli, *Il protomedico napolitano*, p. 48

[6]Jarcho, *Clinical Consultations*, passim.

house-warming. During the fifteen weeks the treatment lasted, he had a woman looking after him, and regular visits from a barber and an apothecary.[7] Italian sufferers also seemed quite matter-of-fact about their treatments. This is the case even when they recounted their disease to the church authorities in the context of canonization processes, in first-person narratives of illness episodes surprisingly free of moralizing.[8] I have found little evidence of Italian healers promoting patient confidentiality and privacy as a way of drumming up business, an approach which seems to have been quite common in early modern London.[9]

Was the pox constructed differently in Italy? The response to venereal disease in Ferrara suggests an early move towards the naturalistic interpretations. Within a few years of its initial outbreak there, venereal disease had apparently 'passed from being a serious and even embarrassing private affair and became just another public calamity.'[10] The medical literature of the time supports this. When writing about the disease, Italian physicians tended to omit the moralising element so prevalent in English treatises of the time.[11] Some, like Ercole Sassonia, adopted an outright secular approach, itself rooted in Galenic medicine. Instead of placing the blame on prostitutes and their sinful ways, for example, Sassonia boasted of his own successful treatment of a well-known Venetian prostitute, Nicoleta, who was able to return to the 'meretricious art.'[12] But even physicians such as Giovanni Battista Sitoni, who wrote for 'all physicians thinking as Catholics' – for whom physical health complimented spiritual health – shied away from an overtly judgemental approach. Sitoni was the first to underline the fact that both men and women could suffer the scourge; it was not simply a matter of women infecting men.[13] A few Italian physicians went so far as so suggest preventative remedies. The mere possibility was too much for the Protestant sensibilities of the Frenchman Henri Estienne. While in Padua Estienne adamantly refused to avail himself of the opportunity of discovering Gabriele Falloppio's promised 'means of womanizing to [one's] heart's content without any fear of Mme. Vérole [Mrs Pox].' Falloppio's students, however, took his lectures all down (or at least one of them did), and his proposed

---

[7]Flood and Shaw, 'The Price of the Pox in 1527.'

[8]Gentilcore, *Healers and Healing*, pp. 179-181.

[9]Siena, 'Foul Disease.'

[10]Arrizabalaga, Henderson, French, *The Great Pox*, p. 47.

[11]Schleiner, *Medical Ethics*, pp. 162-202.

[12]Ercole Sassonia, *Luis venereae perfectissimus tractatus* (Padua, 1644), fol. 4, cit. in Schleiner, *Medical Ethics*, pp. 193-194.

[13]Giovanni Battista Sitoni, *Miscellanea medico-curiosa* (Cologne, 1677), tractatus 45, pp. 288, 294, cit. in Schleiner, *Medical Ethics*, pp. 190, 192.

preservative survives. Falloppio recommended the careful cleaning of the male organ after intercourse, especially by means of an invention of his own. This consisted of a small cloth, cut to the size of one's penis, soaked in particular ointments and then applied to the penis. Falloppio claimed to have tried it out on eleven hundred men. Another professor at Padua, Eustachio Rudio, advised wearing the compress before intercourse as well. Rudio also proposed a preventative for women, consisting of a pessary steeped in a concoction of guaiac, to be worn for a day following intercourse.[14] Both remedies raise the possibility that some of the medicines sold by charlatans, to which I shall turn shortly, may have had a preventative purpose.

The second point concerns the practitioners who treated the disease. It is true that venereal disease straddled the three branches of official medicine – the realms of physicians, surgeons, and apothecaries – thus creating some confusion over whose prerogative it was. This did not mean, however, that charlatans necessarily took up the slack. In fact, there was no slack to take up. The medical marketplace, as closely regulated as it was, provided a range of sources of relief.

Physicians and surgeons specialized in treating venereal patients. In some cases, this could earn them considerable amounts of money, as in the career of the physician and surgeon Berengario da Carpi. They also wrote numerous treatises about both the disease and their procedures in treating it.[15] The physician-surgeon Federico Zerenghi concluded his surgery treatise with a reference to an infallible cure of his own, which promised to work within a few days, without suffering or inconvenience.[16] He promised to publish it in his next book, but this never appeared. Even physicians of the fame of a Giambattista Morgagni – professor at the University of Padua, anatomist and (eventually) author of an influential treatise on disease causation[17] – treated sufferers and gave advice to patients and other physicians, as we know from his many surviving correspondence consultations.[18] Itinerant surgeons like the *norcini* – family dynasties of

---

[14]Henri Estienne, *L'introduction au traitté de la conformité des merveilles anciennes avec les modernes* (Lyon, 1592), book 1, chap. 13, p. 86; Gabriele Falloppio, *De morbo gallico*, in *Opera omnia* (Frankfurt, 1600), vol. 1, p. 737; Eustachio Rudio, *De morbis occultis et venenantis* (Venice, 1610), lib. 5, p. 192, all cit. in Schleiner, *Medical Ethics*, p p. 170–176.

[15]Cellini, *Autobiography*, book xxviii; Bynum, 'Treating the Wages of Sin,' especially pp. 10–12.

[16]Zerenghi, *Breve compendio di cirurgia* (Naples: Costantino Vitale, 1603), p. 52, cit. in Gentilcore, *Healers and Healing*, pp. 118–119.

[17]Giambattista Morgagni, *De causis et sedibus morborum* (Venice: Remondini, 1764); English translation, *The Seats and Causes of Diseases* (London: Millar and Cadell, 1769).

[18]Jarcho, *Clinical Consultations*.

practitioners from the hills around the Umbrian town of Norcia[19] – carried out operations for the removal of the urethral growths associated with venereal disease. This was an extension of their surgical expertise in operations for hernia and bladder stone, which brought them renown and employment in the towns and hospitals of the peninsula well into the eighteenth century.

By 1733 there were so many 'expert practitioners' treating the disease in Venice that the city's health office had the luxury of rejecting a surgeon's proposed remedy as 'something truly common.'[20] These 'experts' included another occupational group: 'those who run the *stufe secche* [hot-houses or heated chambers] and prepare decoctions of holy wood.' By the beginning of the seventeenth century such work had become a recognized occupation in Rome and in most large Italian towns – enough for the Roman *stufaroli* to be denounced for preparing the remedies in the way they wanted 'so as to save costs and effort, with a thousand deceits and very notable harm.'[21] This went on despite a 1595 edict insisting that sellers of guaiac decoctions could prepare them only under a physician's supervision and administer them only with a physician's prescription.[22] Formerly part of the barbers' guild, in 1613 the Roman *stufaroli* achieved guild status on their own.[23] They were thus quite different from charlatans – although both groups were broadly categorized as 'empirics,' in the contemporary sense of 'non-graduate medical practitioners.'[24] ('Empiric' was not coterminous with 'charlatan': although virtually all charlatans could be classed as empirics, according to this definition, not all empirics were charlatans, as we shall see).

In practice the reputation of the *stufaroli* seems to have been higher than that accorded to them by Tomaso Garzoni. He equated the *stufaroli* with go-betweens and brothel-keepers who rented rooms on the sly, thereby 'mixing the cleansing of the exterior [body] with the dirtying of the interior.'[25] The difference between traditional *stufe*, or bathhouses, and

---

[19]Cruciani, *Cerusici e fisici*; Park, 'Stones, Bones and Hernias.'

[20]ASV, *Sanità*, 588, 22/9/1733.

[21]ASR, *Università*, 61, 'Discorso dell'inconvenienti che nascono nella medicina,' 780ʳ.

[22]ASR, *Università*, 217, edict of 1595.

[23]*Statuti, ordini e constitutioni.*

[24]Santorelli, *Il protomedico napolitano*, 45-46.

[25]Garzoni, *Piazza universale*, 'De' stufaroli,' discourse cxxiv, vol. 2, pp. 1322-1323. The bathing/licentiousness and bathhouse/prostitution connections were literary commonplaces. Vigarello, *Concepts of Cleanliness*, 28-37. Hence the insult 'born in the bathhouse' (*nato alla stufa*), directed at the hated Pope Adrian VI. Gnoli, 'Stufe romane,' pp. 404, 406.

the new *stufe secche* (literally, 'dry baths') for the treatment of syphilis is also significant (and Garzoni had in mind the former). The link between the two forms of *stufa* is not hard to find. Several Roman hospitals – among them Santo Spirito in Saxia – owned and operated baths located near their main building. These combined therapeutic with hygienic functions. On the lower floor there were rooms for steam baths; on the upper floor there were dressing rooms and rooms for cosmetic and therapeutic treatments, such as the letting of blood and other minor operations. To obtain the licence of *stufarolo* and be admitted into the guild, the candidate had to pass an anatomy exam conducted by two barbers and two *stufaroli*. The surgical function of baths was one of the reasons why barbers sometimes ran baths of their own or served as partners. In Rome, the census of 1526 makes explicit reference to nine *stufaroli* in the central districts or *rioni*, although there were no doubt others to be found among the ranks of the city's barbers and taverners.[26] By the late sixteenth century, however, public bathhouses and steam-baths were on the wane throughout Europe and with them their associations of impropriety, or what Georges Vigarello has called 'a lost sociability.'[27] They were replaced by the *stufe secche*, which not only corresponded to very different Counter-Reformation sensibilities, but also to the therapeutic needs of the time. Ironically, the very places which so often were described as the site of illicit sexual encounters transformed themselves into the places which treated venereal diseases.

Women like Catherina 'la Siciliana' – as those around her knew her – do not seem to have been regarded as keepers of common stews. Catherina Micheletti offered mercury-based *fumenti*. When asked about herself in a 1674 case, she replied that her 'occupation was to treat the sick, that is, for French disease.' Micheletti claimed her licence to treat people came from the viceroy of Naples and that 'all [her] ancestors [had] practised the same occupation.' She boasted of having 'healed hundreds of people in Naples.' After having lived in Rome for two months, Micheletti was approached by the mother of a sufferer beseeching her to come and see her daughter. The sufferer, Giovanna Prudentia, agreed to undergo Micheletti's treatment after several successive visits by the physician of the

---

[26]Esposito, 'Stufe a bagni pubblici,' p. 83.

[27]Vigarello, *Concepts of Cleanliness*, pp. 22, 29. Their disappearance in Rome can be attributed only in part to increasing difficulties in obtaining sufficient water from the Tiber, the explanation offered by Gnoli, 'Stufe romane,' p. 404. The real reasons have more to do with the sixteenth-century process of 'social discipline,' of which the Counter-Reformation was a part, which resulted in their condemnation by social commentators.

Colonna district, where Prudentia lived. But she was not a model patient. After five days of the smokey hot-house atmosphere, Prudentia 'ran screaming through the house because she felt like she was burning up because of the said *fumenti*.' The fumigations had no effect, Micheletti later remarked, because Prudentia 'wanted to drink all the time ... and she didn't want to stay covered up, but fanned herself instead.' Following Prudentia's death several weeks later, Micheletti was denounced to the Roman Protomedicato by Prudentia's husband, through a 'secret accuser' who singled her out as an unlicensed *medichessa* whose botched fumigations were responsible for Prudentia's death. Micheletti was not charged, however, so the Roman Protomedicato must have been satisfied with her therapeutic abilities, despite the fact that Micheletti had no licence to practice in Rome – although she did make the rather lame claim that she had 'given a few *denari* to her husband to get the said licence.'[28] Women specialists have been documented for early modern London too.[29] While these tended to treat women sufferers, Micheletti named among the other patients she had treated a man (a chaplain named Andrea) and a woman. Indeed little is known about the role of women who treated the pox in early modern Italy. It may be that their role was limited to the administration of fumigations. It is interesting that the only time Prudentia was given any medicines these were administered by Micheletti's husband, Giovanni Battista. This suggests they were a husband and wife team. In any case, as far as the medical authorities were concerned, the practice of any branch of the medical arts was off-limits to women, the only exception being midwifery. At the same time, the authorities recognized that women healers, illicitly practising aspects of physic or surgery in small towns, might be the only source of treatment readily available. In such cases, they might be warned to limit themselves to the practice of midwifery and to become licensed midwives; but they were hardly ever punished.[30]

There were other sources of treatment. Quite early, hospitals intended primarily for sufferers of venereal disease were set up in the main towns of the peninsula. Between the 1490s and 1520s Bologna, Ferrara, Genoa, Rome, Naples, Florence, Brescia, Venice and Padua established what came to be known as Incurables hospitals. Other towns, like Milan, Vicenza, Verona and Orvieto, set aside a ward of an existing hospital for such sufferers. From at least the mid-sixteenth century, and probably earlier, these hospitals were vast consumers of guaiac, as their surviving records

---

[28]ASR, *Università*, 67, 936-944.

[29]Siena, 'Foul Disease.'

[30]Gentilcore, 'Figurations and State Authority,' pp. 368, 377-378.

attest. Guaiac treatment became their mainstay. At the Incurables hospital of San Giacomo in Rome, guaiac was eventually distributed free to thousands of sufferers, at vast expense to the hospital. Bills were even posted on the doors of all the city's churches informing people of admission procedures into the hospital. Here, medical staff visited the sick twice a day. They examined the patients' urine, recommended appropriate food and drink, and prescribed the necessary simples to treat their condition.[31] The treatments provided by the hospitals would then be imitated and practised outside their walls. In 1697 a farm labourer treated a syphilitic acquaintance by spreading sour grapes (*uva agresta*) over his kidneys and genitals. He had seen it done during his five-month stay in hospital in Lecce, where it was used for fever.[32]

Because the treatment was exceedingly costly sufferers might opt to treat themselves, as they so frequently did in a wide range of other diseases, and decide on the appropriate course of action. In the middle years of the eighteenth century a syphilitic named Lodovico Rossa of Brescia had consumed a sarsaparilla tea 'for the last few years' and a wine medicated with sarsaparilla and guaiac, 'which he still takes.'[33] These were standard remedies, as we shall see below; but what is noteworthy is that Rossa took them of his own accord and over a long period of time. In 1532, the goldsmith and sculptor Benvenuto Cellini himself caught the disease, 'from that fine young servant girl I was keeping,' as he wrote. He soon ignored the advice of 'the foremost physicians in Rome,' who had been treating him, and 'took the wood.'[34] The guaiac cure, to which he refers, meant confinement to a closed and heated room for a month or more, all the while keeping to a starvation diet, undergoing daily purges and regular ingestion of a guaiac decoction.

Finally, in a time of medical pluralism, there were also sacred sources of relief, both religious and magical. Common devotions, parish missions, even miracles could be considered treatment. The peasant Donato de Quarto, mentioned above for his hospital-inspired treatment of a syphilitic acquaintance, injected it with the force of the sacred. Before starting the treatment he had two masses said and bought some ribbon blessed in the name of St Francis de Paola, which he also applied to the sick man. De Quarto was a reputed witch, or *magaro*. His patient suspected magic in the ritual and denounced De Quarto to the bishop's court. In his history of

---

31 Arrizabalaga, Henderson, French, *The Great Pox*, pp. 187-189.

32 ADO, *Magia,* I, 'Nicola Gargaro denuncia Donato de Quarto.'

33 Jarcho, *Clinical Consultations*, consultation lxxxiv, undated, pp. 266-267.

34 Cellini, *Autobiography*, book lix.

the Jesuit missions in the kingdom of Naples, Scipione Paolucci recounted the case of a man cured of his venereal disease during the course of a mission. 'He overcame this shame [at his illness] during the course of a mission,' Paolucci wrote, 'and, having vomited all the poison of his soul at the confessor's feet, seemed thenceforth to be healed of every bodily ill as well.'[35] St Job, the Old Testament sufferer raised to sainthood by the Catholic Church, quickly became the patron saint of syphilitics.[36] Of course, any saint – officially recognized or not – would do in a pinch. In 1746, after a fruitless series of interventions by a surgeon, a stay at the Incurables hospital, and a trip to the baths on the island of Ischia, Giuseppe Oreccchio attributed his cure to the miraculous intercession of a recently deceased lay nun.[37]

If the treatment of venereal disease in early modern Italy by a range of practitioners can be seen as a marketplace, it was a regulated one. This regulation was carried out by the medical tribunals, the guilds, and the ecclesiastical authorities. In theory at least it affected physicians and charlatans – indeed all practitioners – in equal measure, to the extent that all were subject to restrictions and controls. We have just seen how guilds examined and oversaw the activities of the *stufaroli*. The peninsula also had a range of medical magistracies: the Protomedicato tribunals, the Colleges of Physicians, and the Health Offices. Although precise jurisdictions varied from state to state, together they licensed and supervised the practice of the 'healing arts.'[38] As part of the 'moral economy,' these magistracies sought to arbitrate between patients and practitioners, respecting the rights of both. Even the fees charged by practitioners for the goods and services they provided corresponded to prevailing notions of the just price. In Sicily, for instance, a standard fee system was in operation, at least as envisioned by the island's Protomedicato tribunal. According to this, the fee charged would depend on the nature and rank of the practitioner (whether physician, surgeon, or mere licensee), the time of the visit (night was more expensive than day), the rank of the patient (and ability to pay), the distance to the sufferer's house (a surcharge was incurred if the

---

35Paolucci, *Missioni*, pp. 88-89, cit. in Gentilcore, *Healers and Healing*, p. 12.

36The Bolognese confrères of Santa Maria dei Guarini dedicated both their confraternity and the hospital they governed – which specialized in treating syphilitics – to St Job. Arrizabalaga, Henderson, and French, *The Great Pox*, p. 52.

37Archivio Segreto del Vaticano, *Sacra Congregazione di Riti*, 1861, 598^r-602^r, cit. in Gentilcore, *Healers and Healing*, pp. 179-180.

38Pomata, *Contracting a Cure*, 1-24; Gentilcore, 'All that Pertains to Medicine'; idem, *Healers and Healing*, pp. 29-55; idem, 'Figurations and State Authority'; Vanzan Marchini, *Mali e rimedi*, pp. 65-102; Palmer, 'Physicians and the State.'

practitioner had to leave the town gates), the seriousness of the illness, the duration of the treatment, and its outcome.[39] The sacred element, like the medical one, was also regulated. A whole range of forces at work in this Counter-Reformation society sought to define and enforce the limitations of orthodoxy regarding both magical and religious beliefs and practices: from tribunals, like the Inquisition and the episcopal courts, to preaching, confessing, and missionary activity.[40]

The third and final criticism against the assertion that 'quack doctors' provided most treatment for venereal disease lies in the various labels applied to the alleged practitioners themselves. The post-modern take on this cluster of terms – charlatan, quack, mountebank, and so on – is quite right to insist on their usage by the medical elites of the time as a way of distinguishing themselves from other, less desirable healers. As such, it is a relational and representational category: the 'other.'[41] The elites depicted charlatans as everything physicians were not: while physicians had imbibed the knowledge of the ancients, charlatans knew only by experience; physicians had a university doctorate, charlatans no formal education; physicians were a part of the divine order of the world, charlatans were menacing and uncontrollable itinerants; physicians were represented in corporations, charlatans were not; physicians practised the noble art of medicine with a sense of decorum, charlatans mixed vulgar commerce with spectacle and histrionic antics; physicians managed the whole individual, in sickness and in health, the charlatan went for the quick fix; and so on.

However, the Italian experience suggests another possible methodology: one that is either bravely 'post-post-modern' or simply old-fashioned, depending on how it is approached and carried out. From the mid-sixteenth century, the various medical magistracies mentioned above required charlatans to submit their wares for inspection and, upon approval, pay a licence fee in order to set up a stage from which to perform and sell them. The licensing of charlatans became an administrative routine. As far as the medical magistracies were concerned, charlatans had a definable identity: they constituted a specific trade or occupation (*professione* in the Italian of the time). In this context, the term 'charlatan' lost some of its bite, becoming less a term of abuse and more a generic, bureaucratic label, identifying a category of healer. The word had a more precise meaning and fewer figurative connotations than it acquired in French and English. More importantly, it was a label the charlatans themselves used. One might

---

39 Ingrassia, *Constitutiones, capitula, iurisdictiones*, pp. 74-90.

40 Gentilcore, *From Bishop to Witch.*

41 Lingo, 'Empirics and Charlatans.'

expect them to be referred to as *ciarlatani* in the licensing records of the medical magistracies. After all, in most cases – with the exception of the health offices of the Venetian republic – the licensers were physicians. What is perhaps more surprising is that when charlatans themselves referred to their occupation, in a variety of non-medical contexts – whether in tax censuses (*catasti*) and registries, or letters and petitions to higher authorities, criminal proceedings, and wills – they invariably put down *ciarlatano* or its equivalents (*ciurmatore, montimbanco, saltimbanco*). Moreover, licensing conferred a degree of status upon them, as well as legality, and this helped compensate for the fact that they lacked a corporation of their own. As a result of both this licensing regime and the notion of charlatanry as an occupational category, Italian charlatans can be studied over the course of the early modern period and their activities, remedies, itineraries, and commercial strategies reconstructed and analysed.[42]

The 'Charlatans Database' I have assembled contains 1,596 licences issued to 1,075 different charlatans the length and breadth of Italy over a period of two and a half centuries. It allows us to understand charlatans and charlatanism 'from the inside.' Applications for licences – few of which were ever turned down – tell us clearly what charlatans wished to sell. The licences in the Database mention 2,716 remedies for sale, made up of some 382 *different* remedies. That said, it is very difficult, if not impossible, to be precise about the number of different remedies, and this for a variety of reasons: human error in recording the licences; remedies with widely varying names might contain the very same, or at least quite similar, ingredients; different remedy names masking identical ingredients; a single remedy but with a variation in the ingredients, either by a single or different charlatans.

In the treatment of venereal disease Italian charlatans – the prototype for the charlatan throughout Europe – are visible by their absence. The handbills, which have proved such a rich source for the exploration of the advertised activities of English practitioners specializing in venereal disease, do not link Italian charlatans with the disease in the same way. There are simply very few handbills from Italian charlatans selling remedies for the disease. It seems that, at least in Italy, charlatans as an occupational category rarely involved themselves in the treatment of venereal disease. By and large, they limited themselves to the sale of remedies for it.

There are exceptions. On 4 May 1671 the Venetian Health Office licensed Carlo Teruggi of Milan, resident in Padua, to 'treat and freely

[42]The subject of my forthcoming book, *Mixing Medicine and Buffoonery: Charlatans and Charlatanism in Early Modern Italy* (Oxford: Oxford University Press).

dispense ... his secret for the French Disease.'[43] This followed the recommendation of the board's protophysician, who wrote that Teruggi should 'not for any reason receive from anyone any kind of molestation.' The licence rendered Teruggi immune from prosecution for any death or harm that might occur as a result of his treatments. And in fact, seven years later, Barbara Como accused Teruggi of having 'reduced [her hausband] to a deplorable condition and to the shape of a skeleton,' despite Teruggi's promises to cure him with his remedy. When the Paduan authorities went to Francesco Como's bedside, they were told that he had been housebound for the previous five months and bedridden for the previous two. He was visited by many surgeons, until one told Como that his haemorrhoids were 'cankered' and that 'there was no further remedy.' At that point Como's mother told him about Teruggi. The treatment was not cheap: Como paid Teruggi ten ducats before starting and agreed to pay him a further five 'if I was cured.' As surety Como also gave Teruggi Barbara's pearl necklace. The treatment began with some 'gross white wine with ingredients' that made Como 'shit his guts' (*mi faceva andare del corpo si può dire le viscere*), followed by an ointment rubbed on his joints for four days, which made him unable to move. Como managed to make his way to see two physicians and both declared that Teruggi had been his ruin. Before the Health Office could take a decision, Como died. However, once they received the licence from the Venetian Health Office, effectively bestowing immunity on Teruggi, their hands were tied. The fact that Teruggi had successfully administered to many other Paduan syphilitics no doubt reinforced his position. This, however, was not enough to protect his associate, Antonio Balegaro. Balegaro had treated sufferers on behalf of Teruggi, but without a licence, so he was fined fifty lire plus costs. His role in the events suggests the high demand for Teruggi's services.

This kind of practice required specialized expertise, which most charlatans simply did not have. However, if Italian charlatans did not generally treat the disease, they did sell medicines for it, most of which were substitutes for mercury. These medicines were chosen for two, related, reasons. First of all, because *stufaroli*, like Rome's Bernardino Fratoddi, tended to specialize in mercury treatments, at least from the seventeenth century onwards.[44] There was no point in operating in an already crowded market. Moreover, the effects of the mercury alternatives were thought

[43] ASPd, *Sanità*, 148, 49–95.

[44] In 1710 Fratoddi accused an aquavite-seller of not paying for his mercury treatment, despite openly walking about without crutches selling his aquavite. ASR, *Università*, 62, 1685.

analogous to mercury's – that of driving the poison out of the body – but without its side-effects. While sweating was deemed crucial to any treatment, mercury's other effects – excessive salivation, loosening of teeth – were less desirable. A Milanese sufferer has left a description of these effects. Rosa Vianelli recounted how after two months' treatment with a 'mercurial ointment,' she felt wretched. 'I could not move for the great weakness,' she continued, 'with my mouth full of sores and all my teeth wobbling, so that when I just tried to swallow liquids they came out my nose, not being able to get them down since my throat was blocked, with a fever that lasted almost two months.'[45]

Although charlatans sold alternatives to mercury, these were not 'alternative medicines' in the sense we mean today – of belonging to a different therapeutic system existing outside the mainstream. The remedies sold by charlatans included decoctions of guaiac and sarsaparilla. In using these plants, they were following the dictates of *official* medicine (just as the hospitals did). Both simples were known sudorifics and both hailed from the New World, like syphilis itself, as it was believed. It made sense that God would place the remedy in proximity to the disease it was to treat: each region produced the antidotes to its own poisons. The fact that they were new and thus unknown to the ancients was also important. 'Ther was never no such dysease knowen,' as Giovanni da Vigo put it in 1525, 'wherefore it was nedefull for the curation of this dysease, to serche out newe remedyes. And to saye the truth, the medicines lately invented are better in thys dysease then the medicines of olde writers.'[46] Guaiac – usually called *legno santo*, or holy wood, in Italy – was first mentioned in 1516.[47] Over the next two and a half centuries it went in and out of fashion among physicians. Although guaiac quickly became *the* treatment for venereal disease, by the middle of the sixteenth century mercury treatment was probably more common. Guaiac then experienced something of a revival, as part of the more generalized shift to 'natural' medicines and therapies during the eighteenth century.[48] Beginning in the 1730s, Giambattista Morgagni was recommending it to his patients, as documented in his clinical consultations. He was of two minds about mercury. On the one hand, he sought to avoid mercurial salivation whenever possible, especially

---

[45]ASPv, *Università*, 890, vol. 5, 10^{v}.

[46]da Vigo, *Workes of Chirurgerye*, clx^{v}–clxi^{r}.

[47]Munger, 'Guaiacum.'

[48]This is traced in McAllister, 'Vegetable Wars,' in a revealing exploration of a single remedy, which is marred only by the author's difficult (and rather dubious) aim of distinguishing 'quacks' from 'honest' practitioners.

that produced by mercury vapour, 'a method almost entirely discarded [he wrote in a consultation of 1739], because it easily harms the head and chest and it often produces horrible swellings in the tongue, throat, gums and cheeks, as well as diarrhea and dysenteries.' On the other hand, Morgagni acknowledged (in a 1746 consultation) that 'it is true that syphilitic infection, when it is established ... requires a strong treatment, and this one in the opinion of the majority [of physicians] requires one of the strongest, namely mercury.' Even in this latter case, however, he preferred to treat it 'palliatively rather than radically.'[49] Mercury remained in European pharmacopoeias throughout the early modern period, as did sarsaparilla.[50]

Charlatans might combine guaiac and sarsaparilla as components in other remedies. An 'antivenereal wine' licensed in Milan contained guaiac (both bark and oil) and sarsaparilla, as well as anise-seed, china root, and senna. China root – cinchona, from which quinine was later derived – was also used as a sudorific to treat syphilis and intermittent fevers. Because senna is a powerful laxative, the wine's effects on the sufferer would certainly have been apparent (similar to that used by Teruggi). The mixture was to be dissolved in half a *brenta* of white wine – a *brenta* being 'a certaine vessell to carrie wyne from place to place, or wine-measurers,'[51] of about fifty litres. The sufferer was to consume a pitcher a day until the supply was consumed, probably about a month. The only reason we have any detailed information about the remedy is because of a campaign undertaken by the newly-instated Milanese commissioners of health in 1767 against the posting of bills and the hanging of signs to advertise medicines. On 17 May 1767 the remedy's originator and manufacturer, Baldassare Garavaglia, was summoned to appear before the commissioners. He had been making and selling it for over forty years. His original patent, issued on 24 July 1726 by the Protofisicato, judged Garavaglia's remedy 'of good quality and helpful for the said venereal disease' so it licensed him 'to prepare, sell and dispense, 4 carried out at the Ospedale Maggiore of Milan,' and he promised he would bring the recipe for the remedy advertised in his handbill. The handbill boasted how

> the said secret was by the above-mentioned Garavaglia tried out in the venerable Ospital Maggiore of this city on a man oppressed because of the

49Jarcho, *Clinical Consultations*, consultations lxxxii and lxxxvii, pp. 264 and 278-281, respectively.

50Sarsaparilla enjoyed a second life as an ingredient in nineteenth-century patent medicines, such as tonics. Estes, 'Public Pharmacology.'

51Florio, *Worlde of Wordes*, p. 49.

> disease by excessive pains, very large gummas and many black sores penetrating deep around his waist (*vita*), and especially on the tip/head (*capo*); and finally he was judged to be near life's end, and therefore unable to receive mercury, given the absence and extenuation of his strength; and from that venerable hospital he has received a very clear testimonial, in addition to various other miraculous experiences worked with the same secret on different people also full of venereal disease, as appears from various other authentic testimonials and attestations, which the above-mentioned Garavaglia has, ready to show to anyone who should wish to see them.

The remedy was unlike any in the official pharmacopoeia, his handbill concluded. It was superior in taste and smell, and did not require bed-rest, a special diet, or any other inconvenience. Garavaglia gave his address, but he did not make a case for secrecy, privacy, or discretion. As promised, Garavaliga produced the recipe (preserving it for posterity in the process). He was told to await the commissioners' decision on the patent's renewal. In the meantime he was to take down the handbill which he had hung up and not to treat any sufferers with the remedy. A month later he had to be threatened with a heavy fine if he did not remove the handbill within twenty-four hours. But the matter ended there.[52]

Little in Garavaglia's remedy differed from those in the official pharmacopoeias, whatever his claims about it. In fact, its similarity was one of the reasons why it was so readily licensed for sale by the medical authorities. For his part, Morgagni was a great believer in these kinds of gentler remedies, even advising patients to avoid strong laxatives. To a sufferer in Gallipoli, he recommended taking 'a simple antisyphilitic decoction' for thirty or forty days in preference to mercury. In this *decoctum lignorum* (literally, 'decoction of woods,' since it contained guaiac, sassafras and licorice, with raisins added) he recommended substituting sarsaparilla for the sassafras and adding half a mountain viper (its flesh having first been made into a paste with the addition of citrus conserve).[53] Morgagni was a strong supporter of both sarsaparilla and viper's flesh in the treatment of venereal disease. The eighteenth century in particular produced an ever-increasing array of medicines for the treatment of syphilis which were subjected to ad hoc trials in the hospitals of Europe.[54] Morgagni supplied one patient with a long list of medicated teas and waters, concluding: 'I could add many other kinds of recommended drugs in the form of waters,

---

[52]ASPv, *Università*, 29.

[53]Jarcho, *Clinical Consultations*, consultation viii, 27 August 1751, pp. 20-23.

[54]Brockliss and Jones, *Medical World*, pp. 633-637, 776-777; Maehle, *Drugs on Trial*, p. 16.

electuaries or tinctures. But, as I have said, I am pleased to hope that time itself will be a sufficient medicine.'[55]

The question remains: how many of these medicines were sold by 'charlatans' (in our more restricted use of this term)? The Database reveals that Italian charlatans also sold a *Panacea Orientale*, pills for gonorrhoea, and various other unidentified remedies. As a proportion of all the remedies for which charlatans were licensed in the period 1550-1800, remedies intended primarily for venereal disease averaged only 2.6% of licensed remedies whose therapeutic function is known. (Therapeutic functions are clearly stated or are known or can be inferred in two-thirds (65.7%) of the remedies licensed for sale in the years 1550-1800.) If we consider all licensed remedies, venereal medicines comprised a mere 1.8%. The results of the Charlatans Database are outlined in the two tables. There is no discernible periodization or pattern in charlatans' licences, with the exception of two peaks in the latter half of the sixteenth century and again in the mid eighteenth century. The low rates overall help explain why so few Italian charlatans' handbills exist advertising venereal remedies and treatments. Does this mean that Italian sufferers were unable to treat themselves in the way that London's population was (where most surviving handbills refer to venereal disease)? Perhaps so, although there were other means of obtaining medicines. Some could be purchased over the apothecary's counter. Francesco Antonio Barra, an apothecary in Naples, advertised his 'miraculous specific' for gonorrhoea in the local press, promising to cure even long-time sufferers with just a few drops, 'and without a prior purge or the need for daily regimen.' Another Neapolitan apothecary sold a pill for the same, promising to supply instructions on how to take it when the sufferer came to buy it.[56] Medicines could also be obtained from monasteries and convents, which were becoming more adept at marketing their own natural medicines. There is certainly no evidence that medical regulation prevented sufferers from exercising their option to choose the source of therapy they preferred, to switch from one to another, or to follow several forms of treatment at once.

One means of testing this hypothesis further would be via the periodical press of the time, particularly in the eighteenth century. While the learned journals offered their well-educated readers discussions on topics like the 'method for giving mercury in syrup form, according to Mr.

---

[55]Jarcho, *Clinical Consultations*, consultation lxxxvi, 18 February 1741, pp. 273-274.

[56]Archivio di Stato, Naples, *Biblioteca, Avvisi di Napoli*, no. 11, 2 March 1734, and *Gazzetta di Napoli*, no. 1, 15 December 1739, in Pizzo, *Informazione medico-scientifica*, pp. 1203-1204.

Table One:
Remedies Licensed for Venereal Disease
as Percentages of Licences Issued per Decade

Veneral Disease Remedies: Percentages	1550 – 1559	1560 – 1569	1570 – 1579	1580 – 1589	1590 – 1599	1600 – 1609	1610 – 1619	1620 – 1629	1630 – 1639	1640 – 1649	1650 – 1659	1660 – 1669	1670 – 1679	1680 – 1689	1690 – 1699	1700 – 1709	1710 – 1719	1720 – 1729	1730 – 1739	1740 – 1749	1750 – 1759	1760 – 1769	1770 – 1779	1780 – 1789	1790 – 1799	Avg.
As a % of all licensed remedies	1.9	3.7	0.0	4.8	6.9	2.8	0.4	0.0	1.4	1.7	0.0	0.0	0.9	1.8	1.0	2.6	0.0	2.1	2.5	2.3	2.6	1.8	2.0	1.9	0.0	1.76
As a % of remedies for which therapeutic function is known	2.6	6.3	6.3	8.3	9.9	5.3	0.5	0.0	1.6	2.1	0.0	0.0	1.6	2.3	1.4	3.6	0.0	3.2	3.7	3.6	4.2	3.2	3.1	2.6	0.0	2.57
Overall % of charlatans' remedies for which therapeutic function is known	71.8	59.2	77.0	57.2	69.3	53.7	76.8	77.2	84.2	82.8	71.8	89.7	68.0	77.0	73.0	72.8	69.5	65.7	68.1	63.5	61.0	58.3	65.5	72.3	69.5	65.5

Table Two:
Types of Remedies Licensed for the Treatment of Venereal Disease

Venereal Disease Remedies	1550 – 1559	1560 – 1569	1570 – 1579	1580 – 1589	1590 – 1599	1600 – 1609	1610 – 1619	1620 – 1629	1630 – 1639	1640 – 1649	1650 – 1659	1660 – 1669	1670 – 1679	1680 – 1689	1690 – 1699	1700 – 1709	1710 – 1719	1720 – 1729	1730 – 1739	1740 – 1749	1750 – 1759	1760 – 1769	1770 – 1779	1780 – 1789	1790 – 1799	Total
decoction, legno santo	1	0	0	0	0	0	0	0	0	0	0	0	0	0	0	0	0	0	0	0	0	0	0	0	0	1
decoction, sarsaparilla	0	0	0	0	0	0	0	0	0	0	0	0	0	0	0	0	0	0	1	0	0	0	0	0	0	1
decoction, wine	0	0	0	1	0	0	0	0	0	0	0	0	0	0	0	0	0	0	0	0	1	0	0	0	0	2
Panacea Orientale	0	0	0	0	0	0	0	0	0	0	0	0	0	0	0	0	0	0	0	1	0	1	0	0	0	2
pills, for gonorrhea	0	0	0	0	0	0	0	0	0	0	0	0	0	0	0	0	0	0	1	0	0	0	0	0	0	1
wine, medicated	0	0	0	0	0	0	0	0	0	0	0	0	0	0	0	1	0	0	2	0	0	0	0	0	0	3
unnamed	0	1	0	0	7	4	1	0	1	1	0	0	1	2	1	1	0	3	5	2	3	2	2	1	0	38
Veneral Disease TOTALS	1	1	0	1	7	4	1	0	1	1	0	0	1	2	1	2	0	3	9	3	4	3	2	1	0	48
Remedy TOTALS (per decade)	53	27	13	21	102	141	253	96	74	58	60	185	107	112	100	77	108	141	362	131	156	163	99	54	23	2716

Bellet,'[57] early newssheets provided a wide range of the population with an equally wide range of therapeutic possibilities. Do the column inches devoted to advertisements for venereal disease cures and curers in Italian newspapers equal those of England and France?[58] To what extent were Italian charlatans able to make use of newspapers to commercialise their activities, effectively bypassing the regulatory bodies? And what about the physicians, surgeons and apothecaries: were they able to advertise their goods and services freely?

Given the present state of knowledge of the history of the Italian periodical press, I am unable to suggest answers to these tantalizing questions.[59] For the time being it remains for me to account for why charlatans sold so few remedies. This low level was due in part to the difficulty charlatans always had in being licensed to prepare and sell internal medicines. Guidelines issued for the deputees of the Milanese Protofisicato in 1675 reminded them of the licensing procedures pertaining to charlatans wishing to make and sell their medicines in the state. These included the standard review of a remedy's ingredients by the officials. The procedures for a remedy to be taken orally were even stricter: the remedy had to be manufactured in the house of the inspector-apothecary, 'so that the ingredients which go into it can be recognized, corrected, or adjusted by the deputees.'[60] Moreover the medical authorities were wary of new medicines. To a certain extent they always had been; but the rise of clinical medicine

---

[57] *Il Magazzino Toscano*, III:2, 1772, pp. 159-160, in Lippi, *Medicina e stampa periodica*, p. 178.

[58] Lawrence Stone noted that advertisements for venereal disease cures accounted for more space in the eighteenth-century English periodical press than any other product (*Family, Sex and Marriage*, p. 600). However, a detailed study of the Bath press during the second half of the eighteenth century found that, of the 302 proprietary medicines advertised, only nineteen (or 6.3%) were for 'the treatment and prevention of venereal disease.' These nineteen appeared in 534 advertisements for proprietary medicines, out of a total of 7,988 (or just 6.7%). Far more significant in terms of the volume of newspaper advertisements were proprietary medicines intended to treat general conditions (1,651 advertisements, or 20.7% of the total), gastro-intestinal disease (1,022, or 12.8%), localized complaints (974, or 12.2%), and a range of dental preparations (825, or 10.3%). Brown, 'Medicines,' p. 158 (although the calculations are my own). This puts remedies for venereal disease in a more realistic context. For Scottish medical advertising, see Dingwall, 'Medical Practitioners'; for France, see Brockliss and Jones, *Medical World*, pp. 646-658.

[59] Italian newspapers have not attracted the sort of interest among social and cultural historians as those of France or England. The few studies available lie within the history of journalism tradition, like Farinelli, *Storia del giornalismo italiano*.

[60] ASPv, *Università*, 43, 'Ordini da osservarsi da SS. Luogo Tenenti eletti & dà eleggersi dal Protofisico Generale nelle città & Luoghi particolari di questo Stato di Milano,' 30/1/1675.

during the eighteenth century made them even more sceptical. In September 1784, as part of an investigation, the protophysician of the Venetian Health Office, Giambattista Paitoni, visited a sick woman whom the charlatan Salvatore Borgia of Palermo boasted of curing with a remedy of his. Alas for Borgia, Paitoni found her 'still sick and covered in sores.'[61]

The low number of remedies may also be a reflection of the continuing high cost of ingredients like guaiac on the world market. Even after 1525, when the Fugger banking family lost its monopoly, the price remained consistently high. In 1687 the price in France was nine *livres* a pound, equivalent to twenty-five days' work for a journeyman tailor.[62] There was thus no direct, immediate relationship between the changing fashions of mercury as a remedy and the charlatans' peddling of guaiac as an alternative to it, as has sometimes been suggested.[63] At the same time, the Database figures may under-represent the number of charlatans' remedies for venereal disease offered for sale in Italy, since other simples with sudorific properties – one example being juniper – might find themselves used in the treatment of venereal disease (sweating being deemed a crucial element). Remedies with a long list of diseases they purported to cure also sometimes included venereal disease. In the 1730s Tommaso Thirocco peddled an unnamed elixir in Turin and Milan, which – his handbill claimed – purified the blood, dried cold humours, and cured scrofula, worms, sciatica, and nerve complaints. It was also good for syphilis:

> Those people who have the *morbo gallico* in any form, even those brought out of their mother's body [with it], without being forced to take to bed or to a room ... in a brief period of time will be cured.[64]

Thirocco, who was a physician from Lyon with a doctorate from Montpellier, also welcomed the sick to his rented accommodation. This invitation was intended for the incredulous who wanted proof of his medicine's efficacy; he makes no mention of his treating the sick. As a physician he would have been able to, but as a foreigner he would have required the special permission of the local College of Physicians in order to practise. Thirocco's case is a sign of how remedy-sellers tended to steer clear of the treatment of venereal disease. This was due in part to the attempts of the medical tribunals to keep separate the various branches of the medical arts

---

61 ASV, *Sanità*, 588, 29/7/1784.

62 Estes, 'European Reception,' pp. 7 and 18, and Vigarello, *Histoire des pratiques*, p. 133.

63 Quétel, *History of Syphilis*, pp. 30, 90.

64 ASPv, *Università*, 29, 'Si fa noto al pubblico ed al privato...,' Brescia, Bergamo, Milano: per Carlo Bolzani, 1731.

and regulate the practice of healing. To sufferers of venereal disease, this meant that they were not consigned to some illicit, back street world in order to get treatment; rather they made the most of a wide variety of sources of treatment openly available in early modern Italy.

University of Leicester
Leicester, United Kingdom

Cited Works

Manuscript Sources

Mantua, Archivio di Stato, *Magistratura sanitaria antica* (ASMa, *Sanitaria*)
Milan, Archivio di Stato, *Studi* (ASMi, *Studi*)
Padua, Archivio di Stato, *Ufficio di Sanità* (ASPd, *Sanità*)
Pavia, Archivio di Stato, *Università: Facoltà Medica* (ASPv, *Università*)
Rome, Archivio di Stato, *Archivio dell'Università* (ASR, *Università*)
Venice, Archivio di Stato, *Provveditori all Sanità* (ASV, *Sanità*)
Oria, Archivio Diocesano, *Magia e stregoneria* (ADO, *Magia*)

Published Sources

Arrizabalaga, Jon, John Henderson, and Roger French. *The Great Pox: The French Disease in Renaissance Europe*. New Haven and London: Yale University Press, 1997.

Brockliss, Laurence and Colin Jones. *The Medical World of Early Modern France*. Oxford: Clarendon Press, 1997.

Brown, P. S. 'Medicines Advertised in Eighteenth-Century Bath Newspapers' *Medical History*, 20 (1976):152-68.

Brown, P. S. 'The Venders of Medicines Advertised in Eighteenth-Century Bath Newspapers' *Medical History*, 19 (1975): 352-369.

Bynum, W. F. 'Treating the Wages of Sin: Venereal Disease and Specialism in Eighteenth-Century Britain' pp. 5-28 in *Medical Fringe and Medical Orthodoxy, 1750-1850*, W. F. Bynum and R. Porter, eds. London: Croom Helm, 1987.

Cellini, Benvenuto. *The Autobiography of Benvenuto Cellini*, trans. J. Symonds. New York: P. F. Collier, 1909-1914.

Cruciani, Gianfranco. *Cerusici e fisici: preciani e nursini dal XIV al XVIII secolo*. Arrone: Thyrus, 1999.

Cunningham, Andrew and Ole Grell. *The Four Horsemen of the Apocalypse: Religion, War, Famine and Death in Reformation Europe*. Cambridge: Cambridge University Press, 2000.

da Vigo, Giovanni. *The Most Excellent Workes of Chirurgerye*. London: Whytchurch, 1543; reprint Amsterdam and New York: Da Capo, 1968.

Dingwall, Helen. '"To Be Insert in the Mercury": Medical Practitioners and the Press in Eighteenth-Century Edinburgh' *Social History of Medicine*, 13 (2000): 23-44.

Estes, J. Worth. 'Public Pharmacology: Modes of Action of 19th-Century 'Patent' Medicines' *Medical Heritage*, 2 (1986): 218-228.

Estes, J. Worth. 'The European Reception of the First Drugs from the New World' *Pharmacy in History*, 37 (1995): 3-23.

Farinelli, Giuseppe. et al., *Storia del giornalismo italiano, dalle origini ai giorni nostri.* Turin: UTET, 1997. pp. 3-82.

Flood, John and David Shaw. 'The Price of the Pox in 1527: Johannes Sinapius and the Guaiac Cure' *Bibliothèque d'Humanisme et Renaissance*, 54 (1992): 691-707.

Florio, John. *A Worlde of Wordes*. London: Blount, 1598; rpt. Hildesheim and New York: Georg Olms Verlag, 1972.

Garzoni, Tomaso, *La piazza universale di tutte le professioni del mondo* (1585), 2 vols. eds. P. Cherchi and B. Collina. Turin: Einaudi, 1996.

Gentilcore, David. '"All that Pertains to Medicine": *Protomedici* and *Protomedicati* in Early Modern Italy' *Medical History*, 38 (1994), pp. 121-142.

Gentilcore, David. 'Figurations and State Authority in Early Modern Italy: The Case of the Sienese Protomedicato' *Canadian Journal of History/Annales canadiennes d'histoire*, XXXIV (1999): 359-383.

Gentilcore, David. *From Bishop to Witch: The System of the Sacred in Early Modern Terra d'Otranto*. Manchester: University Press, 1992.

Gentilcore, David. *Healers and Healing in Early Modern Italy*. Manchester: University Press, 1998.

Gnoli, Umberto. 'Stufe romane della Rinascenza' *Pan: rassegna di lettere, arte e musica*, 2 (1934): 402-408.

Ingrassia, Giovanni Filippo. *Constitutiones, capitula, iurisdictiones, ac pandectae regii protomedicatus officii*. Palermo: Nicola Bua, 1657.

Lingo, Alison. 'Empirics and Charlatans in Early Modern France: The Genesis of the Classification of the "Other" in Medical Practice' *Journal of Social History*, 19 (1986): 583-603.

Lippi, Donatella. 'Medicina e stampa periodica nel Settecento: Il *Magazzino Toscano*' *Rivista di storia della medicina*, 9 (1999): 168-186.

McAllister, Marie E. 'John Burrows and the Vegetable Wars' pp. 85-102 in *The Secret Malady: Venereal Disease in Eighteenth-Century Britain and France*, ed. Linda E. Merians. Lexington: University Press of Kentucky, 1996.

Maehle, Andreas-Holger. *Drugs on Trial: Experimental Pharmacology and Therapeutic Innovation in the Eighteenth Century*. Amsterdam: Rodopi, 1999.

Morgagni, Giambattista. *The Clinical Consultations of Giambattista Morgagni*, trans. and ed., Saul Jarcho. Boston: Countway Library of Medicine, 1984.

Munger, Robert. 'Guaiacum, the Holy Wood from the New World' *Journal of the History of Medicine*, 4 (1949): 196-229.

Palmer, Richard. 'Physicians and the State in Post-Medieval Italy' pp. 47-61 in *The Town and State Physician in Europe from the Middle Ages to the Enlightenment*, ed. A. Russell. Wolfenbüttel: Herzog August Bibliothek, 1981.

Paolucci, Scipione. *Missioni de Padri della Compagnia di Giesù nel Regno di Napoli* Naples: Secondino Roncagliolo, 1651.

Park, Katherine. 'Stones, Bones and Hernias: Surgical Specialists in Fourteenth- and Fifteenth-Century Italy' pp. 110-130 in *Medicine from the Black Death to the French Disease*, eds. Roger French, Jon Arrizabalaga, Andrew Cunningham and Luis Garcia-Ballester. Aldershot: Ashgate, 1998.

Pizzo, Antonietta. 'L'informazione medico-scientifica a Napoli nel Settecento. Rilievi dalla stampa periodica e da alcuni saggi' pp. 1199-1221 in *Gli archivi per la storia della scienza e della tecnica*, vol. 2, ed. G. Paoloni. Rome: Ministero per i Beni Culturali e Ambientali, 1995.

Pomata, Gianna. *Contracting a Cure: Patients, Healers, and the Law in Early Modern Bologna*. Baltimore: The Johns Hopkins University Press, 1998.

Porter, Roy. *Health for Sale: Quackery in England, 1660-1850*. Manchester: University Press, 1989.

Quétel, Claude. *History of Syphilis*, trans. Judith Braddock and Brian Pike. Cambridge: Polity, 1992.

Santorelli, Antonio. *Il protomedico napolitano, ovvero dell'autorità di esso. Dialogo raccolto da un discepolo ... e data in luce dal signor Fabio Cava*. Naples: Roberto Mollo, 1652.

Schleiner, Winfried. *Medical Ethics in the Renaissance*. Washington DC: Georgetown University Press, 1995.

Siena, Kevin. 'The "Foul Disease" and Privacy: The Effects of Venereal Disease and Patient Demand on the Medical Marketplace in Early Modern London' *Bulletin of the History of Medicine*, 75 (2001): 199-224.

Statuti, ordini e constitutioni della università de barbieri e stufaroli dell'alma città di Roma Rome: Blado, 1559; reissued and reprinted in 1613. Copy in the Biblioteca del Senato della Repubblica, Rome, *Statuti*, 609.

Stone, Lawrence. *Family, Sex and Marriage in England, 1500-1800*. New York: Harper and Row, 1977.

Vanzan Marchini, Nelli-Elena. *I mali e i rimedi della Serenissima*. Vicenza: Neri Pozza, 1995.

Vigarello, Georges. *Concepts of Cleanliness: Changing Attitudes in France since the Middle Ages*, trans. J. Birrell. Cambridge: University Press, 1988.

Vigarello, Georges. *Histoire des pratiques de santé: le sain et le malsain depuis le Moyen Age*. Paris: Seuil, 1999.

Zerenghi, Federico, *Breve compendio di cirurgia*. Naples: Costantino Vitale, 1603.

Joseph Grünpeck's Astrological Explanation of the French Disease

Darin Hayton

Responses to the French Disease varied widely, depending on social status, education, profession, and political commitments.[1] Physicians tried to incorporate the new sickness into existing categories in an effort to naturalize and control it. Empirics saw in it the opportunity to extend their own authority by encroaching on territory normally held by learned doctors. Religious and political reformers seized the opportunity to call for social and religious reform. Each group made sense of the French Disease in light of its own intellectual commitments and goals, and each offered a different interpretation of what was really occurring. For Joseph Grünpeck, who produced the first German tract on the pox, the advent of the French Disease was both terrifying and promising. He was more of a political propagandist than a physician, so his works on the French Disease were more than mere medical tracts. Combining his training in medicine and astrology with his search for a powerful patron, Grünpeck interpreted the advent and spread of the pox in political and social terms and incorporated it into his own career ambitions.

Joseph Grünpeck's early career was unremarkable. In 1487 he was admitted as a *pauper* to the University of Ingolstadt, where he studied rhetoric with Conrad Celtis and medicine with Wolfgang Peyser.[2] After obtaining his M.A. in 1491, he joined his many countrymen who went to Pavia to study medicine.[3] When his friend and traveling companion Bernhard von Waldkirch was appointed canon of the cathedral in Augsburg, in

[1]The best recent study of these responses is Arrizabalaga, Henderson and French, *The Great Pox*. See also French and Arrizabalaga, 'Coping with the French Disease,' pp. 248–287.

[2]The best biography of Grünpeck remains Czerny, 'Der Humanist und Historiograph Kaiser Maximilians I,' pp. 315–364. More recently, Russell, 'Astrology as Popular Propaganda,' pp. 165–195.

[3]On the German preference for the University of Pavia, see Grendler, *The Universities of the Italian Renaissance*, pp. 82–93.

the summer of 1494, Grünpeck left Pavia and relocated to the University of Krakow to combine his study of medicine with astrology. Because it was the only university in Central Europe at that time to have chairs in both astrology and medicine, Krakow attracted many students who hoped to become court physicians and advisors at one of the many local and regional courts.[4] Grünpeck remained in Krakow only a short time before returning to Ingolstadt in early 1495, where he began tutoring to students at the University of Ingolstadt in Latin rhetoric.

When the plague broke out in Ingolstadt that summer, Grünpeck was already convinced that he deserved a position at the imperial court. Accordingly, he fled Ingolstadt and returned to Italy, where he hoped to meet Emperor Maximilian I, who was leading the imperial troops back onto the peninsula in an effort to expel the French. However, when he encountered the imperial troops in Tuscany, he did not find the emperor but the French Disease raging through the army. Like his contemporaries, Grünpeck was terrified of this new epidemic that he could neither understand nor explain. Rather than remain in Italy, Grünpeck returned to Augsburg, resumed his job as Latin tutor to the now exiled Ingolstadt students, and redoubled his efforts to find a rich patron. In early 1496, Grünpeck capitalized on the emperor's visits to Augsburg in April, May, and June to cultivate his relationships with influential members of Maximilian's court, including his friend Waldkirch and the humanists Conrad Celtis and Conrad Peutinger. Grünpeck was, no doubt, hoping for the opportunity to secure a career in the imperial bureaucracy. In the autumn of 1496, Grünpeck produced two works on the advent and spread of the French Disease and used them to create the opportunity that he needed finally to attract the attention of Emperor Maximilian I.

MAXIMILIAN'S 'BLASPHEMY EDICT'

The appearance of the French Disease among the imperial troops and its continued spread into Austria and southern Germany was the source of great concern for Maximilian I. On the one hand, he took an immediate and pragmatic interest in the pox that was decimating his army in Italy and threatening to unravel his plans to expel the French from the peninsula. On the other hand, and more importantly, Maximilian saw the French Disease as a symbolic threat to his larger political ambitions, a threat that required immediate and official attention.

---

[4]Markowski, 'Die Astrologie an der Krakauer Universität in den Jahren 1450–1550,' pp. 83–89.

Maximilian became the *de facto* Holy Roman Emperor upon the death of his father, Frederick III, in 1493. His claim to the title, however, did not go unchallenged, and he had to struggle constantly to reassert his authority. Indeed, his massive propaganda campaigns were intended to legitimate his position as emperor.[5] A key component in these efforts was Maximilian's attempt to portray himself as the prophetic, universal emperor who would reform the church, unite Europe, expel the Ottoman threat, and lead a crusade to retake the Holy Land.[6] Maximilian's conviction that he was the prophetic emperor was shared by many imperial propagandists. As early as 1488, Johannes Lichtenberger had predicted that Maximilian would lead a unified Christian army against the infidels, vanquish the Ottoman threat, and usher in a Golden Age before handing the imperial insignia back to God in Jerusalem.[7] As suggested by Lichtenberger's prediction, Maximilian was thought to enjoy a particularly close relationship with God that required him to surpass all his predecessors as well as his contemporaries in honour and piety and to defend the Christian faith. Indeed, the guiding model for Maximilian's life was that of the pious knight, a model that he drew from the courtly romances and Arthurian legends he avidly collected and read.[8] At the end of the fifteenth century, with the Turkish armies on Europe's eastern borders and deep divisions between the emperor and his allies as well as his enemies, this image of the ideal knight and prophetic emperor became a powerful vehicle of imperial propaganda. Consequently, Maximilian could not allow the advent of the French Disease – which he, like most people, believed to have been sent from God as a punishment for human sin – to escape notice.

At the imperial Diet in Worms in 1495, Maximilian focused on imperial reform, addressing social and political issues in most of his edicts.[9] On 7 August, in the closing session of the Reichstag, he addressed the problem of the French Disease in his edict against blasphemy, published almost immediately in both Latin and German and circulated widely throughout the

---

[5]Diederichs, *Kaiser Maximilian I. als politischer Publizist.*

[6]The best introduction to the tradition of the last emperor is Reeves, *The Influence of Prophecy in the Later Middle Ages*. See also the discussion in Tanner, *The Last Descendant of Aeneas*.

[7]Lichtenberger, *Prognosticatio Ioannis Liechtenbergers*. The other popular prophecy in the late fifteenth century, the pseudo-Methodian prophecies, also looked to Maximilian as the prophetic emperor. See *Opusculum divinarum revelationum sancti Methodij*.

[8]A catalog of Maximilian's books is found in Gottlieb, *Büchersammlung Kaiser Maximilians*, p. 101. See Williams, 'The Arthurian Model in Emperor Maximilian's Autobiographic Writings,' pp. 3–22; Waas, *The Legendary Character of Maximilian*.

[9]See Wiesflecker, *Kaiser Maximilian I*, pp. 217–249.

empire.[10] In this 'Blasphemy Edict,' Maximilian called on the citizens of the empire to reform their religious practices, claiming that the decline in religious observation along with an increase in sinning had caused innumerable ailments in the civic body. Maximilian pointed out that just as in the past, God had again sent famine, earthquakes, diseases, and other plagues as punishments for the irreligious behaviour of the citizenry.[11] However, contemporary conditions were worse than ever, and consequently God had sent a more severe plague: 'especially these days the severe disease and human plague, named the evil pox, which previously had never existed or been heard of in human memory.'[12] To encourage the citizens of the Empire to reform their blasphemous ways, Maximilian established a system of fines for anyone who succumbed to the heat of passion and lust, public drunkenness, or similar offences.[13] This was not simply a form of social control or policing of his citizenry; it was also an attempt to bolster his economic reforms and establish a fiscal hierarchy that culminated with the emperor – Maximilian's system of fines placed the burden on local authorities to collect the fines and remit them to the emperor.[14] For Maximilian, the French Disease was a social problem that he consciously linked to his political and social reform projects. Maximilian's 'Blasphemy Edict' would provide the impetus and context for Grünpeck's works on the French Disease.

---

[10]The text of the edict is found in a number places. I have used the copy in *Deutsche Reichstagsakten unter Maximilian I*, pp. 575–577. A Latin version is available in Fuchs, *Die ältesten Schriftsteller*, pp. 305–306. There is some question to the actual date of composition. Hans Haustein suggested that it was written in 1497 and predated to 1495. Paul A. Russell originally accepted this dating, but then seemed to reject it a few years later. Cunningham and Grell echo Russell's claim. The Reichstagakten and Hermann Wiesflecker have adopted 1495 as the date of composition. Along with French and Arrizabalaga, I accept the earlier date as more likely. See Haustein, *Die Frühgeschichte der Syphilis*, pp. 300–301; Russell, 'Syphilis, God's Scourge or Nature's Vengeance?,' p. 290; Russell, 'Astrology as Popular Propaganda,' p. 173; Cunningham and Grell, *The Four Horsemen of the Apocalypse*, pp. 253, 342 note 12; French and Arrizabalaga, 'Coping with the French Disease,' p. 249.

[11]Escatological fears were wide-spread in late fifteenth- and early sixteenth-century Europe. See, for example, Cunningham and Grell, *The Four Horsemen of the Apocalypse*, chaps. 4 and 5.

[12]Maximilian, *Deutsche Reichstagsakten*, p. 576.

[13]'nemlich wo solichs aus bewegter hitz des zorns, aus trunkenheit oder dergleichen zufall unbedacht beschehe, umb 1 mark lötigs goldes, ... in der gebiete solich mißhandlung getan wurdet.' Maximilian, *Deutsche Reichstagsakten*, p. 577.

[14]At the same time, Maximilian was struggling to bring about a variety of tax reforms that would have relied on a similar structure of collection and payment. Wiesflecker, *Kaiser Maximilian I*, pp. 189–190, 223.

When he produced his tracts on the French Disease, Grünpeck captured the spirit of Maximilian's 'Blasphemy Edict.' His Latin *Tractatus de pestilentiali scorra sive mala franzos* appeared in mid-November, followed a couple of weeks later by the German version, *Ein hübscher Tractat von dem Ursprung des bösen Franzos.*[15] These two booklets explain the advent, spread, and symptoms of the French Disease within an astrological framework, and both served Grünpeck's political goals as much as they offered a medical account of the disease. Both their similarities and differences reflect the contours of Grünpeck's larger political and social project.

GRÜNPECK'S ASTROLOGICAL EXPLANATION

Like all his contemporaries, Grünpeck was baffled and frightened by the French Disease and admitted that standard medicine had trouble explaining its appearance. Although Grünpeck claimed that physicians' inability to account for the pox was one of the primary reasons for publishing his texts, he could nevertheless draw on a number of tools and models when composing his tracts. In response to the frequent plague outbreaks the plague tractate, or plague concilia, had developed by the late fifteenth century into a popular genre of medical writing. Plague concilia shared common characteristics and explanatory categories. Physically, they were short, rarely more than a handful of pages, and printed in a small format, often in Latin and the vernacular. This helped keep costs low for both printer and consumer and ensured a wide reading public. Their content included explanations of the source and causes of the plague, usually a mixture of natural, astrological, and supernatural causality. Plague concilia concluded with advice on how to avoid the disease and dietary regimens for maintaining and recovering health.[16] The most famous of these concilia was written by the renowned Italian physician Gentile da Foligno, but this was just one of many such works circulating throughout Europe in the late fifteenth century.[17] When Grünpeck wrote his works, he adopted both the format and the content of the plague concilia to fit the French Disease.

15Russell claims that the German tract preceeded the Latin. The internal dates suggest the opposite order, which I have accepted here. See Russell, 'Syphilis, God's Scourge or Nature's Vengeance?,' p. 293.

16Siraisi, *Medieval and Early Renaissance Medicine*, pp. 128–129. For an analysis of the contents of some early plague tractates, see Campbell, *The Black Death and Men of Learning*, pp. 34–92.

17Russell likens Grünpeck's work to Gentile's. While this is true, it undervalues the importance of the entire genre of writing represented by the plague tractates. Russell, 'God's Scourge or Nature's Vengeance,' pp. 290–291. On Gentile, see the recent work: French, *Canonical Medicine*.

Grünpeck distinguished two causes for the French Disease, a first cause or source and a secondary or physical cause. He had no doubt that the first cause or source of this new plague was the will of God. As everybody knew, during times of increased blasphemy and sinning, God sent down a series of punishments. In particular, He punished the sins of pride, greed, and lust with pestilences, bloodshed, and famine.[18] As Grünpeck reminded his reader, this was well attested in the Holy Scriptures. It should come as no surprise then, Grünpeck claimed, that God had sent the French Disease now, when these and worse sins are common amongst people:

> Hence all those torments, which lay hidden in former ages, are now frightfully on the increase. Therefore it is clear that these ills are sent down by the will of God to terrify men. For such reasons this filth, which they call the French Disease, clearly emanates from divine vengeance.[19]

The echoes of Maximilian's 'Blasphemy Edict' were not accidental. In Grünpeck's explanation, just as in Maximilian's, God's will was the source of this horrible illness.[20]

At the same time, he needed to explain the secondary or physical cause of the French Disease. Sensing no tension in his account, Grünpeck explained to his reader how the motions of the planets, especially planetary conjunctions, caused all manner of physical change on earth.[21] Although he points to Aristotle as his authority for this position, he also borrows from the Arab astrologers Albumasar and Messahalla when he claims that 'the death of races, which have passed away, and the desolation of kingdoms are due to the conjunctions of two stars, Saturn and Jupiter.'[22] For Grünpeck,

---

[18] Grünpeck, *Ein hübscher Tractat von dem Ursprung des bösen Franzos*, sign. A7^{v}. Grünpeck, *Tractatus de pestilentiali Scorra sive mala de Franzos*, sign. A6^{r-v}.

[19] 'Unde hec etiam. que superioribus etatibus latuerunt. plage horribilissime ingruunt. Quare haud clam est, hec flagicia e deifica voluntate in terram ad terrorem hominum demittti. Quam ob rem etiam hec colluvies. quam malum de Franzos vocant. ex superna vindicta demergi par videri potest.' Grünpeck, *Tractatus*, sign. A6^{v}.

[20] On the necessary religious aspect of the French Disease, see French and Arrizabalaga, 'Coping with the French Disease,' pp. 249–250.

[21] For a lucid discussion of how the plague could be seen both as a punishment from God and a product of natural causes, see Esser, 'Die Pest—Strafe Gottes oder Naturphänomen?,' pp. 32–57. Esser, however, mischaracterizes Grünpeck's tracts as about the plague: 'Der Traktat handelt nicht, wie der Titel vermuten ließe, nur von der Franzosenkrannkheit (Syphilis), sondern auch von der Pest.' Esser, 'Die Pest,' p. 39.

[22] 'Anni ubertas et sterilitas fiunt per stellarum mutationem in signis diversis super climata septem, et mortalitas gentium praeteritarum, atque regna vacua fiunt apud coitum stellarum duarum, Saturni et Jovis. Per eorum etenim mutationem de triplicitate ad triplicitatem accidunt accidentia magna, praeterea Martis cum praefatis planetis congres-

all plagues shared a divine first cause and an astrological secondary or physical cause; the French Disease was no exception.[23] Although a proper account had to incorporate both, Grünpeck concentrated on the astrological causation.

Central to Grünpeck's idea of astrological causation was the theory of great conjunctions, which had been developed most fully by the Arab astrologers Albumasar and Messahalla. According to this theory, conjunctions of the outer planets, especially Jupiter and Saturn, correlated with significant and wide-scale changes on earth. Albumasar had distinguished three types of conjunctions based on their frequency – *conjunctio magna*, *conjunctio major*, and *conjunctio maxima*. Following the first conjunction of Saturn and Jupiter in the sign of Aries, minor conjunctions occurred every twenty years as the two planets came together in the different the signs of the first triplicity – a trio of zodiacal signs related by the primary quality they were thought to share, either fire, air, water, or earth.[24] In sixty years, the planets again met in Aries, producing a *conjunctio magna*. The fourth such conjunction, 240 years after the initial one, shifts out of the first triplicity, and Jupiter and Saturn meet in the first sign of a new triplicity. This conjunction was called a *conjunctio major*. Saturn and Jupiter repeat this through the four triplicities until finally, after 960 years, the two planets come together once again in the original sign of Aries. This was a *conjunctio maxima*. With its convenient periods of 60, 240, and 960 years, the theory of great conjunctions became a common tool for understanding history in the medieval and Renaissance periods.[25] By the time Grünpeck was writing, it had become a set piece in the popular plague tractates, and Grünpeck simply adapted it to fit his contemporary situation.

However, in order to employ the theory of great conjunctions, Grünpeck had to establish two important conditions. First, he had to

---

sus in casibus eorum significabit terrae siccitatem.' Grünpeck, *Tractatus*, sign. A7^{r-v}. In the German version, Grünpeck truncates this discussion to just a few lines at the end of a chapter. In the Latin edition, his discussion of planetary causes includes humoural theory and a more detailed discussion of Aristotle and occupies an entire chapter.

23 'darumb nachvolget. das dise plagen auß der ersten und meysten ursach kommen auß dem willen gottes, ... Darnach die annder ursache diser geyseln von gott kommende. ist ein teyl natürlich, ein teyl kummt sy auß den züsammenfügungen der planeten.' Grünpeck, *Ein hübscher Tractat*, sign. A8^{r}.

24 The best discussion of this remains North, 'Astrology and the Fortune of Churches,' pp. 181–211.

25 Albumasar's text is available in a modern edition and translation, see Albumasar, *Liber introductorii maioris ad scientiam judiciorum astrorum*; Albumasar, *Abu Ma'Sar. The Abbreviation of the Introduction to Astrology*. For a detailed analysis of how this could be used as a tool for understanding history, see Smoller, *History, Prophecy and the Stars*, and Veenstra, *Magic and Divination at the Courts of Burgundy and France*, chap. 4.

determine the horoscope for the earth, or the configuration of the heavens at the moment of its creation. From this he could then calculate when the first Saturn-Jupiter conjunction had occurred in Aries. Second, he needed to establish the age of the earth, which would enable him to calculate the number of years that had elapsed from that first conjunction until the present. Only then could he use this theory to account for the most important feature of the French Disease – its appearance.

There was a long tradition of trying to establish the horoscope for creation, the *thema mundi*, stretching back at least to the fourth century. Julius Firmicus Maternus used the astrological assumption that a planet's exaltation – the portion of the zodiac in which the planet was considered particularly efficacious – corresponded to its location in the zodiac at the moment of creation.[26] Maternus and those who followed his example placed Aries at the important *medium coelum* and the sun in Leo. Opposed to this was the Christian tradition that placed the sun near the beginning of Aries, the vernal equinox, so that the Creation, Annunciation, and Crucifixion could occur on the same day. An important variation from these two traditions arose out of the writings of Pierre d'Ailly.[27] Basing his work on Albumasar, he combined the Christian and Arab traditions and ultimately arrived at a unique *thema mundi*, which he published in his *Concordantia astronomie cum theologia*. Grünpeck was probably familiar with much of this tradition. Because he was not a first-rate astrologer or mathematician, he preferred to borrow from it rather than calculate his own *thema mundi*. Without bothering to acknowledge it, he used d'Ailly's *Concordantia* as the source of his own horoscope for Creation. Grünpeck apparently did not read the text very carefully, relying instead on the illustrations in d'Ailly's book. Grünpeck's horoscope for Creation and his explanatory text both reproduced the two errors from d'Ailly's illustration.[28] Nevertheless, he used this erroneous horoscope as the point from which to calculate the first great conjunction and all subsequent conjunctions.

Grünpeck now needed to establish the age of the earth. Here again he relied heavily on d'Ailly's work. Throughout the medieval period, St. Augustine was clearly the most authoritative Christian source on the age of the earth. Building on an analogy to the six days of creation, he had divided history into six ages, delimited by significant historical events. In the fifteenth century, this framework for understanding history acquired in-

---

[26]Maternus, *Matheseos libri VIII*, bk. 3, chap. 1.

[27]For a fuller account of d'Ailly's *thema mundi*, see Smoller, *History, Prophecy and the Stars*, pp. 65–67.

[28]On the errors in the figure, see Smoller, *History, Prophecy and the Stars*, p. 67.

creased significance, particularly after d'Ailly used these divisions to warn that the Day of Judgment threatened if the Church did not mend the Great Schism.[29] At the end of the century, as millennial fears increased, Augustine's model of history had lost none of its impact. Grünpeck recognized this fact when he adapted d'Ailly's presentation for his own contemporary situation. Indeed, Grünpeck's account of the history of the earth apes d'Ailly's in every detail.

The key problem in calculating the age of the earth, Grünpeck claimed, was to determine the length of the first era, from the creation to the Flood. Despite disagreement amongst the most important chroniclers, Grünpeck assures his reader that they all affirm that 2,242 years elapsed between the moment of creation and the Flood.[30] Grünpeck offered no explanation for this value and perhaps did not understand how d'Ailly had calculated it. For his own purposes, d'Ailly's calculations were best ignored, and he quickly moved on, filling in the remainder of his chronology: Flood to Abraham, 942 years; Abraham to Kind David, 940 years; King David to expulsion from Babylon, 485 years; Expulsion from Babylon to Christ, 590 years.[31] He apparently did not notice or, more likely, did not care that these values did not equal the accepted duration for the period from the Flood to Christ – 3,101 years and 10 months, a value both he and d'Ailly had quoted from the Alphonsine Tables. It is characteristic that neither this discrepancy nor the other details of his explanation troubled Grünpeck, as he was more concerned with establishing the proper astrological model for his explanation and feigning authority and knowledge than with the minutia of his account. Indeed, he could confidently expect to impress his readers with this show of erudition and technical expertise because most of them would not have recognized his borrowings from d'Ailly, whose *Concordantia astrologiae cum theologia* was a daunting and expensive text that had only recently been printed.

Grünpeck's façade of expertise ran into its first problem when he hinted at the correlation between *conjunctiones magnae* and significant historical events. He listed the seven *conjunctiones maximae* that had occurred in history, from 320 years after the creation of the earth to the most recent, 735 years after the birth of Christ.[32] His assertion that these conjunctions had signaled

---

29 See Smoller, *History, Prophecy, and the Stars*, pp. 85–101.

30 Grünpeck, *Ein hübscher Tractat*, sign. B3^r^. D'Ailly had arrived at this figure by assuming that the great conjunction 2,240 years after creation had preceded the Flood by two years. On d'Ailly's calculations, see Smoller, *History, Prophecy, and the Stars*, pp. 65–67.

31 Grünpeck, *Ein hübscher Tractat*, sign. B3^r^; Grünpeck, *Tractatus*, sign. B1^v^–B2^r^.

disasters, plagues, and the downfall of kingdoms rang hollow, as he was unable to point to any such correlations.[33] Once again undaunted by this hurdle, he simply shifted the burden of proof from the *conjunctiones maximae* to the more frequent *conjunctiones magnae* and *conjunctiones majores*:

> Although the general changes and the great miracles always come during the *conjunctiones maximae*, and have always done so, as one finds in all histories filling the chronicles that have been written from beginning of the world up to this time, still stranger things have always happened during the times of *conjunctiones magnae* of the two planets Saturn and Jupiter.[34]

This argument was essential for he wanted to trace the advent of the French Disease to the most recent Saturn-Jupiter conjunction, a *conjunctio major* that had occurred in the evening of 25 November 1484.

This was a clear attempt to overcome the difficulty posed by the more than seven centuries between the last *conjunctio maxima* and the advent of the pox. However, even the most recent *conjunctio major* had occurred ten years prior to the initial outbreak of the pox, and as Grünpeck had reminded his reader, *conjunctiones majores* portended changes in kingdoms and increased power and riches for the nobles. This left him wanting a convenient explanation for natural disasters and the advent of plagues, preferably one that would help him bridge the ten-year gap. For this he relied on two further forms of astrological causation. First, Saturn-Mars conjunctions, which occurred every 30 years, signaled both famine and war.[35] Finally, again borrowing from Albumasar, Grünpeck pointed to the theory of ten revolutions of Saturn. Together, these different types of celestial causation all played a role in Grünpeck's account of the advent and spread of the pox, an account that was much more sophisticated and nuanced than those that simply referred to the theory of great conjunctions.[36]

32Again, he borrowed this list from d'Ailly. Owing to the errors he imported from d'Ailly in his *thema mundi*, Grünpeck could not have calculated these values.

33Grünpeck, *Ein hübscher Tractat*, sign. B5ᵛ–B6ʳ; Grünpeck, *Tractatus*, sign. B3ʳ.

34'Nach dem aber die gemein veränderung unnd grosse wunderwerck kommen allzeyte zü den größten züsamenfügungen. unnd allzey geschehen sind als man in alen hystorien fynndet Auch alle bücher erfüllet sint die man vomm anfang der welt biß auff dise zeyt von den geschehnenn dingen geschriben hat. Sind allweg wunderlichere ding geschehen zu den zeyten der grossen züsamenfuugung der zweyer Planeten Saturni und des Jupiter.' Grünpeck, *Ein hübscher Tractat*, sign. B4ʳ.

35Grünpeck, *Ein hübscher Tractat*, sign. B7ʳ.

36Many of Grünpeck's contemporaries simply glossed over the ten-year gap between the last greater conjunction and the advent of the pox and made little attempt to account

The bulk of Grünpeck's work was consumed in laying out his theory; proving its validity required only that Grünpeck fill in the historical events, which he did in meticulous detail on a single page. The primary cause of the French Disease was a series of planetary conjunctions. The first of these was the *conjunctio major* at 6:04 PM on 25 November 1484, when Saturn and Jupiter had met at 23°43' of Scorpio, a sign ruled by Mars. The solar eclipse that followed on 25 March 1485 was the second conjunction, whose effects were made worse by its proximity to the *conjunctio major.* Finally, Saturn and Mars came together at 9° of Scorpio on 30 November 1485. Like the eclipse, this conjunction was under the malevolent influence of the preceding *conjunctio major.*[37] These phenomena had a cumulative effect and indicated a period of increasingly dire catastrophes, including plagues, famines, war, and natural disasters. Grünpeck reminds his reader that this is exactly what had come to pass: Germany had been suffering from droughts and famines since the middle of the previous decade; war between the Empire and Charles VIII of France was raging in Italy; the plague had become endemic in many southern German cities, breaking out each summer; and a number of earthquakes had occurred in the early 1490s. Worst of all, 'in addition to all this there came the cruel and unheard of and unseen sickness, the French Disease, which also the aforementioned conjunction has brought here from France into Italy, and after that into Germany.'[38] On this account, the pox was the culmination of dire consequences springing from the series of conjunctions in the mid-1480s.

Grünpeck still had to confront the decade-long gap between this series of conjunctions and the advent of the pox. He recognized that this was the weakest part of his argument and attempted to reinforce it at every turn. At this point, he introduced the ten revolutions of Saturn precisely to address the gap between the conjunctions and the advent of the pox. Like the theory of great conjunctions, the ten revolutions of Saturn was an Arab contribution to Western astrology. According to this theory, every tenth revolution of Saturn was correlated to significant changes on earth, including the advent of pestilences and death.[39] This gave a period of roughly 300 years and

---

for the spread and symptoms of the disease. See, for example, the works in Fuchs, *Die ältesten Schriftsteller*, and Sudhoff, *Zehn Syphilis-Drucke*.

37 Grünpeck, *Ein hübscher Tractat*, sign. B8^{r}; Grünpeck, *Tractatus*, sign. C2^{r-v}.

38 'über die all ist kommen dise grausame unerhörte und ungesehne kranckeyt. das böß Franzos. Das auch dise vorgemeldte Coniunction hat hieher gefügt von den Franzosen in Wälhischeland. darnach in teütsche.' Grünpeck, *Ein hübscher Tractat*, sign. B8^{v}.

39 'Es sind auch über das mer zehen umbleüffe Saturni Von wölchen do sagt Albumasar. die all haben gar ein grosse bedütnuß in der verwandlung der reych und der gesez. auch anderer grossenwürkung nach der lere der grossen Sternseher wölchen dingen

another way of dividing history. In his most detailed list yet, which he again lifted from d'Ailly, Grünpeck correlated every tenth revolution of Saturn with some important historical event from the time of Alexander the Great to the most recent in 1489.[40] This last one was followed by

> numerous great evils, at first the great famine, which lasted for a full seven years and has not finished yet. After that the cruel pestilence, which also still rages, and the great war with the King of France. Beyond these ills, there now comes the fearfully cruel sickness, and the aforementioned French Disease.[41]

Introducing the influence of the ten revolutions of Saturn helped Grünpeck attribute the advent of the pox to a more recent celestial phenomenon and account for at least part of the ten-year gap. Moreover, it allowed him to draw direct connections between celestial phenomena and plagues.

The spread of the disease was easier to explain. Here, Grünpeck relied on the primary qualities of the planets and zodiacal signs, and the belief that these planets and signs affected the people who shared those characteristics. Jupiter, normally a beneficial planet, was a hot and moist planet and ruled over France. However, in the 1484 conjunction, Jupiter's influence had been negated by two facts. First, the malevolent Saturn had suppressed Jupiter in the conjunction, and second, Mars, the other malevolent planet, had been Lord of the conjunction. Here Grünpeck's politics begin to appear. Just as Jupiter, France's ruling planet, had been overcome by the other planets during this conjunction, so too were the French the first to be oppressed by the pox, for their normally fit complexion had a natural abundance of blood, moisture, and saturation, all of which were prone to rotting.[42] In a thinly veiled political statement, Grünpeck implied that the Italians were no better than the French and thus were particularly susceptible to the French Disease, a conclusion he arrived at by pointing to the similar odour that accompanied both the pox and the Italians. Finally, he treats rather summarily the pox's spread into the Germanies and England. Mars's role in the conjunction, along with its

---

auch nachvolgen pestilenz. sterben und ander groß krankkeyt.' Grünpeck, *Ein hübscher Tractat*, sign. $B7^{r-v}$.

[40]On d'Ailly, see Smoller, *History, Prophecy, and the Stars*, pp. 68–69.

[41]'... die grossen übel. amm ersten des groẞs hunger. der wol siben jar geweret hat und noch kein ennde hat. Darnach die grawẞam pestilenz. die auch noch regiret. Und der groß kryeg mit dem künige auß Franckreych. über die übel alle kommet nun die erschrockenlich grawẞam krankeyt das vorgemelt böß Franzos.' Grünpeck, *Ein hübscher Tractat*, sign. $C2^{v}$.

[42]Grünpeck, *Ein hübscher Tractat*, sign. $B8^{v}$; Grünpeck, *Tractatus*, sign. $C2^{v}$.

influence over the similarly warlike and fierce Germans, explained the spread of the pox into the empire.[43]

The last piece of Grünpeck's explanation, which cemented its validity, was its account of the pox's symptoms. Like all writers of the period, Grünpeck had to address the question: why did the pox strike the genitals?[44] Once again he turned to astrology. The latest *conjunctio major* had occurred in Scorpio, which in accepted medical theory ruled the sexual organs. Consequently, this conjunction portended some horrible disease afflicting the genitals. Scorpio was also the house of the malevolent Mars, indicating that this affliction would be particularly severe. Grünpeck could, however, make his explanation more specific than this. Nobody doubted that the French Disease resulted from an excess of the two humours melancholy and cholera, as confirmed by the disease's symptoms: black, oozing sores that produced a rancid stench; fevers and burning in the limbs and joints.[45] According to Galenic medicine, Saturn influenced the production and expulsion of melancholy, while Mars exercised similar control over cholera. This relationship was essential to Grünpeck's explanation. Drawing on both the *conjunctio major* and, more importantly, the subsequent conjunction of Saturn and Mars, Grünpeck pointed out how the main symptoms of the pox were derived from these two planets. To explain the final characteristic symptom of the French Disease, the concentration of the black pustules on and around the genitals, Grünpeck needed only to point to the fact that all the conjunctions had occurred in the sign of Scorpio. Nature, he claimed, tries to relieve the excess of melancholy and cholera by expelling them where there is a concentration of veins, heat, and moisture, that is, the genital area, which Scorpio ruled.[46]

Although Grünpeck saw the French Disease as a new, unique, and historically significant disease, he offered little in the way of novel advice for its treatment or prevention. When Grünpeck offered his reader advice on how to avoid contracting the French Disease, he actually relied on quite standard precautions proffered for every plague. Despite his laments that standard medicine had trouble explaining the pox – making necessary his erudite astrological theorizing – he readily fell back on highly traditional

43The last planet to play a significant role in the conjunction had been Saturn, which ruled over England. This accounted for the disease's subsequent spread into that country. Grünpeck, *Ein hübscher Tractat*, sign. $C1^{r-v}$; Grünpeck, *Tractatus*, sign. $C3^{r-v}$.

44See Jon Arrizabalaga's contribution to this volume for fuller discussion of this question.

45On humours in treating diseases, see Siraisi, *Medieval and Early Renaissance Medicine*, pp. 115–152.

46Grünpeck, *Ein hübscher Tractat*, sign. $B8^{v}$–$C1^{v}$; Grünpeck, *Tractatus*, sign. $C2^{v}$–$C3^{r}$.

advice, which he copied from the popular plague tractates that served as models for his entire text. The best way to avoid the pox was flight combined with proper dietary practices and a cheerful disposition, for depression fosters sickness. Astrology was curiously absent. There was, however, one piece of advice specific to the French Disease. Grünpeck suggested that 'one should keep away from women, because this sickness is aroused by that.'[47] Although Grünpeck seemed to link sexual activity with contracting the pox, it is not clear that he understood sexual contact as the mechanism for catching the disease. Rather, he thought sexual arousal would increase a person's chances of falling ill. Moreover, he assumed a male patient and placed women in the role of infecting agent. This assumption informed the title-page illustration, which depicts a group of infected women and the male corpse of their most recent victim. This dynamic, which colours much medical writing on the disease for centuries to come, can be detected in the earliest recorded responses. Grünpeck's advice, with its moralizing overtones, fit neatly with Maximilian's intent in his 'Blasphemy Edict.'

The French Disease as Political Tool

Grünpeck's *Tractatus de pestilentiali scorra* and his *Ein hübscher Tractat* were more than just his attempt to account for the French Disease. They shared a basic astrological framework and capitalized on the fact that the French Disease was a serious social problem. Further, they both borrowed extensively from the popular plague tractates and thus reflect common late fifteenth-century practices. Yet in their presentation, scope, and reliance on textual authorities these two works show important differences beyond the linguistic one, differences which reveal the contours of Grünpeck's various goals and expectations.

His Latin *Tractatus de pestilentiali scorra* was obviously beyond the reach of the vast majority of people. Indeed, Grünpeck used this tract as an opportunity to display his erudition to a very select audience, one centred on the imperial court. The first hint of this comes in the dedicatory letter written to Grünpeck's long-time friend Bernard von Waldkirch. By late 1496, Waldkirch had become a familiar figure amongst Maximilian's courtiers and had recently been appointed canon of the Augsburg cathedral. Waldkirch had facilitated Grünpeck's entrance into Conrad Celtis's Danubian Literary Sodality and was certainly an important friend.[48] He now hoped that Waldkirch

---

[47]Grünpeck, *Ein hübscher Tractat*, sign. $C4^v$.

[48]Shortly before Grünpeck dedicated his *Tractatus* to Waldkirch, the two of them

could help him move into imperial service. This was, however, just Grünpeck's opening salvo. Taking advantage of a fortuitous conjunction of events – Maximilian's recent 'Blasphemy Edict,' Grünpeck's own experience with the pox in Italy, and his recent contact with the court as it passed through Augsburg – Grünpeck hoped to secure a lucrative position, preferably one at the imperial court. He recognized that to accomplish this he would have to demonstrate his erudition and eloquence, and display talents that the emperor valued. Laden with classical allusions and learned digressions, his *Tractatus de pestilentiali* was intended to accomplish these goals. At the same time, Grünpeck argued openly that his talents would be a service to any court.

In the late 1480s and early 1490s, the University of Ingolstadt became a centre for humanist education and learning. This thrust was centred around Conrad Celtis and his efforts to improve the educational standards at the university by introducing humanist scholarly techniques and to establish the first of his many sodalities.[49] These efforts were instrumental in Celtis's efforts to gain imperial favour, which led to his crowning as *poeta laureatus* in 1487. It is no surprise then, to see Grünpeck larding his text with classical allusions and indications of his own humanist talents. Xenophilus, the long-lived musician, and the Praenestine oracles along with Egyptian sages, Greek gods, and the Roman author Valerius Maximus all play important supporting roles in Grünpeck's work, alongside more typical sources such as the Bible, Aristotle, Galen, and Ptolemy.[50] Grünpeck mixes

---

wrote a letter to Celtis, expressing pleasure at his recovering health and claiming that it was thanks to Jupiter that the recent bad weather had abated. See Celtis, *Der Briefwechsel des Konrad Celtis*, pp. 224–225.

[49]For the introduction of humanist studies to Ingolstadt, see the now dated but still useful Bauch, *Die Anfänge des Humanismus in Ingolstadt*. See also Schöner, *Mathematik und Astronomie an der Universität Ingolstadt im 15. und 16. Jahrhundert*. On Celtis in general, see Spitz, *Conrad Celtis*.

[50]Xenophilus enjoyed considerable fame in the Renaissance, probably due to Pliny the Elder's claim that he lived 105 years without ever being sick. Indeed, Grünpeck quotes Pliny in his reference to Xenophilus: 'Xenophilius Musicum centum et quinque annis sine ullo corporis incomodo vixisse.' Cf. C. Pliny, *Naturalis historia*, VII, 50. The most famous use of Xenophilus is probably Montaigne's essay, 'Que philosopher, c'est apprendre à mourir,' where he makes the same claim. In Grünpeck's Latin texts the Praenestine oracles are referred to as the 'praenestine sorores,' surely an error either on his part or that of the printer for *sortes Praenstinae*, which Roman emperors and foreign potentates consulted. Grünpeck surely knew of these through Virgil's *Aeneid*, VII, 678, and perhaps Valerius Flaccus, who reportedly came from there. Once again, Grünpeck is quoting from a classical source when he mentions Valerius: '...testis est Valerius, qui nullam ait esse tantam felicitatem que malignitatis dentes vitare possit.' Compare with Valerius Maximus' *Factorum et dictorum memorabilium*, IV, 7, ext. 2.

classical allegory with astrology, humoural medicine, and physiology without distinction. Indeed, his primary insight into the causes of the French Disease came in an allegorical dream:

> On the thirteenth of last November, I was trying to hurry across an Egyptian stream that springs, so they say, from the centre of the philosopher's fountain. I was persistently running back and forth consulting with and intently asking not only philosophers and physicians but also other learned persons, all the while contemplating what this disease might be, this disease that now so miserably assails, torments, irritates, and scorches human bodies and afflicts them with itching. Due to my extreme efforts, which caused me to sweat profusely, I was overwhelmed by a deep sleep. However, when everyone confessed to be ignorant of the origin of this disease, I immediately decided to go to the schools of the Egyptians. When I had feasted my eyes on the pellucid waters of that most lovely river and was gazing at the older men refreshing themselves there, who likewise looked back at me in the most encouraging way, I decided to sit down and conversed with them. I was eager to know what sorts of people they might be. Then one of them whispered in my right ear that Hippocrates, Galen, Avicenna, Plato, Aristotle, Ptolemy – and he listed innumerable other astrologers – were discussing their opinions about terrestrial and celestial matters. A few were discussing among other things the cause of this French Disease. Some claimed it was the plant of the night, others the mentagra, others still a species of leprosy, and they cured it with the remedies by which these other diseases are healed. ... When at last, as happens with impetuous youth, always eager for distinction, I found myself compelled to say and prove by various arguments that this conjunction of planets that occurred a few years ago was definitely the cause of this disease. Everybody agreed with this. But now they had to leave. They said that they had been sent by immortal Jove from the underworld to this little stream only to do good for mankind. In a sealed letter they gave me the results of their supreme assembly so that I would publish them throughout the world. They then vanished with a sigh, and I, as if in a dream, returned to town and composed what follows on this disease of the French.[51]

---

[51] 'Proximis idibus Novembris Egyptiacum quendam rivulum, scaturientem e medio, ut aiunt, philosophorum fonte celeri cursu traijcere conabar. Nam et assidue cursitando cum phylosophos atque medicos, tum omnes etiam sapientes, consulendo. Sedulo inquirendo intentissimeque cogitando, quidnam id mali esst. Quod tam misere premit urget, inflammat, torquet, prurit, incalescitque mortalium corpora. Sudorifero nimio labores, usque sopore profligatus fueram. Quum autem unusquique se illius rei originem ignorare fateretur, illico statui Egypciorum gymnaisia adire. Cumque pavissem oculos in cristallina illius fluvij amenissimi unda, intuererque maiores natu viros illic sese recreantes,

Modeling himself after Celtis, Grünpeck hoped that his combination of disciplines and eloquence would appeal to Maximilian.

Fearing that he had been too subtle, Grünpeck made his desire for a position at court more explicit at other places in his *Tractatus de pestilentiali*. Although he was quick to point out that he had not wasted his 'youth in sluggishness and stupid luxury without useful study,' he was nevertheless hesitant to put pen to paper, fearing that he would be harshly judged.[52] He marshaled the courage to publish only after suggesting that he would be the harshest critic of his own work. He compared himself to the most eminent authors, who had been ridiculed by the ignorant masses, and implied that whatever criticisms his work may evoke, he still deserved a place amongst 'the most distinguished men, endowed with the highest learning, virtue, and wisdom.'[53] At the end of his work, Grünpeck again praised his own work by placing it in the company of some of the greatest works of antiquity.

> In my meagre judgment, admittedly that of a novice, you have before you, Bernard of Waldkirch, a useful little work written on 5 November, which seems to explain the cause of this sickness that assails us now. ... If however, it is not expounded with the skill of a master, in the manner of the Minerva of Phidias or the Venus of Apelles, nevertheless it will be a useful gift from a friend to you. For I do not ask that you place it in a golden chest, nor prize and value it as much as Ptolemy Philadelphus did his library, replete with every sort of book, nor hold it in such honour as

---

qui rursum amicabilissimos vultus in me conijcerent, consedi, confabulavique. Avidus vero sciendi quos se gererent, tum unus qui aderat dexteram in aurem mihi susurrebat, Eosdem esse Hyppocratem Galienum Avicennam Platonem Aristotlem Ptolomeum. Aliosque ferme innumeros astrologos recensebat, qui dererum naturalium celestiumque contemplatone dissererent. Inter cetera quidam huius mali de Franzos causam discutere elaborabant asserentes id esse plantam noctis. Alij mentagoram. Alij lepre speciem, eisdem quibus hee egritudines sanantur, remedijs mederi. ... Unde quum postremo, ut mos est ferventis novitatumque avide adolescentie, verba premere propria nequirem, in eum prorupi planetarum coitum, qui paucis exactis annis fulxit, eundem esse huius morbi proprijssimam causam varijs argumentatoniubs ostendens, a singular mihi assensum fuit., interim abire coacti sunt. Nanque ses ab inferis ab immortali Jove, in fluuiolum hunc missos fuisse, ad hominum falutem fatebantur ea qui summo consilio conclusissent. Obsignata charta mihi dradidere, quo per orbem terrarum disseminarm. Sic e conspectu meo evanuerunt magno edito gemitu. Ego veluti stupefactus in urbem redij, hancque subiunxi huius mali de Franzos causam que sequitur.' Grünpeck, *Tractatus*, sign. B4^{v}–C1^{v}.

52'adolescentiam ignavia luxuque inerti sine bonis leteris traduxisse.' Grünpeck, *Tractatus*, sign. C2^{r}.

53'cum dignissimi viri, omni virtute, sapientia atque doctrina praediti,' Grünpeck, *Tractatus*, sign. C2^{r}.

> Darius did the books of Homer, which he kept in a chest with the spoils of war; this was adorned with gold, gems, and pearls, and he ordered that it protect Homer's poems. Nor will I prevent you from throwing it into the flames after you have read it, since it is not one of Virgil's works, which despite the poet's protests, the deified Augustus forbade burning.[54]

Grünpeck clearly esteemed his *Tractatus de pestilentiali* rather highly, and the implication was obvious: Grünpeck and his texts were worthy of the highest accolades.

Grünpeck's title-page woodcut further supported his attempts to flatter the emperor and secure a position at his court. The woodcut shows the baby Jesus sitting on the Virgin's lap and healing a pair of infected but suppliant women. The corpse of an infected man, one who presumably did not observe the appropriate degree of piety, lies in the foreground. Maximilian kneels to the Virgin's right, where he is receiving the imperial crown from her. This woodcut served Grünpeck's goals in two ways. First, in the manner of Maximilian's 'Blasphemy Edict,' it suggested that even those afflicted with the French Disease could be cured through proper religious devotion. Second, Maximilian is depicted as the divinely chosen emperor, pure in his devotion and thus in his right to lead the Holy Roman Empire. Grünpeck was not alone in his belief that Maximilian occupied a special place, nor was this the only place that he expressed this conviction.[55] In his 'Prognosticon für 1496–1499,' which he dedicated to Hans Langenmantel, the Burgermeister of Augsburg, Grünpeck claimed that it was through the emperor that Jesus would bring peace to the empire.[56] Furthermore, although the imperial armies

[54]'Habes, Bernard de Waltkirch meo iuditio licet minus gravi sed simpllici sinceroque et hominis, at ita dicam, tyronis opusculum utile lucubratum proximis Nonis Novembribus, quod causam huius elluviunois que iam ingruit explicare videtur. ... Si tamen non est elaboratum subtili artificio, quemadmodum minerva phidie, seu Venus appellis, tamen gratum tibi erit amici munus. Nam non postulo ut in archam auream reponas, et tanti facias quani Ptolomeus philadelphus bibliothecam suam omnis generis librorum refertissimam estimavit. Neque ut tanto in hornore reservandum putes, quanto Darius libros Homeri retinendos duxit cum scrinio capto inter spolia quoad erat auro gemmisque ac margaritis praeciosum custodie voluminum homeri dare praecipit. Neque inhibeo posteaquam sedulo perlegeris ut igni non credes, quam non sunt Virgilij Codices quos divus Augustus contra voluntatem eius cremari vetuit.' Grünpeck, *Tractatus*, sign. C_4^v.

[55]Following Frederick III's death, Maximilian became the object of much prophetic literature produced in the Germanies. Johannes Lichtenberger's work enjoyed the widest popularity but was just part of a larger tradition that existed in both manuscript and print.

[56]'Wann unser herr Ihesus xpus do er eingieng in die welt do hat er geeret das römisch reych zü den zeiten seiner zükunfft, Wann durch den keyser Augustus er fridsam machet, die welt do mit in seiner heiligen gegenwürtigkait frid wär.' Joseph Grünpeck, 'Prognosticon für 1496–1499,' Bayerische Staatsbibliothek, Cgm 3042, f. 9^r.

were presently embroiled in wars with the French and plagues were raging in many southern German cities, Grünpeck was convinced that the situation would improve dramatically after Maximilian's fortieth birthday in 1499.[57]

Emperor Maximilian I certainly appreciated Grünpeck's efforts. The emperor was constantly beset with domestic unrest and foreign struggles that threatened his authority and claim to the title of emperor. His successes at the imperial Diet in Worms in 1495 had, by early 1496, largely evaporated as the princes and electors co-opted his political and financial reforms. Moreover, Maximilian was still bogged down fighting the French in Italy, a struggle precipitated by the duplicity of Pope Alexander VI. Although the pope had recently renewed his alliance with the emperor, Maximilian was constantly wary of the pope, who had notoriously switched allegiance between the French and the empire. In Grünpeck's opinion, which he shared with many of his German contemporaries, Alexander VI was in part responsible for the advent of the French Disease and its subsequent spread up the peninsula and over the Alps.[58] In this context, Grünpeck's derogatory comments about the French and the stinking Italians must have resonated with the emperor and the population more broadly. Further, Maximilian would have been happy to appropriate Grünpeck's implication that the French and Italians are, in the end, going to be overwhelmed by the Germans, just as Jupiter had been subsumed under the power of Mars.

Grünpeck's vernacular treatise differed in some important aspects; nonetheless, it functioned in similar ways. He pruned *Ein hübscher Tractat* of all extraneous material, particularly the more learned allusions and discussions found in his Latin text. Consonant with his goals and the purpose of the text, this version is a much simpler handbook on the source and cause of the French Disease and conformed to the patterns and expectations of the late fifteenth-century vernacular plague tractates, which were responses to the recurring plague outbreaks and quickly adopted a common format and content.[59] When Grünpeck wrote his *Ein hübscher Tractat*, he simply adapted this literature to fit his immediate context.

An important aspect of most vernacular plague tractates was their connection to the local city councils or princes.[60] As the plague became

[57]Grünpeck, *Prognosticon sive (ut alij volunt) Judicium Ex Conjunctione Saturni & Jovis Decenalis et revolutione Saturni Ortu* (Vienna, 1496), n.p. Unfortunately, Grünpeck does not explain why he thought matters would improve.

[58]Grünpeck did not name the pope in his tracts on the French Disease. However, in his 1496 prognostication that he produced for the Burgermeister of Augsburg he identified the pope and his duplicity as largely responsible for the various plagues currently afflicting the Germanies. See Grünpeck, 'Prognostikon für 1496–1499,' fol. 4^{v}.

[59]On the plague tractates in general, see Campbell, *The Black Death*.

increasingly common, and as physicians continued to flee from infected areas along with everybody else who could, local authorities realized that they needed to do something to assuage the fears and concerns of many people who were forced to remain in the city and infected areas. Their attempts to compel physicians to stay, either through higher payments or threats of punishment, generally failed. They did succeed in persuading town physicians to write short, vernacular treatises on the origins, spread, and prevention of the disease. These sold for little money so that they could be widely available and would enable people to treat themselves during plague outbreaks. In this way, plague tractates were linked to the local political authorities and associated with a position as a town physician. Further, town councils and local princes used them to show the citizenry that they were concerned for the general welfare, turning plague tractates into political tools aimed at consoling the fears of the populace and thus quelling any unrest that might accompany plague outbreaks.

Grünpeck intended his *Ein hübscher Tractat* to function in the same way as the plague tractates. He offered his reader a description in simple German of the origins and causes of the French Disease. Moreover, he suggested a variety of precautions for avoiding the disease – these precautions were exactly those presented in the plague tractates. Grünpeck might have viewed this text as a secondary plan, should his attempt to find a position in the imperial bureaucracy fail. It served as a kind of application to the city fathers in Augsburg, advertising Grünpeck's ability to be town physician. Indeed, he seems to have anticipated a practice that became more common in the sixteenth century, when city councils retained physicians specifically to treat the French Disease.[61] It was certainly no accident that Grünpeck dedicated his German text to Hans Langenmantel, the Burgermeister of Augsburg. However, this text also supported Grünpeck's efforts to secure his ideal position. Emperor Maximilian I was constantly struggling to build cohesion and support amongst his German subjects. While Grünpeck's *Ein hübscher Tractat* lacked the eloquent digressions of his Latin *Tractatus*, it retained all the political, pro-imperial implications of that more elite text, including the disparaging references to the French and Italians, and the title-page woodcut showing Maximilian as saviour. In other words, Grünpeck's *Ein hübscher tractat* could function as a yet another tool in Maximilian's political agenda. It helped

---

[60]The most important of these plague tractates was Gentile da Foligno's *Concilia*. Indeed, Gentile's text gives its name to this entire genre of medical texts. See French, *Canonical Medicine*, pp. 274–296. See also Siraisi, *Medieval and Early Renaissance Medicine*, p. 148, and Giralt, 'The *Consilia* Attributed to Arnau de Vilanova.'

[61]French and Arrizabalaga, 'Coping with the French Disease,' p. 251.

to portray Maximilian as concerned for his subjects health and welfare. And unlike the plague tractates, which were at least initially grounded in particular locales, Grünpeck's *Ein hübscher Tractat* was simultaneously printed in Augsburg, Cologne, Leipzig, and Nürnberg, thereby spreading Grünpeck's pro-Habsburg message across much of southern Germany. It was, in this way, yet another piece of pro-imperial propaganda.

Conclusion

Grünpeck's attempts to secure a position at the imperial court were successful, due in no small part to his two works on the French Disease. Because the French Disease was a sensitive and important issue for Maximilian, Grünpeck seized on it to bring himself to the emperor's attention. Moreover, although Grünpeck explained the French Disease within an astrological framework, he interpreted the pox within the political and social terms that resonated with Maximilian's larger efforts to build cohesion and support for a pan-German ideal. The disease and Grünpeck's account of it, thus, became part of Maximilian's political propaganda. Shortly after Grünpeck's *Tractatus de pestilentiali* and *Ein hübscher Tractat* appeared he was invited to perform in front of the emperor and his family. A few months later, at the imperial Diet in 1497, he was crowned poet laureate. By the end of the Diet he had been appointed Maximilian's personal secretary and was working on the emperor's biography.

Unfortunately, Grünpeck's meteoric rise was cut short when he contracted the pox in 1501 after attending a dinner party hosted by his friend Celtis. Moments after leaving the city of Augsburg he was assailed by the pox's deadly arrows, which pierced his genitalia and caused them to ulcerate and swell so large that his two hands could scarcely conceal them. Terrified and despondent, Grünpeck skulked back home and remained isolated for some time. Although shame prompted him to suffer the disease in silence, when he returned to his duties and was again amongst his friends, his sickly pallor betrayed his condition and forced him to confess that he too had caught the French Disease. He was immediately ostracized from the court and even from his circle of closest friends while he struggled with the disease for the next two years.[62] He recounts in often gruesome detail his symptoms – for nearly four months a thousand abscesses appeared around his genitalia before spreading to other parts of his body – and the agonizing treatments he endured in the hopes of finding a cure. As he had in his earlier works, Grünpeck again dismissed learned medicine, which had been entirely

[62]Grünpeck, *Libellus*, sign. 7r.

ineffectual at reducing even the severity of the symptoms. Instead, he turned to empirics, quacks, and charlatans, before he stumbled upon a treatment that seemed to work.[63] In 1503, a healthy and slightly more humble Grünpeck published a short work, *Libellus de mentulagra alias morbo gallico*, in which he detailed his sufferings and eventual cure.

Although now himself a survivor of the pox, Grünpeck's understanding of the French Disease had changed little in the seven years since he first published his thoughts on the pox. In general, he still associated it with sexual activity – he tells us that not only Ceres and Bacchus but also Venus had attended Celtis's dinner party – and genitalia, where according to him the disease always appeared first and most virulently. He did not, however, understand sexual contact as a mechanism for catching the French Disease.[64] Except for his one brief comment about Venus, Grünpeck makes no further reference to women, sexual intercourse, or even loose sexual mores. Remarkably absent is any mention of sin, lust, or blasphemy, which had at least provided the context for his earlier *Tractatus de pestilentiali*. Perhaps sensing his own culpability and hoping to avoid the charge of hypocrisy, he eschewed all moralizing and concentrated instead on describing the disease and various remedies. He returned to his earlier conviction that the advent of the French Disease was caused by the planetary conjunctions in 1484. Indeed, he offers the same explanation in the opening pages of his *Libellus de mentulagra*, once again relying on the celestial influences, the association between Scorpio and the genitalia, and the affiliations between planetary qualities and human complexions to explain the appearance and spread of the pox as well as its symptoms.[65]

Throughout his *Libellus de mentulagra*, Grünpeck carefully separated his explanations of the French Disease's cause from his account of its treatment. Nowhere does he suggest that he used astrology in treating his disease. In fact, the cesspool emptiers, tailors, cobblers, rubbish collectors, and other quacks and empirics who lanced Grünpeck's tubercles, smeared him with stinking ointments and encouraged him to ingest bizarre pills and medicaments,

---

[63] Grünpeck, *Libellus*, sign. 12^{v}–14^{r}.

[64] 'Verumquidem cum paulopost Augustensis in oppido rogatu quorundam sodalium et commilitonum meorum quodam die convivium instituissem: cui non solum bachus et ceres sed etiam venus intererat: medie voluptati sese ingessit infensa humanarum pestium nutrix contagio innumera istius infectionis spicula gerents: cuius horrore territi relictis epulis omnes aufugimus: sed vix pedes extra portas Augustensis in agrum emovi: dum terrorem per frigida membra fusum aliarum rerum obiectis expellere elaborarem: infelix numen me a tergo ex improviso adortum gravissime sauciavit: quo vulnere totus infectus duobus fere annis a cesaris consuetudine:' Grünpeck, *Libellus*, sign. 2^{v}.

[65] Grünpeck, *Libellus*, sign. 2^{v}–3^{v}, 9^{r}–10^{r}.

probably knew little astrology and less learned medicine. Grünpeck turned to them out of desperation, hoping to find the cure that would allow him to return to his position at the court, a return that was made possible by Maximilian's increasingly ambivalent attitude toward the pox. Sometime between his 'Blasphemy Edict' in 1495 and the early sixteenth century, the emperor softened his stance on the French Disease. He ceased to condemn those suffering from it and instead demanded simply that they excuse themselves from the court until they were cured. This was, no doubt, a pragmatic decision – Grünpeck and Celtis are just two of the more famous courtiers within Maximilian's inner circles who suffered from the pox, and Maximilian himself reportedly contracted the disease a few years later.[66] Although Grünpeck certainly had not wished for the disease, he turned his experiences and frenetic search for a cure to his advantage. Having tried various available treatments without success, Grünpeck concluded on a positive note by offering the one remedy that seemed to work. Making this remedy available for other people, he claimed, had motivated him to publish his *Libellus de mentulagra*.[67] More importantly, he also used the opportunity to show publicly that he was now cured and was prepared to resume his duties as Maximilian's personal secretary.

For Grünpeck, the pro-imperial propagandist and avid courtier, astrology was not a tool of medicine, but rather a political and social tool. In his hands, it provided a means of explaining the advent, spread, and symptoms of the French Disease. Astrology also allowed him to capitalize on the emperor's larger political agenda. Grünpeck recast Maximilian's concerns about lust, loose sexual practices, and blasphemy in an astrological framework at precisely the right moment to ingratiate himself to emperor. Seven years later, after having endured and overcome the French Disease, Grünpeck still relied on astrology to describe it. This time, however, he shifted the astrology into the background in order to emphasize his experiences, treatment, and eventual cure that enabled him to return to the imperial court.

Haverford College
Haverford, Pennsylvania

[66] French and Arrizabalaga, 'Coping with the French Disease,' p. 257.
[67] Grünpeck, *Libellus*, sign. 3^v.

Cited Works

Manuscript Sources

Munich. Bayerische Staatsbibliothek Cgm. 3042, Joseph Grünpeck 'Prognostikon für 1496–1499.'

Published Sources

Albumasar. *Liber introductorii maioris ad scientiam judiciorum astrorum*, 9 vols. ed. Richard Lemay. Naples: Insituto Universitario Orientale, 1995.

Albumasar. *Abu Ma'Sar. The Abbreviation of the Introduction to Astrology. Together with the Medieval Latin Translation of Adelard of Bath*, ed. Charles Burnett, Keiji Yamamoto, and Michio Yano. Leiden: Brill, 1994.

Anonymous. *Opusculum divinarum revelationum sancti Methodij*. Basel: Michael Furter, 1498.

Arrizabalaga, Jon, John Henderson, and Roger French. *The Great Pox: The French Disease in Renaissance Europe*. New Haven: Yale University Press, 1997.

Bauch, Gustav. *Die Anfänge des Humanismus in Ingolstadt. Eine litterarische Studie zur deutschen Universitätsgeschichte*. Munich: R. Oldenbourg, 1901.

Campbell, Anna Montgomery. *The Black Death and Men of Learning*. New York: Columbia University Press, 1931.

Celtis, Conrad. *Der Briefwechsel des Konrad Celtis*, ed. Hans Rupprich. Munich: C. H. Beck'sche Verlagsbuchhandlung, 1934.

Cunningham, Andrew and Ole Peter Grell. *The Four Horsemen of the Apocalypse: Religion, War, Famine and Death in Reformation Europe*. Cambridge: Cambridge University Press, 2000.

Czerny, Albin. 'Der Humanist und Historiograph Kaiser Maximilians I. Joseph Grünpeck' *Archiv für österreichische Geschichte,* 73 (1888): 315–364.

Deutsche Reichstagsakten unter Maximilian I. Fünfter Band, Reichstag von Worms 1495. Vol. 1, pt. 1. ed. Heinz Angermeier, Göttingen: Vandenhoeck & Ruprecht, 1981.

Diederichs, Peter. *Kaiser Maximilian I. als politischer Publizist*. Jena: Eugen Diederichs Verlag, 1933.

Esser, Thilo. 'Die Pest—Strafe Gottes oder Naturphänomen? Eine frömmigkeitsgeschichtliche Untersuchung zu Pesttraktaten des 15. Jahrhunderts' *Zeitschrift für Kirchengeschichte,* 108 (1997): 32–57.

French, Roger. *Canonical Medicine: Gentile da Foglio and Scholasticism*. Leiden: Brill, 2001.

French, Roger and Jon Arrizabalaga. 'Coping with the French Disease: University Practitioners' Strategies and Tactics in the Transition from the Fifteenth to the Sixteenth Century' pp. 248–287 in *Medicine from the Black Death to the French Disease*, eds. Roger French, Jon Arrizabalaga, Andrew Cunningham, and Luis García Ballester. Aldershot: Ashgate, 1998.

Fuchs, C. H. *Die ältesten Schriftsteller über die Lustseuche in Deutschland, von 1495 bis 1510*. Göttingen: Verlag der Dieterichschen Buchhandlung, 1843.

Giralt, Sebatià. 'The *Consilia* Attributed to Arnau de Vilanova' *Early Science and Medicine,* 7 (2001): 311–356.

Gottlieb, Theodor. *Büchersammlung Kaiser Maximilians.* Amsterdam: G.T. van Heusden, 1968.

Grendler, Paul F. *The Universities of the Italian Renaissance.* Baltimore: The Johns Hopkins University Press, 2002.

Grünpeck, Joseph. *Ein hübscher Tractat von dem ursprung des bösen Franzos. das man nennet die Wylden wärzen. Auch ein Regiment wie man sich regiren soll in diser zeyt.* Ausgburg: Hans Schauer, 1496.

Grünpeck, Joseph. *Prognosticon sive (ut alij volunt) Judicium Ex Conjunctione Saturni & Jovis Decenalis et revolutione Saturni Ortu.* Vienna: Johannes Winterburg, 1496.

Grünpeck, Joseph. *Tractatus de pestilentiali Scorra sive mala de Franzos. Originem. Remediaque eiusdem continens.* Augsburg: Hans Schauer, 1496.

Grünpeck, Joseph. *Libellus de Mentulagra alias morbo gallico.* Memmingen: Albrecht Kunne, 1503.

Haustein, Hans. *Die Frühgeschichte der Syphilis, 1495–1498.* Vienna: [n.s.], 1930.

Lichtenberger, Johannes. *Prognosticatio Ioannis Liechtenbergers.* Heidelberg: H. Knoblochtzer, 1488.

Markowski, Mieczslaw. 'Die Astrologie an der Krakauer Universität in den Jahren 1450–1550' pp. 83–89 in *Magia, Astrologia e Religione nel Rinascimento: convegno polacco-italiano, Varsavia, 25–27 settembre 1972.* Wroclaw: Zaklad Narodowy im. Ossolinskich, 1974.

Maternus, Julius Firmicus. *Matheseos libri VIII.* Stuttgart: B.G. Teubner, 1968.

North, J. D. 'Astrology and the Fortune of Churches' *Centaurus,* 24 (1980): 181–211.

C. Pliny Secundi. *Naturalis historiae libri XXXVII.* Stuttgart: B.G. Teubner, 1967–70.

Reeves, Majorie Hope. *The Influence of Prophecy in the Later Middle Ages: A Study of Joachimism,* 2nd ed. Notre Dame, IN: University of Notre Dame Press, 1993.

Russell, Paul Albert. 'Syphilis, God's Scourge or Nature's Vengeance? The German Printed Response to a Public Problem in the Early Sixteenth Century' *Archiv für Reformationsgeschichte,* 80 (1989): 286–306.

Russell, Paul Albert. 'Astrology as Popular Propaganda: Expectations of the End in the German Pamphlets of Joseph Grünpeck († 1533?)' pp. 165–195 in *Forme e destinazione del messaggio religioso. Aspetti della propaganda religiosa nel cinquecento,* ed. Antonio Rotondò. Florence: Leo S. Olschki, 1991.

Siraisi, Nancy. *Medieval and Early Renaissance Medicine.* Chicago: University of Chicago Press, 1990.

Smoller, Laura Ackerman. *History, Prophecy and the Stars: The Christian Astrology of Pierre diAilly, 1350–1420.* Princeton, NJ: Princeton University Press, 1994.

Schöner, Christopher. *Mathematik und Astronomie an der Universität Ingolstadt im 15. und 16. Jahrhundert.* Berlin: Duncker & Humblot, 1994.

Spitz, Lewis. *Conrad Celtis: The German Arch-Humanist.* Cambridge, MA: Harvard University Press, 1957.

Tanner, Marie. *The Last Descendant of Aeneas: The Habsburgs and the Mythic Image of the Emperor.* New Haven: Yale University Press, 1993.

Valerius Maximus. *Factorum et dictorum memorabilium.* Stuttgart: B.G. Teubner, 1998.

Veenstra, Jan. *Magic and Divination at the Courts of Burgundy and France: Text and Context of Laurent Pignon's* Contre led divineurs *(1411).* Leiden: Brill, 1998.

Waas, Glenn Elwood. *The Legendary Character of Maximilian.* New York: Columbia University Press, 1941.
Wiesflecker, Hermann. *Kaiser Maximilian I. Das Reich, Österreich und Europa an der Wende zur Neuzeit.* Vol. 2. Vienna: Verlag für Geschichte und Politik, 1975.
Williams, Gerhild S. 'The Arthurian Model in Emperor Maximilian's Autobiographic Writings *Weisskunic* and *Theuerdank*' *Sixteenth Century Journal*, 11 (1980): 3–22.

Literary and Metaphoric Responses

(Po)X Marks the Spot: How to 'Read' 'Early Modern' 'Syphilis' in *The Three Ladies of London*

Jonathan Gil Harris

How do we 'read' 'early modern' 'syphilis'? I employ this somewhat clumsy sequence of quotes to put pressure on my question's literary verb, historical adjective, and pathological noun. Those parts of speech give some indication of the linked though potentially disparate scholarly disciplines – English, History, Medicine – that have greatly enriched recent understandings of venereal disease in sixteenth-century Europe. Yet there is much in this pox-pourri that invites more extensive theorization. In particular, I would argue that literary scholars might make a significant contribution to the dialogue by teasing out the textual dimensions of 'early modern syphilis': which is to say, by theorizing not just the relationship between syphilis and early modern texts, but also the diverse strategies of *reading* – symptomatic, metaphoric, historicist – that have conspired to generate such pre-textual effects as 'early modernity' and 'syphilis.'

In this essay, I question the persistent, if often unwitting tendency to locate early modern syphilis in any one of a variety of supposedly extra-textual spaces. These spaces have been customarily limned by means of what might be termed 'symptomatic reading,' a process that paradoxically requires texts to produce the effect of a reality resolutely prior to, and constitutive of, them. The early modern physician was trained to 'read' through a process of diagnostic translation the symptoms of pox writ large on the body's surface – skin lesions and chancres, genital suppuration, nasal decay, alopecia, madness, etc. – in order to acquire certainty about 'that within which passeth show.' Similarly, the medical historian now subjects early modern literary texts to symptomatic reading in order to arrive at otherwise elusive knowledge about the nature, incidence, and transmission of the disease in late fifteenth and sixteenth-century Europe. In the process, however, symptomatic readings of early modern syphilis reify their object. These readings assume that there *is* an entity outside the sphere of textuality or culture that we can safely know as 'syphilis.'[1] The term, devised by the Veronese physician Girolamo Fracastoro in 1530 but not in common usage till the eighteenth century, often tends to be regarded as less a coined name than a physical fact – a fact that is confidently posited as the extra-textual referent for a set of bodily and linguistic signs that date back to the last decade of the fifteenth century.[2]

My goal in this essay is not to suggest that there was no such thing as syphilis, however, but to underscore the primacy of its textuality. In doing so, I may seem to follow the lead of many literary and cultural historians, who have tended to focus less on syphilis as a specific pathological condition and more on the ways it was represented, particularly with respect to its implication within a widespread European discourse of cultural and national othering.[3] But such studies, invaluable as they have been, have often replicated the tendency to reify a knowable disease that precedes its diverse textual mediations. By contrast, Jon Arrizabalaga, John Henderson, and Roger French have argued that syphilis has no timeless essence, but is rather a changing object of discourse diversely constituted within different knowledge systems.[4] Following their lead, I shall insist that early modern syphilis, even in its most 'scientific' accounts, is a persistent effect of textuality. As Bruce Boehrer has noted, medical treatises of the period – including Fracastoro's poem – consistently construct the disease by means of 'elaborate fictional narrative.'[5] In its early modern literary and medical narrations alike, the disease is what I call a 'pathotext': an inscription rather than re-presentation of sickness that incarnates the Latin etymological root of 'text' – *texere*, to weave, twine together, or plait. Syphilis, I shall argue, is not a simple pathological fact outside of and prior to language (even if that is one of the

[1]See, for example, Fabricius, *Syphilis in Shakespeare's England*. In an intriguing if not entirely convincing analysis of what he terms Shakespeare's 'midlife crisis,' Fabricius examines the recurrent images of prostitution, infection and corruption in Shakespeare's so-called problem plays, and draws from these the conclusion that Shakespeare contracted syphilis in about 1601.

[2]See Fracastoro, *Syyphilis sive Morbus Gallicus*. According to the OED, the earliest recorded English usage of 'syphilis' dates to 1718.

[3]As Claude Quétel notes, 'Each newly affected country lost no time naming the disease after the neighbor which it suspected ... of having been the source of contamination.' *History of Syphilis*, p. 16. For more extensive discussions of the presumption that the disease always came from elsewhere, see Foa, 'The New and the Old,' Nelkin and Gilman, 'Placing the Blame for Devastating Disease,' and Arrizabalaga, Henderson, and French, *The Great Pox*. See also my *Foreign Bodies and the Body Politic*, especially chap. 3, and *Sick Economies*, especially chap. 2.

[4]Arrizabalaga, Henderson, and French, *The Great Pox*, chap. 1.

[5]Boehrer, 'Early Modern Syphilis,' p. 206.

principal effects produced by the language used to speak about it), but a textual palimpsest that splices together many strands of discourse – strands that include not only the physiological and the pathological, but also the religious and the economic.

To the extent that syphilis might be read as a pathotext, however, I shall also argue that, as such, it represents less a synchronic cultural moment or historical period than an anachronistic yoking of different temporalities. Much scholarship on syphilis has tended to reify historical period as well as disease, viewing sixteenth-century attitudes to the pox as univocally representative of a larger 'early modernity.' The customary view is that, medically, socially, or culturally, syphilis embodies something unmistakably new. Because syphilis has been conventionally narrated as first appearing in the aftermath of the momentous year of 1492, the disease has even become a metonymy for the European 'discovery' of a New World, and hence for a new epoch of global modernity separated irrevocably from the more insular medieval period that preceded it.[6] At the same time, medical historians have increasingly insisted on an impermeable historical divide between the sixteenth-century and the present, arguing that 'early modern' pox is an entirely different construct from 'modern' syphilis.[7] Yet once we start regarding pox or syphilis as a palimpsest, it becomes difficult to see either as representative of any one period. Palimpsests, after all, are not the product of a single moment; they are sites of diachronic textual production that cannot erase the traces of earlier inscriptions. My coinage, 'pathotext,' suggests not only the textuality of pathology, but also the diachronic and even anachronistic dimension of the palimpsest, deriving as it does from

---

[6]In making such connections, scholars of early modern syphilis have followed Fracastoro, who in his poem *Syphilis* suggests that the disease 'from the Western Climes 'twas wafted o'er,/ When daring Spaniards left their Native shore' (I, 34–35). But there is also a widespread tendency to identify syphilis with 'newness' in a variety of other forms. Karl Sudhoff, for example, associates knowledge of syphilis with the rise of new print technologies that are themselves metonymies for modernity: 'the newly recognized scourge of humanity … illustrate[s] too how the new art of reduplication – for which the world was indebted to Coster and to Gutenberg – had become an instrument for the advancement of knowledge.' *Earliest Printed Literature on Syphilis*, p. x. For a discussion of the antinomies of 'new' and 'old' in writing about syphilis, see Foa, 'The New and the Old.'

[7]See Arrizabalaga, Henderson, and French, *The Great Pox*. The authors follow Andrew Cunningham in asserting that the history of diseases prior to their definition in the modern laboratory is wholly inaccessible. To avoid the pitfalls of anachronism, the name 'syphilis' – which was not favoured until the eighteenth century – is omitted from the book's title. As much as I admire this argument, and have been greatly influenced by it, I am drawn to the anachronism of 'syphilis' if only because, as I shall argue, there is something anachronistic about *any* textual production of disease.

the Latin 'textum' and the earlier Greek 'pathos.' In the pathotext of early modern syphilis, I shall argue, we can see the palimpsested traces of not only multiple discourses, but also multiple historical moments.

To understand syphilis as a palimpsest, moreover, is also to embrace a different mode of reading disease – one that proceeds less through the diagnostic translation of various symptoms into a reified, extra-textual thing (be it a disease or a historical period), than from the recognition that history lies not *outside* the pathotext as a knowable synchronic moment, but *inside* it as a diachronic assemblage of competing forms. If the first mode of reading is 'symptomatic,' the second might be labeled 'formalist' – though not in the traditional, ahistorical sense of that term. Noting the propensity of literature to resist any univocal reflection of the material circumstances of its production, Fredric Jameson writes how 'form, secreted like a shell or exoskeleton, continues to emit its ideological message long after the extinction of its host.'[8] With this assessment, Jameson introduces a diachronic, historical dimension to his theorization of literary form. Just as importantly, his pathological metaphor offers the scholar of early modern syphilis a highly suggestive hermeneutic with which to begin theorizing how we read sixteenth-century pathotexts. If what we have come to call 'early modern syphilis' is a textual organism comprising many such historical exoskeletons, I shall argue that each exoskeleton makes itself legible through a mode of reading distinctive to it: medical, metaphoric, or historicist. Despite their apparent differences, the three modes each ground meaning in a space supposedly external to textuality, whether corporeal, spiritual, or epochal, and to that extent can be seen as a logocentric process of translation for which symptomatic reading provides the template. A historical formalist reading, by contrast, attends to the intra-textual relations between the pathotext's layers and the modes by which we read them. Far from entailing period-specific cultural redactions of a knowable disease, then, literary treatments of the pox can help the formalist reader illuminate the pathotextuality and diachronic historicity of 'early modern syphilis' in all its inscriptions.

The literary text in which I shall ground my argument is Robert Wilson's play, *The Three Ladies of London* (c. 1580). The latter is in no sense

---

[8]Jameson, *The Political Unconscious*, p. 151. It is worth noting that the well-known imperative with which Jameson commences his study, 'Always historicize!' (p. 1), has been repeatedly misunderstood by so-called historicists; the latter have tended to understand the project of 'historicizing' as a matter of simply reading a literary text in relation to synchronic historical co-texts external to it rather than recognizing the diachronic, and often anachronistic, competing forms *within* it.

a work about syphilis; it does not dramatize a case of syphilis; and it does not even make a single explicit reference to syphilis or its synonyms. But the play does offer an excellent case study of the kind of palimpsested pathotext that I have sketched above. In one significant episode, Wilson seems to literalize Jameson's metaphor of the exoskeleton, staging the production upon a body's exterior of an outer crust – or, in this case, a collection of 'spots' – that threatens the health and integrity of its host organism.[9] As I shall show, there are a number of ways to read these spots. Perhaps most strikingly, they seem to draw on early modern discourses of syphilitic infection. However, to read the spots simply as symptoms of early modern pox is to neglect their polyvalent signifying power. The spots participate just as much within putatively medieval literary traditions of representing the sinful soul and Elizabethan understandings of transnational commerce. As a consequence, the spots are pathotexts in which can be read not just the extra-textual 'facts' of syphilis or early modernity, but also multiple historical forms. The spots promise a veritable treasure of signification. But it might be fairer to say, adapting both the old saw of pirate literature and the indeterminate shorthand of algebra, that X Marks the Spot in *The Three Ladies of London*, inasmuch as the spots cannot be univocally reduced to any single referent. Perhaps paradoxically, it is in that very textual over-determinacy that 'early modern syphilis' is most visible – albeit as an anachronistic palimpsest rather than a positive fact.

SPOTTING SYPHILIS: MEDICAL READING AND THE CHRONOTOPE OF NATURAL HISTORY

The Three Ladies of London is, in many respects, a medieval morality play *après la lettre*. Written in the early 1580s, and thus possibly performed in London's new commercial playhouses, it nonetheless harks back to the allegorical frame of reference of earlier morality plays like *Everyman* by staging the triumph of the wicked Lady Lucre over the good Ladies Love and Conscience (the

---

[9]Wilson, *Three Ladies of London*, in Hazlitt, *A Select Collection of Old English Plays*, VI. p. 368. All further references are cited in the text. In early modern England, the lesions of the pox were often regarded as a crust or 'tetter'; see Dennie, *A History of Syphilis*, p. 36. One might compare the Ghost's account in *Hamlet* of how Claudius's poison coated his body with a 'tetter' or 'vile and loathsome crust' (1.5.69–70), which Fabricius diagnoses as syphilis, *Syphilis in Shakespeare's England*, p. 45. It cannot escape attention, though, that the Ghost twice connects his symptoms to leprosy: he refers to the 'leprous distilment' of Claudius's poison (1.5.62) and the 'lazar-like' quality of his 'crust' (1.5.70). This underlines the point I make in the essay – i.e. the extent to which 'syphilis' is a palimpsest in which multiple discourses, pathological and otherwise, are visible.

eponymous three figures of the play's title).[10] Lucre is aided and abetted by a gang of sinister characters, including Dissimulation and Usury. She and her henchmen successfully conspire to have Love married off to Dissimulation; the fate that she inflicts on Conscience, however, is more dramatically spectacular. Towards the end of the play, Lucre commands Usury to fetch the instrument with which she will inflict Conscience's ruination:

> ... Usury, step in,
> And bring me the box of all abhomination, that stands in the window:
> It is little and round, painted with divers colours, and is pretty to the show. (337)

An extraordinary scene is then enacted, as outlined in the stage directions. First Usury enters 'with a painted box of ink in his hand' (337); then the play-text directs the actors to 'let LUCRE open the box, and sip her finger in it, and spot CONSCIENCE's face' (338), after which Lucre announces ceremoniously: 'I have spotted Conscience with all abhomination' (339).

It is hard not to submit the 'spotting' of Conscience to the kind of symptomatic reading I outlined in the previous section. Despite the absence of any explicit reference to syphilis in this or any other episode, Conscience's spots invite identification with the disease. For one, her affliction is coded pathologically. When she is tried before the Judge at play's end for deceiving people under the 'colour' of her name, he associates her spots with epidemic contagion:

> Declare the cause, Conscience, at large how thou comest so spotted,
> Whereby many by thee hath been greatly infected ...
> Why wast thou then corrupted so, and spotted on thy face? (368)

Even without the Judge's pathological prompting, Conscience's spots invite identification with venereal disease, inasmuch as the most conventional sign of infection by the pox in late fifteenth- and early sixteenth-century print culture was the eruption of visible stains or spots upon the skin, especially the face.

This is particularly apparent in the earliest printed images of the French pox. In what may be the oldest surviving pictorial rendering of the disease, dating from approximately 1495, the German woodcarver Wolfgang Hamer depicts a group of men and women whose faces are covered with black spots or 'blattern' (blisters) kneeling before St. Minus, one of the patron saints of the so-called French Disease.[11] The 'blattern'

---

[10]For a useful discussion of the conditions of the first stage productions of Wilson's play, see Kermode, 'The Playwright's Prophecy.'

[11]The image is reproduced in Fabricius, *Syphilis in Shakespeare's England*, p. xv (fig. 2).

quickly became a conventional detail in early German images of the pox. In September of 1496, the satirist and professor of jurisprudence Sebastian Brant published a broadsheet in verse, *De Pestilentiali Scorra siue Mala de Franzos Eulogium*, which features a woodcut depicting the Virgin Mary with the baby Jesus in her left arm. From his hands pass rays that alight on one woman and three men who, in various poses of abjection or supplication, are covered with small black spots.[12] Two months later, the layman Joseph Grünpeck of Burckhausen published a commentary on Brant's poem in which he adapted the illustration to the latter.[13] Once again, the victims of what he calls the *mala de Franzos* are coated with black spots. But whereas Brant's woodcut had represented the rays emanating from the baby Jesus as the agents of infection, in Grünpeck's tract the illustration presents the rays as healing the black spots of those who pray to him. A spotty corpse, however, has not been so lucky, the implication being that those victims who fail to petition God for mercy will die. Such primarily religious images of the healing of the pox quickly became part of the medical canon as well. The frontispiece to a short tract published in 1498 by the Viennese physician Bartholomaeus Steber likewise depicts a scene of healing the 'morbus gallorum,' though in this case the treatment of a man and a woman – both of whom are coated with black spots – is undertaken by physicians with potions.[14] And the frontispiece to William Clowes's 1579 English treatise on the 'morbus gallicus,' which reproduces the coat of arms granted to the Company of Barber Surgeons in 1569, speckles the two hounds that hold up the heraldic shield with seemingly poxy spots.[15]

If spots are a common detail in early modern pictorial renderings of the illness, they feature less prominently in written narratives. The latter foreground, by contrast, symptoms that are not publicly visible, such as genital suppuration and bone decay.[16] Nevertheless, the term 'spots' appears in both specialist and lay descriptions of the pox. In his English translation of John de Vigo's medical writings, Robert Traheron speculates that Augustus Caesar had contracted a disease with an uncanny resemblance to

---

[12]The woodcut is reproduced by Sudhoff in *The Earliest Printed Literature on Syphilis*, p. xxiii (fig. 3), and in Fabricius, *Syphilis in Shakespeare's England*, p. 11 (fig. 7).

[13]Grünpeck, *Tractatus de pestilentiali scorra sive Mala de Franzos*, sign. a1.

[14]Steber of Vienna, *A malafranczos, morbo gallorum, praeservatio ac cura*, frontispiece.

[15]Clowes, *A Short and Profitable Treatise*, frontispiece. See also Fabricius, *Syphilis in Shakespeare's England*, p. 194.

[16]Indeed, 'bone ache' is often employed as a synonym for syphilis in early modern literary texts; see, for example, Shakespeare's *Troilus and Cressida*, 2.3.20 and 5.1.26. See also Lucio's quips about 'hollow bones' in *Measure for Measure*, 1.2.56.

the French pox, the chief symptom being that 'he had spots, dispersed upon the breast and belly.'[17] And a satirical poem called *The Hunting of the Pox* claims that 'The Scots ... when they have met, some part of this disease,/ They use in jest to say that they are bit with Spanish Fleas,/ Because they leave red spots behinde, as fleas used to doe.' [18] Indeed, early modern descriptions of the spots of pox – which medical writers also dubbed 'boils,' 'chancres,' 'knobs,' 'postumes,' 'pustules,' 'scabs,' 'scales,' and 'tetters' – present, in stark contrast to the monochromatic 'blattern' of the early German woodcuts, a rainbow of colourful hues. An English translation of Ulrich von Hutten's treatise on the French Disease, for example, asserts that the victims of the disease acquire acorn-like 'Boils' which, unlike the red spots of *The Hunting of the Pox*, are 'a dark Green.'[19] Conscience's spots in Wilson's play, derived as they are from a paint-box, may have been equally colourful.

A symptomatic medical reading of Conscience's spots might view them through the prism of modern pathology and its understanding of the natural history of syphilis. According to the latter, the symptoms of syphilis vary over the course of the disease's spread through the body, which is conventionally divided into three and sometimes four phases. In the primary phase, which spans the four weeks following infection by the parasitic spirochete *Treponema pallidum*, the victim develops a lesion at the inoculation site, usually in the region of the genitalia. In the secondary phase, four to ten weeks after infection, more lesions appear, most commonly in the flexar and volar body surfaces (the palms and soles). Though hyper-pigmentation, or darkening, of the lesions can occur, they are equally prone to hypo-pigmentation, or lightening. Papules frequently appear in the microcutaneous junctions and moist areas of the skin; these tend to be dull pink or grey hypertrophic lesions. In the tertiary and quaternary stages of the disease, to which only a minority of victims proceed, granulomas appear in the nose and eyes, and encephalitis is a liability. For the symptomatic reader of early modern writing about the pox, then, spots readily correspond to the hyper-pigmented lesions of syphilis. Similarly, a symptomatic reading of *The Three Ladies of London* might see Lady Conscience's painted spots, like the psychedelic boils and tetters of early modern medical literature, as a theatrical version of the multi-coloured flexar, volar and other cutaneous papules of secondary-stage syphilis.[20]

---

[17]Traheron, *Workes of Ioan de Vigo*, p. 254.

[18]J. T. of Westminster, sign. B1.

[19]Hutten, *A Treatise of the French Disease*, p. 3.

[20]What modern physicians might recognize as other symptoms of tertiary-stage syphilis – including loss of hair, decay of the nose, and madness – feature prominently

This medical mode of symptomatic reading diagnostically translates sixteenth-century literary spots into the afflictions of a universal, pre-textual syphilitic body. In doing so, it also presumes a distinctive conceptual organization of space and time or, to use Mikhail Bakhtin's term, 'chronotope.'[21] This particular chronotope informs what modern physicians call natural history – the medical narrative that explains the course of a disease. In early modern treatises on the pox, as much as modern natural histories of syphilis, space and time are dynamic, but in the domain of *physis* rather than of culture, society, or economy. Narrating the course of the *lues venerea*, for example, Clowes speaks of how 'any outward part being once infected, the disease immediately entreth into the blood, and so creepeth on like a canker from part to part, until it commeth to the liuer, where being once entred, it corrupteth the fountaine of the blood.'[22] As Clowes's narrative makes clear, the supposedly pre-textual space of disease is one that conforms to a 'first ... and then' temporality of causation: the pox enters the body and then slowly but lethally changes it. Although Clowes comes close to articulating a modern notion of disease as an invasive entity rather than a state of humoral imbalance, the chronotope of natural history that his narrative assumes reproduces the structuring principle of classical Hippocratic and Galenic pathology, according to which disease is not a static event, but a causal sequence of bodily developments.[23] A symptomatic reading that would seek to translate Conscience's marks into the lesions of 'secondary' syphilis thus renders her spots as the signs of but one 'stage' in a universal, medically predictable process that unfolds both prior and subsequent to the spots' appearance.

What this mode of reading cannot explain, however, is how the spots of early modern writing are laden with symbolic freight that exceeds the medical chronotope of natural history. Why are these spots repeatedly

---

in later literary fantasies of the pox, especially Shakespeare's. Shakespeare speaks of 'tetters' in *Hamlet* and *Troilus and Cressida*; but he is more inclined to joke anxiously about nasal decay – see, for example, the Clown's gags on whistling through the nose in *Othello*, 3.1.4 – or alopecia, as is shown by his many quips about bald French crowns (see *A Midsummer Night's Dream*, 1.2.37-8, or *Measure for Measure*, 1.2.28) and the extended discussion of hair in *The Comedy of Errors*, 2.2.61–84. For discussions of Shakespeare's use of syphilis imagery, see Bentley, *Shakespeare and the New Disease*, Fabricius, *Syphilis in Shakespeare's England*, and my *Sick Economies*, chaps. 2 and 4.

21 Bakhtin, *The Dialogic Imagination*, passim.

22 Clowes, *Briefe and Necessary Treatise*, p. 153.

23 For the emergence of new conceptions of disease as an invasive thing rather than a humoral state, see Nutton, 'The Seeds of Disease.' See also my *Foreign Bodies and the Body Politic*, passim, and *Sick Economies*, chap. 1.

presented as uniformly dark, or luridly colourful, when the modern narratives of pathological medicine insist that the lesions of syphilis are equally prone to hypo-pigmentation? Why are spots early sixteenth-century visual culture's favoured metonymy for infection by the pox, when there are so many other visible symptoms that could have been made representative of the disease, and indeed later *did* become representative (e.g. alopecia, nose decay and madness)? And why, indeed, were they even called 'spots'? I would argue that the recurrence of spots – both symptom and term – in early modern narratives of the pox has less to do with the physiological 'facts' of syphilis, than with the persistence of another textual tradition that dates back to Scripture. Lurking in this other tradition is a second chronotope, one that presumes – at least in Wilson's play and its scriptural pretexts – a metaphoric mode of reading somewhat different from, even as it came to be subtly accommodated by, the medical mode of symptomatic reading.

SPOTTING SIN: METAPHORIC READING AND THE CHRONOTOPE OF PROVIDENTIAL JUDGMENT

The spots of early modern literature are by no means reliable signs of pox. The Old Testament provides a very different template for reading spots when, in Jeremiah 13:23, the prophet asks: 'Can the Ethiopian change his skin, or the leopard his spots?' Here Jeremiah refers to the entrenched wickedness of his fellow Jews, whom he regards as beyond reformation. The leopard's black spots are read by the prophet as metaphors for the wicked soul, and specifically the sexually transgressive soul: in a gloss that recalls the language of Lucre's 'box of abhomination,' Jeremiah imagines God declaring to the Jews, 'I have seen thine adulteries, and thy neighings, the lewdness of thy whoredom, and thine abominations on the hills in the fields' (13:26). This Jeremiac tradition of reading spots survived well into the seventeenth century. Shakespeare draws on it repeatedly – for example, when Richard II rebukes Bushy, Bagot, Wiltshire, and Green for 'their spotted souls' (3.1.134), when Gertrude claims to see in her soul 'such black and grained spots' (3.4.90), or when Timon tells Apemantus that 'wert thou a leopard, /... the spots of thy kindred were jurors on thy life' (4.3.335-336).[24] Like Jeremiah's question, such pronouncements presume a mode of reading that interprets spots not as physical expressions of a pathological process, but as graphic metaphors for both spiritual turpitude

[24]In this context, of course, one cannot help but think also of Lady Macbeth's 'damned spot,' which no amount of washing can erase (*Macbeth*, 5.1.30).

and the moral verdict ('the spots of thy kindred were jurors on thy life') that such turpitude occasions.

If the medical reading of spots illuminates the chronotope of natural history, the metaphoric reading illuminates the chronotope of providential judgment. While natural history is sequential and grounded in corporeality, providential judgment is instantaneous and of no fixed abode, as the very term 'metaphoric' implies. The latter derives from the Greek 'metaphorein,' to transfer; but while in rhetoric the transfer promised by metaphor takes the form of a linguistic condensation of terms for two unlike things, the metaphoric reading performs a transfer between two or more unlike *locations*. The medical reading of syphilitic spots, therefore, is not metaphoric in the specific sense I have sketched above: although the chronotope of natural history demands the translation of a body's symptoms into truths about that body, the resulting narrative remains grounded in the same corporeal location even as it transforms the latter into something knowable. The spots of metaphoric reading, by contrast, demand several transfers between different, and even opposed, locations. As Jeremiah's gloss on the leopard's spots suggests, the chronotope of providential judgment requires not only a primary image of bodily spots, but also an interpretive explication that transfers meaning from the body to a different, spiritual space – the invisibly 'spotted' soul of the sinner – which may not even inhabit that body. This space is in turn transferred to the sign of an omnipresent, omniscient God who alone 'sees' and judges the invisible marks of sin.

The locus classicus of the metaphoric reading of spots – or loci classici, given that such reading always entails transfers from a visible body to invisible spiritual locations – is furnished by the vulgate cycle of Arthurian legends. During the quest by the Knights of the Round Table for the Holy Grail, Gawain has a dream:

> What Gawain saw in his sleep was a vision of himself in a meadow of green grass and many flowers. In the meadow there was a rack where one hundred and fifty bulls were feeding. The bulls were fierce, and all but three of them were spotted. ... You should understand these bulls to be the members of the Round Table who, in their pride and lust, fell into such mortal sin that sins could not be concealed within them, but were forced to the surface, making them spotted and stained as the bulls were, that is to say, vile and hideous. ... There were three unstained bulls, those without sin. Two were perfectly fair and pure, while the third had a trace of spots. The two perfect ones represent Galahad and Perceval, who are fairer and purer than anyone. They are fair indeed, being perfect in all virtues. And they are pure without blemish or stain, which is almost impossible to find in a human being. The third one, bearing the trace of a blemish, is Bors, who once lost his virginity. But since then he has made such amends through a life of chastity that his sin has been pardoned.[25]

This passage neatly illustrates the multiple locative transfers that I have identified as the hallmark of metaphoric reading. An incarnated image of spotted and spotless bulls is translated by Gawain's gloss into an index of the divergent yet invisible spiritual complexions of the Knights of the Round Table. Their unseen souls then become the second-order signs of a providential will that sees and judges (or in the case of Bors, 'pardons') all souls. In Jeremiac fashion, then, Gawain's dream reads spots as both signifiers of and divine punishment for sin, specifically lechery.

The metaphoric tradition of reading spots instanced by Gawain's dream entails an intriguing dialectic of visibility and invisibility. The marks of sin are legible only to divine providence; as Thomas Becon writes in his *New Catechism* (1559), 'all creatures were found spotted in the sight of God.'[26] Yet the spots of sin become visible also to the Christian reader by a process of metaphoric substitution. A stand-in, whether Jeremiah's leopard or Gawain's bulls, is needed to incarnate the immateriality of sinful desire. Such a substitution is performed in Cesare Ripa's *Iconographia* of 1593, whose gloss on the figure of Penance makes visible what only God can see: 'an old grey woman; clothed in white, yet full of spots ... her years are already worn out by age, lamenting over the ill spent time: which is expressed by the spots upon the white garment. The same being the innocence which is given us by the holy Baptism.'[27] Here Ripa follows Jeremiah by making Penance's dark spots, visible on her garment if not her body, incarnate the otherwise invisible state of the baptized Christian's fallen soul.

A metaphoric reading of Conscience's spots in *The Three Ladies of London* would likewise follow Jeremiah by transferring the materiality of her visible blemishes to the invisible marks of sin, specifically lechery, and the power of divine will. According to such a reading, Wilson's Conscience is not a naturalistic case study of the symptoms of syphilis, but an allegorical stand-in for the universal soul pledged to lechery yet susceptible to the all-seeing judgment of Providence. This reading is emphasized within the play by the character of Judge Nemo. He claims that

> ... under the colour of Conscience thou deceived'st many,
> Causing thee, to defile the temple of God, which is man's body.
> A clean conscience is a sacrifice, God's own resting place:
> Why wast thou then corrupted so, and spotted thy face? (368)

---

25 *Lancelot-Grail*, pp. 155–156, 161.

26 Becon, *The Worckes*, I. fol. 445b.

27 Ripa, 'Penitenza,' British Library Ms. Add 23195.

The Judge has already answered his question. Conscience, he proclaims, stands accused as a lustful 'bawd unto Lucre, ... spotted with all abhomination' (366). The word 'abomination' derives from the Latin 'ab-ominari,' to deprecate as an ill omen; but its homonym 'abhomination,' as the matter of Conscience's spots is termed, derives from 'ab-homine,' a deviation away from man. This sheds light on the Judge's claim that Conscience did 'defile the temple of God, which is man's body ... A clean conscience is a sacrifice, God's own resting place.' Conscience's 'ab-homination' is thus both cause and effect of God's judgment. Her spiritual uncleanness ensures that God has departed her body. At the same time, her spots are God's instantaneous visible punishment for the invisible sin of lechery. The Judge's remark models the metaphoric transfer of meaning from incarnated mark to absent spiritual marker. As if to illustrate this process further, the 'abhomination' with which Conscience is spotted is not just a bodily deformity, but also doubles as an unseen allegorical personage literally wedded to carnal sin: the audience hears about, but never lays eyes upon, a certain 'Master Abomination and Mistress Fornication his wife' (341). By invoking yet deferring this concupiscent 'Master,' the play offers another instance of metaphoric transfer. Just as the matter of Conscience's 'abhomination' gestures in the direction of an invisible God who has relocated *ab homine*, so does the locative and lexical shift from onstage spotty 'abhomination' to offstage Master 'Abomination' involve a transfer from visible matter to invisible sin.

Yet to subject Conscience and her spots to an exclusively metaphoric reading is to ignore the extent to which the chronotope of providential judgment was always already palimpsested with that of natural history. For millennia, the symptoms of disease have been interpreted by various religious communities as signs of divine punishment. Pathological spots figure prominently in the Judeo-Christian iconography of God's scourging of innocent as well as sinful souls. The catch-all term 'plague,' deriving from the Latin 'plaga,' strike or blow, was employed as a conventional figure for God's punishment of individual and communal sins; with the epidemics of bubonic plague that swept through Europe in the Middle Ages and Renaissance, this punishment was incarnated for writers like Thomas Lodge in 'spottes, which the common people call Gods tokens.'[28] The 'spottes' of plague were often metaphorically linked to those of another disease. Accounting for the horrific plague epidemic of 1603, for

[28]Lodge, *A Treatise of the Plague*, sign. B2 ^{v}. On the epistemological implications of the etymology of plague, see Sontag, *AIDS and its Metaphors*, passim, and Healy, *Fictions of Disease in Early Modern England,* pp. 58–64. See also my *Sick Economies*, chap. 5.

example, Thomas Dekker wrote that 'Our heauenly parts are plaguy sick/ And there such leaprous spots do stick.'[29] Dekker's vision of plague – a disease that he moralizes as the product of 'Luxury,' 'Stewes,' and 'Sodomy'[30] – draws on the medieval convention of reading leprosy and its spots as divine punishment for the sin of lechery. Thus in Robert Henryson's fifteenth-century sequel to Chaucer's poem 'Troilus and Criseyde,' Cresseid is punished by Saturn for her 'wantoun blude' with the symptoms of leprosy, including 'spottis blak.'[31]

Henryson's Cresseid is but one local expression of an archetype visible not only in Ripa's Penance, but also in Wilson's Conscience: the woman of 'spotted fame' whose pathological marks are signs of both her lecherous soul and the certainty of providential judgment. This archetype has a particular power in early modern literature, where it is made to lend voice to fears about the pox. John Lane's poem 'Tom Tel-Troths Message' (1600), for example, alludes to '*spotless* Chastitie' as the virtuous antithesis of the sinful woman infected with 'the French Disease.'[32] The pox, like plague and leprosy before it, thus occasioned an adaptation of the metaphoric mode of reading. Rather than providing *metaphors* for the state of the unseen soul, the spots of pox became actual *symptoms* of sin. This is most apparent in the early German woodcuts that, by depicting the baby Jesus both causing and healing the black spots of pox-ridden sinners, borrow from the providential iconography of 'spotted' leprosy – a tendency that, as Anna Foa has noted, is recurrent in early modern narrations of syphilis.[33]

The German woodcuts also demonstrate how, in the palimpsested narratives of providential judgment and natural history, the specific identity of the spot-causing sickness is in a very real sense immaterial. For in medieval and early modern writing, venereal disease – a category in which we can also place Henryson's leprosy and Dekker's plague – is less a physiological than a spiritual condition. It does not matter if this condition is explicitly named leprosy, plague, or pox; indeed, as Dekker's 'leaprous spots' of plague suggest, the afflictions were interchangeable.[34] What matters instead are the physical marks that provide both the metaphoric

---

[29] *The Plague Pamphlets of Thomas Dekker*, ed. Wilson, pp. 85–86.

[30] *The Plague Pamphlets of Thomas Dekker*, ed. Wilson, p. 87.

[31] Henryson, *The Testament of Cresseid*, lines 314, 341. For a study of moral readings of leprosy in the Middle Ages, see Brody, *Disease of the Soul*.

[32] See *Tell Trothes New Yerres Gift*, ed. Furnivall, p. 133.

[33] See Foa, 'The New and the Old.'

[34] In *The Epicurean*, Erasmus refers to the 'scabbes of Naples' as 'the new leprosie'; see *Tudor Translations of the Colloquies of Erasmus*, ed. Spurgeon, p. 149.

incarnation and the pathological symptoms of the soul sick with the sin of lechery. Even when they do not refer to spots, sixteenth-century etiologies of the pox repeatedly fasten onto physical symptoms such as the stench of suppurating flesh to signify, in the words of Clowes, the 'stinking sinne that is the originall cause of this infection.'[35] Clowes's remark underscores the utter old-fangledness of the supposedly 'new' disease. Like the 'medieval' Henryson, the 'early modern' Clowes cross-hatches the signs of medical infection and moral infraction, creating a pathotext that is legible also in Conscience's spots.[36]

When employed in tandem, the medical and metaphoric modes of reading can help unravel the entwined pathological and religious strands of Robert Wilson's syphilitic pathotext. Neither mode, however, can explain the significance within the play of Lady Lucre and Usury, the agents of Conscience's spotting. These characters' centrality hints at yet another strand in the pathotext of syphilis: the economic. Teasing out the latter demands a third type of reading – the historicist – which, like medical and metaphoric reading, generates the effect of a pre-textual ground for meaning. Like medical and metaphoric reading too, historicist reading presumes its own distinctive chronotope. However, whereas natural history was formulated by 'classical' physicians like Galen, and providential judgment received its literary elaboration in the work of 'medieval' writers like Henryson, this third chronotope is a recognizably 'early modern' development. It is of special interest to this essay, moreover, as it is also the dominant conceptual organization of space and time underwriting contemporary scholarship on early modern literature and culture.

Spotting Economy: Historicist Reading and the Chronotope of Mercantile Space

The Three Ladies of London is, I have suggested, a morality play. Yet that generic classification sits uncomfortably with aspects of Wilson's drama. In contrast to precursor moralities such as *Everyman* or *The Castle of Perseverance*, which stage allegorical battles waged between virtue and sin for a universal soul, Wilson's play at crucial moments locates itself in geographi-

---

35Clowes, *Short and Profitable Treatise*, sign. A3 v. For an invaluable discussion of religious etiologies of syphilis, see Schleiner, 'Moral Attitudes toward Syphilis and its Prevention in the Renaissance.'

36This pathotext, moreover, haunts 'modern' medical knowledge of syphilis. An echo of Jeremiah's reading of the leopard's spots resonates in the condition called 'Leopard Spot Hypofluorescence,' one of the clinical syndromes associated with secondary and tertiary-stage syphilis.

cal space and historical time. Characters such as Lucre and Usury vacillate between being placeless embodiments of sin and geographically specific instances of vice. Usury, we learn, has come to England from Venice (268); and although Lucre is the object of universal lust – 'men come from Italy, Barbary, Turkey [and] Jewry' to win her (250) – she is likewise given a Venetian pedigree (268). Into this Mediterranean mix Wilson also adds a scheming Italian merchant, Mercatore, and a Jewish merchant resident in Turkey, Gerontus. Wilson's insistence on locating his characters geographically, as the play's title also indicates, ultimately results in his dramatizing less the perils of universal sin than economic issues specific to late sixteenth-century London: rent-racking, overcrowding in slums, immigrant artisanal labour, new modes of commerce and credit, and the rise of consumer culture.[37]

In the process, the play subscribes at least in part to a chronotope of mercantile space. The latter is glimpsed when the Italian merchant Mercatore claims to ship English commodities such as 'corn, leader/ beef and bacon' to his own country (277) and to sell English consumers 'new toys' from 'Barbary and ... Turkey' (308). Indeed, the circulation of goods and characters between the Turkish east, the Romish south, and the English north provides much of the impetus for the play's plot. This traffic presumes a conception of space and time different from those produced in medical and metaphoric readings of Conscience and her spots. Whereas natural history subordinates bodily space to the diachronic course of a disease and providential judgment subordinates space to the instantaneity of divine will, mercantile space subsumes time within a geographical plane. For all the dynamic hustle and bustle of the mercantile chronotope, its movements characteristically describe and solidify the boundaries of nations. To read this chronotope, then, entails positing synchronic relations of exchange and circulation between discrete if connected domains.

In *Shakespearean Negotiations* (1988), Stephen Greenblatt outlines the praxis of reading that underwrites his well-known theory, integral to the new historicism, of the circulation of social energy:

> The textual traces that have survived from the Renaissance and that are at the center of our literary interest in Shakespeare are the products of extended borrowings, collective exchanges, and mutual enchantments. They were made by moving certain things – principally ordinary language but also metaphors, ceremonies, dances, emblems, items of clothing, well-worn stories, and so forth – from one culturally demarcated zone to another. We need to

[37]See Kermode, 'The Playwright's Prophecy,' pp. 60–87.

> understand not only the construction of these zones but also the process of movement across the shifting boundaries between them.[38]

Greenblatt's mode of reading eerily replicates that presumed by the early modern chronotope of mercantile space. Like the latter, Greenblatt's 'understanding' of space and time is predicated on economically coded 'movement' – 'borrowings, collective exchanges,' and so on – but ultimately works to map the 'boundaries' between discrete 'culturally demarcated zones.' Although Greenblatt acknowledges that these boundaries may shift over time, a possibility that would introduce a diachronic dimension into his analysis of the circulation of social energy, the mode of reading that he practices in *Shakespearean Negotiations* – and which mainstream historicist criticism has subsequently reproduced – overwhelmingly focuses on the synchronic relations between 'culturally demarcated zones.' Plotting the movement of symbolic entities between those zones works to map a grid of 'early modernity' which is then metaleptically refashioned as the pre-textual ground of historicist reading.

Greenblatt's theorization of historicist reading is only partial, inasmuch as it neglects how its own critical vocabulary has been enabled by, and anachronistically reiterates, early modern textual productions of mercantile space. These productions include accounts of the transnational circulation of goods, as instanced by Mercatore's description of his 'new toys' from Barbary and Turkey. They also include narrations of the pox, particularly those in which the name for the disease is prefixed with a national adjective. Unlike Clowes's narration of the *lues venerea*, which describes only the history of the disease once it 'entreth the body,' accounts of the 'Neapolitan disease' or the 'French pox' frequently offer an extra-corporeal history that illuminates the boundaries of what Greenblatt calls 'culturally demarcated zones.' Rather than simply being a universal affliction that runs its course within the body (as per natural history), or a condition of the sick soul incarnated in spots (as per providential judgment), the disease becomes instead a traveler, migrating across national borders. In his *Tractado contra el mal serpentino* (1539), for example, the Spanish physician Ruy Díaz de Isla asserts that

> The French called it the *Disease of Naples*. And the Italians and Neapolitans, as they had never been acquainted with such a disease, called it the *French Disease*. From that time on as it continued to spread, they gave it a name, each one according to his opinion as to how the disease had its origin. In

38Greenblatt, *Shakespearean Negotiations*, p. 7.

> Castilia they call it *Bubes,* and in Portugal the *Castilian Disease,* and in Portuguese India they call it the *Portuguese Disease.*[39]

English writers produced their own narratives about pox's transnational migration. Robert Greene offered the standard nationalized etiology of the 'French pox' in 1590, claiming 'that villainie, lept from *Naples* into *Fraunce* and from *Fraunce* into England.'[40] And the physician Philip Barrough, in his treatise on the 'morbus gallicus' (1596), elaborated further on the pox's history prior to its emergence in Italy: 'First, the Spaniardes borrowed it of the Indians, and brought it home in stead of their gold,' after which it was spread 'to Rome and Naples.'[41]

To see these narratives simply as xenophobic reactions to the infectious 'villainie' of other nations neglects how their accounts of pox's global spread often has an economic dimension, one that is particularly explicit in Barrough's sardonic conversion of gold into disease. This shows how the pox was coming to be regarded as less an internal state of humoral imbalance or *dyskrasia* than a transnational migratory entity analogous to commodities and specie. Such a recoding can be glimpsed in Shakespeare's *Comedy of Errors.* In an extended set-piece, Dromio of Syracuse maps the nations of the globe onto the body of a diseased woman. The latter has, in Dromio's description, recognizable marks of the pox: 'France,' he claims in a punning reference to alopecia, is 'in her forehead ... making war against her heir' (3.2.109–111). It is in Dromio's description of the location of Spain and the Americas, however, that pox emerges as a migratory commodity. 'Spain' is felt 'hot in her breath,' and 'America, the Indies,' is 'upon her nose, all o'er embellished with rubies, carbuncles, sapphires, declining their rich aspect to the hot breath of Spain' (3.2.116–121). This image conflates the wealth of the American Indies, appropriated by Spain, with symptoms of the pox – 'rubies' and 'carbuncles' being but two synonyms for the red spots associated with the disease.[42]

Dromio's analogy suggests how the enormous growth of global trade in the sixteenth century affected understandings of sexually transmitted disease. The pathological machinations and movements of the Italian Lucre and Usury in *The Three Ladies of London* likewise hint at an increasing

---

[39]Díaz de Isla, *Tractado contra el mal serpentino*, p. 181; translation from Fabricius, *Syphilis in Shakespeare's England*, pp. 6–7.

[40]Robert Greene, *A Disputation Between a Hee and a Shee Cony Catcher*, in *The Life and Complete Works in Prose and Verse of Robert Greene*, ed. Grosart, vol. 10, p. 198.

[41]Barrough, *Methode of Phisicke*, p. 361. See also Schleiner, 'Moral Attitudes toward Syphils and its Prevention in the Renaissance,' p. 391.

[42]See my *Sick Economies*, chap. 2.

tendency to situate venereal disease within mercantile space. It is thus almost surprising that a play about transnational migration should make no explicit reference to the 'French' pox. Inasmuch as Wilson's play palimpsests mercantile space with natural history and providential judgment, however, I shall argue that it is exemplary of the syphilitic pathotext. This palimpsest can be glimpsed in one keyword employed toward the end of the play: 'canker.'

In the final courtroom scene, the Judge makes explicit the commercial dimension of Conscience's 'abhomination' by asking: 'O Conscience, shall cankered coin corrupt thy heart?' (369). The Judge's phrasing derives from Saint James's complaint that rich men's 'gold and siluer is cankred' (James 5:3). However, 'canker' was also associated with the pox: the French term for canker, 'chancre,' was a common synonym for the poxy spot.[43] As such, 'canker' participated in all the chronotopes I have outlined. It featured in natural histories of the disease's course: Hutten asserts that 'there will appear small Holes and Sores, turning cankerous and fistulous,'[44] and Clowes claims that the disease, once it has entered the body, 'creepeth like a canker from part to part.'[45] 'Canker' was also used to invoke the chronotope of providential judgment: in language that recalls Conscience's 'abhomination,' Traheron lists 'lothsome cankers' as one of the prime symptoms of that 'most filthy, pestiferous, & abominable disease.'[46] Yet other instances of 'canker' suggest the contours of mercantile space: in his play *The Three Lords and Ladies of London* – the 1588 sequel to *The Three Ladies of London* – Robert Wilson recognizably conflates the term with pox when Simplicity wishes that Pleasure be consumed by 'the French canker.'[47] Here canker does not simply creep, as it does for Clowes, *within* the body; instead it creeps *between* bodies and, importantly, between nations.

If the English Conscience is 'cankered' by the continental Lucre and Usury, then, the term suggests not only syphilitic or providential marking, but also a mercantile understanding of commercial transactions across national borders. To this extent, Wilson's rhetoric anticipates that of the English mercantilist, Gerard Malynes. In *The Canker of England's Commonwealth* (1601), Malynes employs the disease as a metaphor that suggests both cankered coin and the chancres of pox. The treatise endeavours to explain

---

43 See Keil, 'The Evolution of the Term Chancre and its Relation to the History of Syphilis.'

44 Hutten, *Treatise of the French Disease*, sign. C2.

45 Clowes, *Briefe and Necessary Treatise*, sign. U1.

46 Traheron, *Workes of Ioan de Vigo*, sign. +ii.

47 Wilson, *Three Ladies and Lords of London*, in *Select Collection of Old English Plays*, ed. Hazlitt, VI. p. 499.

the causes of England's economic crisis, which Malynes attributes partly to the scheming machinations of the continental banker – a figure whose name entails a serendipitous rhyme with 'canker.' The continental banker deliberately undervalues English currency, rendering the pound sterling's international exchange rates far poorer than the value of its component metals. English merchants thus save more by sending their coin directly to overseas factors instead of buying foreign currency at present exchange rates, and so the nation's supply of treasure cannot help but haemorrhage – a depletion that, Malynes argues, is the 'unknowne disease of the politicke body.'[48] This is more than a diagnostic reading of a sick body. In his account of the foreign 'canker' of offshore specie-flow, Malynes engages in the kind of historicist reading advocated by Greenblatt, delineating the boundaries between discrete zones or nations by observing the processes of 'exchange' and 'movement' of specie between England and continental nations. That we can now also read in Malynes's tract an additional exchange, the circulation between economic and medical 'zones' of a discourse of foreign migration and infection, only goes to show how pervasive the mercantile chronotope and its historicist mode of reading has become.

Malynes's narration of England's infection by the dangerous continental Banker Canker resonates powerfully with Wilson's fantasy of the Italian Lady Lucre cankering Conscience. Although the pox may be made legible in *The Three Ladies of London* through medical and metaphoric readings of Conscience's spots, it is equally produced by a strategy of historicist reading like Malynes's, which plots the homologous movements of disease and coin across national borders. I would even argue that the chronotope of mercantile space and the historicist reading it demands are what distinguish the syphilitic pathotext from its close cousin the leprous pathotext, with which it shares the layers of natural history and providential judgment. In her important study of syphilis, Anna Foa rightly notes the extent to which the early modern iconography of the pox overlaps with medieval representations of leprosy as divine punishment for sin. Yet even as she acknowledges the widespread xenophobic assumption that syphilis always came from foreign countries, Foa overlooks how this assumption also worked to locate the disease within a mercantile as much as a religious framework. Hence her largely metaphoric reading of disease neglects the emergent mode of historicist reading that helped transform the leprous into the syphilitic pathotext.[49]

---

[48]Malynes, *Treatise of the Canker of Englands Commonwealth*, sign. B2. For an extended reading of Malynes's 'canker,' see my essay 'The Canker of England's Commonwealth.'

[49]See Foa, 'The New and the Old.' It must be noted that although Foa writes cannily

To privilege *solely* the historicist reading of the syphilitic pathotext, however, is to risk naturalizing synchronic analysis by assuming that only within the larger 'fact' of early modernity – imaged by Greenblatt as a kind of cultural stock exchange governing the transactions between various 'zones' in Shakespeare's historical moment – can the disease really be understood. This is the trap stumbled into by some scholars who would have us historicize 'early modern' venereal disease by replacing the anachronism of 'syphilis' with the more historically correct 'pox.' Such an exchange assumes that any object of knowledge is produced entirely within the epistemological or discursive horizons of a historical moment. As I have argued, however, objects of knowledge need to be seen equally as diachronic reworkings of older modes of knowing and reading that, as such, render anachronism unavoidable. This is why I not only distinguish between the historically correct 'pox' and the anachronistic 'syphilis'; I actively prefer 'syphilis' inasmuch as it has the power to redirect attention to the diverse historical forms – what Jameson would call the 'exoskeletons' – that constitute the multi-layered textuality of pathology. When used to describe early modern pox, 'syphilis' does not so much essentialize a disease prior to language as foreground the anachronism of *any* pathotext. To theorize the pathotext, then, we need to be more attentive to the palimpsests of textuality in general. In this regard, *The Three Ladies of London* is particularly illuminating, for it insists on both the *writing* and the *overwriting* of Conscience's spots.

Conscience's spots, I have argued, are pathotexts that serve as turnstiles between not only multiple discourses, but also multiple chronotopes and their distinctive modes of reading. Which mode of reading we privilege is largely dependent on our particular investment in an extra-textual ground of meaning – whether Biology, God, or Historical Moment. All these transcendental signifieds, I have argued, are generated through different processes of symptomatic reading. A historical formalist reading, by contrast, attends to Conscience's spots not for a single reality external to them, but for the skein of intratextual relations embedded in them. In this respect, what is most striking about Conscience's spots is their metonymic association with writing. Wilson's stage direction specifies that Conscience's colourful spots derive from 'a painted box of ink,' about which Usury asks Lady Lucre: 'is there any superscription thereon?' (337).

---

about the interplay of 'new' and 'old' in early modern representations of the disease – and to that extent appears to gesture toward an understanding of its diachronic textuality – she repeatedly presumes that syphilis is *not* a textual effect, but a real entity that precedes its textual mediations.

Both the 'painted box' and its questionable 'superscription' emphasize how Conscience's spots are inked palimpsests produced through a process of super-scription, or writing over writing. In *The Three Ladies of London*, then, syphilis is an anachronistic palimpsest rather than a corporeal, spiritual, or historicist fact prior to textuality. That pathotext is haunted by, but can never be fully reduced to, 'early modern pox.' For that reason, in Wilson's play as in other early modern syphilitic pathotexts, (po)X marks the spot.

George Washington University
Washington D. C.

Cited Works

Manuscript Sources

London, British Library, Ms. Add 23195, Ripa, Cesare. 'Penitenza.'

Published Sources

Arrizabalaga, Jon, John Henderson, and Roger French. *The Great Pox: The French Disease in Early Modern Europe*. New Haven: Yale University Press, 1997.

Bakhtin, Mikhail. *The Dialogic Imagination: Four Essays*, trans. Caryl Emerson and Michael Holquist. Austin: University of Texas Press, 1981.

Barrough, Philip. *The Methode of Phisicke*. London: Richard Field, 1596.

Becon, Thomas. *The Worckes of Thomas Becon*. 3 vols. London, Iohn Day, 1564.

Bentley, Greg W. *Shakespeare and the New Disease: The Dramatic Function of Syphilis in 'Troilus and Cressida,' 'Measure for Measure' and 'Timon of Athens'*. New York: Peter Lang, 1989.

Boehrer, Bruce T. 'Early Modern Syphilis' *Journal of the History of Sexuality*, 1:2 (1990): 197–214.

Brody, Saul Nathaniel. *The Disease of the Soul: Leprosy in Medieval Literature*. Ithaca: Cornell University Press, 1974.

Clowes, William. *A Short and Profitable Treatise Touching the Cure of the Disease Called Morbus Gallicus by Unctions*. London: I. Daye, 1579.

Clowes, William. *A Briefe and Necessary Treatise, Touching the Cure of the Disease Now Usually Called Lues Venerea, by Unctions and Other Approued Waies of Curing: Newly Corrected and Augmented*. London: Edm. Bollifant, 1596.

Cunningham, Andrew. 'Transforming Plague: Laboratory Medicine and the Identity of Infectious Disease' pp. 209–244 in *The Laboratory Revolution in Medicine*, ed. Andrew Cunningham and Perry Williams. Cambridge: Cambridge University Press, 1992.

Dennie, C. C. *A History of Syphilis*. Springfield, IL: C. C. Thomas, 1962.

Isla, Ruy Díaz de. *Tractado contra el mal serpentino: que vulgarmente en Espana es llamado bubas*. Seville, 1539.

Fabricius, Johannes. *Syphilis in Shakespeare's England.* London: Jessica Kingsley, 1994.

Foa Anna. 'The New and the Old: The Spread of Syphilis (1494–1530)' pp. 26–45 in *Sex and Gender in Historical Perspective,* eds. Edward Muir and Guido Ruggiero. Baltimore: The Johns Hopkins University Press, 1990.

Fracastoro, Girolamo. *Syphilis sive Morbus Gallicus,* trans. Heneage Wynne-Finch London: Heinemann, 1935.

Greenblatt, Stephen. *Shakespearean Negotiations: The Circulation of Social Energy in Renaissance England.* Berkeley: University of California Press, 1988.

Grünpeck, Joseph. *Tractatus de pestilentiali scorra sive Mala de Franzos.* Augsburg: Hans Schauer, 1496.

Harris, Jonathan Gil. ''The Canker of England's Commonwealth': Gerard de Malynes and the Origins of Economic Pathology' *Textual Practice,* 13 (1999): 311–328.

Harris, Jonathan Gil. *Foreign Bodies and the Politic: Discourses of Social Pathology in Early Modern England.* Cambridge: Cambridge University Press, 1998.

Harris, Jonathan Gil. *Sick Economies: Drama, Mercantilism and Disease in Shakespeare's England.* Philadelphia: University of Pennsylvania Press, 2004.

Healy, Margaret. *Fictions of Disease in Early Modern England: Bodies, Plagues and Politics.* New York: Palgrave, 2002.

Henryson, Robert. *The Testament of Cresseid,* ed. Denton Fox. London: Nelson's Medieval and Renaissance Library, 1968.

Hutten, Ulrich von. *A Treatise of the French Disease, Publish'd above 200 Years Past,* trans. Daniel Turner. London: John Clarke 1730.

Jameson, Fredric. *The Political Unconscious: Narrative as Socially Symbolic Act.* New York: Methuen, 1981.

Keil, Harry. 'The Evolution of the Term Chancre and its Relation to the History of Syphilis' *Journal of the History of Medicine,* 4 (1949): 407–416.

Kermode, Lloyd Edward. 'The Playwright's Prophecy: Robert Wilson's *The Three Ladies of London* and the 'Alienation' of the English' *Medieval and Renaissance Drama in England* 11 (1999): 60–87.

Lancelot-Grail: The Old French Arthurian Vulgate and Post-Vulgate in Translation, 5 vols., ed. Norris J. Lacy. New York: Garland Publishing, Inc., 1993–1996, vol. 1., trans. E. Jane Burns.

The Life and Complete Works in Prose and Verse of Robert Greene, ed. Alexander B. Grosart. 10 vols. New York: Russell and Russell, 1886.

Lodge, Thomas. *A Treatise of the Plague: Containing the Nature, Signes, and Accidents of the Same.* London: Thomas Creede and Valentine Simmes, 1603.

Malynes, Gerard. *A Treatise of the Canker of Englands Commonwealth.* London: Richard Field, 1601.

Nelkin Dorothy, and Sander L. Gilman. 'Placing the Blame for Devastating Disease' pp. 39–56 in *In Time of Plague,* ed. Arien Mack. New York: New York University Press, 1991.

Nutton, Vivian. 'The Seeds of Disease: An Explanation of Contagion and Infection from the Greeks to the Renaissance' *Medical History,* 27 (1983): 1–34.

The Plague Pamphlets of Thomas Dekker, ed. F. P. Wilson. Oxford: Clarendon Press, 1925.

Quétel, Claude. *History of Syphilis*, trans. Judith Braddock and Brian Pike. Baltimore: The Johns Hopkins University Press, 1990.

Schleiner, Winfried. 'Moral Attitudes toward Syphilis and Its Prevention in the Renaissance' *Bulletin of the History of Medicine,* 68 (1994): 389–410.

Shakespeare, William. *The Norton Shakespeare*, ed. Stephen Greenblatt et al. New York: Norton, 1997.

Sontag, Susan. *AIDS and Its Metaphors*. New York: Farrar, Straus & Giroux, 1989.

Steber, Bartholomaeus. *A malafranczos, morbo gallorum, praeservatio ac cura*. Vienna: Johannes Winterburg, 1498.

J. T. of Westminster, *The Hunting of the Pox*. London: I. White, 1619.

Tell Trothes New Yerres Gift: Shakespeare's England, ed. F. J. Furnivall. Series 6, vol. 2. London: New Shakespeare Society,1876.

The Earliest Printed Literature on Syphilis: Being Ten Tractates from the Years 1495 1498, ed. Karl Sudhoff. Florence: R. Lier & Co, 1925.

Traheron, Richard. *Workes of Ioan de Vigo*. London: Edward Whytchurch, 1543.

Tudor Translations of the Colloquies of Erasmus (1536–1584), ed. Dickie Spurgeon. New York: Scholars' Facsimiles and Reprints, 1972.

Wilson, Robert. *The Three Ladies of London*, in vol. 6 of *A Select Collection of Old English Plays*, ed. W. Carew Hazlitt. 15 vols. London: Reeves and Turner, 1874.

Wilson, Robert. *The Three Lords and Ladies of London*, in vol. 6 of *A Select Collection of Old English Plays*, ed. W. Carew Hazlitt. 15 vols. London: Reeves and Turner, 1874.

Luxury and Lechery: Hunting the French Pox in Early Modern England

Roze Hentschell

In 1585, the surgeon William Clowes bewailed the rampant spread in England of what later became known as syphilis: 'it is wonderfull to consider the huge multitudes of such as be infected with it, and that dayly increase, to the great daunger of the common wealth, & the staine of the whole nation.'[1] At the heart of Clowes's complaint is the damage that has been inflicted, not on the individuals with the disease, but rather on England itself. Clowes regards individual cases as a national crisis; the physical decay of the infirm body comes to symbolize the moral decay of a country that has opened itself to foreign iniquities. Even as surgeons and satirists acknowledged that the disease most likely spread through sexual contact, this lasciviousness was viewed as the result of the influence of strangers and blame for the disease was routinely placed on foreigners. Sixteenth and early seventeenth-century medical manuals in particular, while explicitly concerned with the identification of and treatment for the pox, are also preoccupied with the foreign origin of the disease. While acknowledging that this malady was now England's problem, English writers took great pains to distance the disease from their isolated nation, thereby constructing England as a previously untainted island that had been infected through no fault of its own.

This essay is concerned with the English discourse surrounding the pox. I posit that the textual explanation of the origins and spread of the 'new' disease coincides with a more general rhetoric of blame in England, both in non-fiction and imaginative works, wherein England's social ills – especially vanity and lechery – are deflected onto other nations, particularly France, England's longtime enemy. As Jonathan Gil Harris asserts, the 'radical conceptions of disease as an exogenous, invading entity' allowed for the rhetorical construction of social ills as foreign: 'the body politic no

---

[1] Clowes, *A Brief and Necessary Treatise*, sign. A1^{v}.

longer became diseased because problems generated within its internal systems of organization or its hegemonic fractions . . . but as a result of infiltration by hostile, foreign bodies.'[2] The pox was seen both as a metaphor for and an indicator of a larger breakdown of morals, a symptom of the deadly sins that infected the nation with increased contact with the French, through both martial conflict and travel. *Morbus Gallicus* was regarded as both a venereal disease and an obsession with French clothing and manners. Often these two 'maladies' were seen as one; overt preoccupation with French fashions was taken as a symptom of the disease and vice versa; vanity and venery were thus interchangeable.[3] In the popular English imagination, the desire for French luxury goods is the medium through which the vice of pride associated with this disease penetrates England. Thus, as we see in Clowes' statement, textual discourse about the disease relocates the French pox from the body to the nation.

WHAT'S IN A NAME? BLAME

Both the naming of the disease and the desire to identify its origin, perhaps above all, give us insights into the complex ways that blame is assigned textually.[4] Contemporaries vigorously debated the origins of the disease and, indeed, medical historians and scientists still keep the issue alive, as the question of the role of Columbus and the famed siege at Naples remains unsolved. It is not the accuracy of historical events, however, that interests me here. Rather, the multiple readings of the same moment, and the persistent impulse to explain the disease *away* from England are at the heart of this rhetoric of blame. While recent scholars have focused on the way that the blame for the disease has been placed on prostitutes and contact with 'unclean' women, in much of the primary literature the disease is dislocated from the body of those afflicted to the perceived countries of origin.[5] Virtually all medical manuals that give sustained attention to the

---

[2]Harris, *Foreign Bodies*, p. 14.

[3]As a literary scholar, I am interested in the discourse of all types of printed texts, both imaginative and 'non-fiction.' However, I resist drawing a clear line between the literary and non-literary. Just as 'fictional' texts involving the pox rely on medical information and historical narratives, medical manuals offer writing that is imaginative, highly crafted, and operating within rhetorical conventions that assume a particular audience. As Bruce Boehrer asserts, there is a tendency for early modern doctors 'to deal with syphilis in elaborate fictional narrative.' Boehrer, 'Early Modern Syphilis,' p. 206.

[4]See Bentley, *Shakespeare and the New Disease*, chap. 3, for a discussion of the pox's relationship to slander.

[5]For helpful discussions of the vilification of women in relation to the pox see

new disease are preoccupied with the various names ascribed to the pox. An early tract on the disease, Ulrich von Hutten's *De medicina guaici, et morbo gallico*, printed in English in 1533, demonstrates the interest in giving the disease a name based on its locus of origin, while also acknowledging that there is no one name to attach to it:

> In the yere of Christ 1493 or there about, this pestiferus evyll creped amongst the people, not only in Fraunce, but fyrst appeered at Naples, in the frenchemennes hoste, (wherof it toke his name) whiche kept warre under the french kyng Charles, before hit appered in any other place. By which occasion the french men puttynge from them this abhorred name, calle it not the frenche pockes / but the evyl of Naples / reckenynge it to theyr rebuke, if this pestilent disease shulde be named the french pockes. (A1[r])

Although Hutten clearly identifies the disease as *morbo gallico* in his title, because the disease first seemed to appear in the French camps, he acknowledges that the moniker was anathema for the French, who in turn associated it with Naples where the French had laid siege. In *The Method of Physick*, Philip Barrough discusses the naming of the disease as it reflected changing notions of its origin:

> First, the Italians call it Morbus Gallicus . . . because it first appeared among the Frenchmen at the siege before named. The French call it Scabiem, or Morbum Italicum, because they had the victory, and for that they had this sicknes. And they also called it Scabiem Hispanicam because the Spanish first brought it out of the Indies. The Germans call it Menium to signifie the privy parts infected with this disease. Some of them call it Scabiem Hispanicum. In Spain they name it Morbum Neapolitanum, the cause I told you before. They of Naples call it also Patnysa paradneptur, that is, the proper name at home in India . . . and we in our countrey call it, the French disease. But however it bee called it skilleth not, so that we knowe how to helpe it, which I minde to declare hereafter by God's grace. (362)

As much as Barrough would like to claim that 'it skilleth,' or matters, 'not' just what the disease is called, the long list detailing all the names indicates an impulse to locate the disease outside the boundaries of the nation in which it appears. As Winfried Schleiner has observed, the desire to name is 'a traditional rhetorical strategy dating from the time when the etymology of a word . . . was thought to reveal some part of the truth of what it named.'[6]

Fabricius, *Syphilis in Shakespeare's England*, especially chaps. 5 and 6; Siena, 'Pollution, Promiscuity, and the Pox;' and Schleiner, 'Infection and Cure through Women.'

[6]Schleiner, 'Moral Attitudes,' p. 393. Also see French and Arrizabalaga, 'Coping with the French Disease,' p. 253.

Thus, attaching the name to a particular country was in part an effort to get at the essence of the disease itself.

This impulse to name via location of origin is again revealed or, perhaps more accurately, satirized in a 1616 text called *The Hunting of the Pox* by J.T. of Westminster. This long poem describes the author's encounter with 'Pild-Garlicke' a man with whom he discusses the disease by describing the life and death of Morbus Gallicus, an Englishman infected with the French pox.[7] Part didactic text (the author provides both a glossary of medical terms and a bibliography), part allegorical morality tale (Morbus Gallicus's shameful death is recounted), and part satire of foppish London gallants, *The Hunting of the Pox* imitates the medical manuals that insist on naming the disease:

> the *French* did put the blame
> Upon the *Spaniards*, that brought it to *Naples* when they came;
> The *Neapolitans* did say, the *French* did bring it them,
> For they this painfull sore disease, did never know till then:
> The *Flemmings* call it *Spanish* Pox, and sure they brought it first
> To Christiandome, as you have heard, and therefore more are curst:
> The *Scots* likewise, when they have met, some part of this disease,
> They use in jest to say that they are bit with *Spanish Fleas*,
> Because they leave red spots behinde, as fleas doe used to doe,
> And sure this jest is used in France, belike they use it too.
> . . . .
> The *English* they in plaine good troth, will swear it came to us
> From France, and therefore takes the name of *Morbus Gallicus*. (B1^{r-v})

While serving as a sort of mnemonic, the rhythm of the iambics in this poem also works to poke fun perhaps at the insistence of other authors fixing the disease to a particular locus. The light-hearted tone and the acknowledgement that many of these names are said in 'jest' show that the interest in naming is arbitrary – there is no way to *know* the disease's true essence if the essence depends upon one's own physical location.

William Clowes, the doctor most closely associated with the treatment and discussion of this disease in late sixteenth-century England, recognized the disease as retribution for immorality in England, but locates the disease elsewhere. The disease he names as 'morbus gallicus,' or 'lues venerea' is 'a

---

[7]The name 'Pild-Garlicke' has many connotations, all related to the French Disease. 'Pild' might mean 'piled,' referring to 'piles' or hemorrhoids, which were regarded as symptoms of the pox. 'Garlicke,' is obviously the bulbous root; sometimes bulbous sores would appear on the skin of the infected. Most likely, however, 'Pild' denoted 'pilled.' To 'pill' meant to strip the skin off something, such as a fruit or garlic. It also meant to make bald, a symptom famously associated with the pox.

notable testimony of the just wrath of God against the filthie sinne, which at this daie [1596], not only infecteth Naples, Spain, and France' . . . but has spread 'itself throughout all England.'[8] Interestingly, the disease 'spreads itself,' indicating a lack of agency on the part of any individual. However, the insistence on relating the disease to Italy, Spain, and France works to undermine the moralistic shaming of the English who did not contract the disease by their own volition. The ambiguous language – it is the 'filthie sinne' of venery rather than the disease itself that has 'spread' into England – indicates that moral laxity is an infectious disease stemming from the Continent.

While the assignment of origin in these texts seems to be relatively innocuous, the name does tell us about the attitude of those who are doing the naming towards the country with which they associate the pox. Anna Foa asserts that no matter who was doing the naming, the pox always came 'from a neighboring country or, better yet, from the country of the enemy.'[9] So, if ascribing the name of the pox to *different* countries invariably disrupted a notion that there was *one* particular essence, what it did do was emphasize one epistemological 'truth': that the disease was *not* part of 'us,' whoever 'we' were. As the French author of the late seventeenth-century text, *A New Method of Curing the French Pox*, observed, man, 'to excuse himself, is forward to ascribe to his Neighbour the Sources and Original of this Distemper.'[10] And this, perhaps, is the key to understanding the show of xenophobia so ingrained in a disease whose origins were not (and perhaps may never be) known. The terrifying and grotesque new disease, one that was almost immediately moralized as a mark of sexual transgression, could not possibly have come from a nation as pure as 'ours.' Susan Sontag articulates this logic when she describes the pervasive link between illness and the other: 'It lies perhaps in the very concept of wrong, which is archaically identical with the non-us, the alien.'[11] This desire to project blame onto the other, however, is not simply one of cavalier chauvinism. It reveals a sense that there is something real to fear and loathe. In the desire to clarify a name for the disease in print – what Sander Gilman would call

---

[8]Clowes, *A Brief and Necessary . . . newly corrected*, sign. A3r. Clowes initially called it 'Morbus Gallicus, or Lues Venerea' in his 1585 treatise on the subject. In his revised 1596 treatise he drops the association with the French and indicates in the title that it is 'now usually called Lues Venerea.' I would suggest that this change is less a desire to exonerate the French than an attempt to highlight the immorality associated with the pox, a theme he develops in both texts.

[9]Foa, 'The New and Old,' p. 26.

[10]*A New Method of Curing the French Pox*, sign. B1r. The English translator of the text refers to the fact that the original author is French, but does not name him.

[11]Sontag, *AIDS and Its Metaphors*, pp. 47–48.

the 'carnival' of 'fixed structures of art' – what is revealed is the authors' (or the culture's) terror and repulsion of infection: 'The sense of the carnivalesque provides us with exactly the missing fixity for our understanding of the world which the reality of disease denies. For illness is a real loss of control that results in our becoming the Other whom we feared, whom we have projected onto the world.'[12]

By the late sixteenth century the pox had spread all over northern and eastern Europe, yet the disease was persistently identified with the Catholic countries of France, Spain, and Italy. The association of the pox with papist nations underscores an English Protestant agenda to decry these countries by associating them with lascivious diseases. Philip Massinger's *Emperor of the East* makes the association clear: 'The pox sir / Though falsely nam'd the Sciatica, or Goute, / Is the more Catholick sickeness' (IV.iii.88–90). The disease's connection to Catholicism is no where more explicit than in *The Whore of Babylon's Pocky Priest*, an anti-papist tract wherein the author describes a recently arrested priest who is also afflicted with the pox. Ostensibly written as a pamphlet describing the case of one Catholic man, the piece offers biting invective against all papists whose very religion is capable of spreading sexual disease. Catholic priests, the author argues, allow 'themselves a Liberty of all kind of Debaucheries' even though they 'make such a noise of *Single Life* and *Chastity*' (2). The detained priest, 'tainted with *Uncleanness*, and filthy Diseases' is also guilty of the deadly sin of vanity. When he was informed of the disgrace that would fall upon him when his disease is made public, his purported reply was simply, '*I care not, The World will count me a more modish well-bred Gentleman*' (9,10). Catholic vanity, a stereotype reaching at least as far back as Chaucer's 'religious' pilgrims, is underscored by the fact the priest has the disease. Luxury and lechery, located in the body of the priest, show the pox as foreign, even in England.[13] The force of anti-Catholic sentiment in early modern England has been well demonstrated.[14] Indeed, *The Whore of Babylon's Pocky Priest* was published in 1680, in the midst of the Exclusion Crisis when anti-popish anxiety was particularly intense. The link between the pox and papistry – or at least popish nations – further exonerates England and works to organize sentiments of Protestant nationalism through the vilification of Catholic countries.

---

[12] Gilman, *Disease and Representation*, p. 3.

[13] As Winfried Schleiner reminds us, 'anti-Roman sentiment (and the link with syphilis) was not limited to England but expressed in other Protestant countries as well." Schleiner, 'Moral Attitudes,' p. 391.

[14] See Miller, *Popery and Politics*. See Siena, 'Pollution, Promiscuity, and the Pox,' p. 554, for a discussion of *The Whore of Babylon's Pocky Priest*.

Despite the common association of the disease with Catholic countries in general, the other with whom authors most often associated the pox needed to be fixed textually in the French in order to help make sense of this disease. If we return to Barroughs's long parade of names for the pox, it is significant that 'the French Disease' is that which punctuates the list, thus lending it privilege and permanence. This is what 'we' English people call it. As the author of *The Hunting of the Pox* asserts, the English (i.e. 'we') 'will swear it came to us / from France.' The insistence on blaming France (even though the author admits the Spanish brought the disease into Europe) points to the desire to locate what was ultimately unlocatable in an obvious enemy. While there were dozens of names associated with the pox in early modern England, in both didactic and imaginative texts the 'French Disease' or 'Morbus Gallicus' attached itself to the culture like the disease itself.

One notable exception to the desire to attach the disease to France is to be found in the work of Peter Lowe, a Scottish surgeon. In his tract, *An Easy, Certain, and Perfect Method to Cure and Prevent the Spanish Disease*, Lowe derides those who insist on calling the disease Morbus Gallicus:

> There are some ignorant malicious people, who call it the French sicknes, without any cause or reason. The most part call it the Venerian sicknes, because most commonly, it procedeth of the act of venus . . . Now it may be called generall sicknes, because it is generally spred throughout all the world: but for that these things, concerning the originall and names, are not greatly materiall, I will pass them over. (B2^{r})

Like Barrough, Lowe insists that the name itself does not particularly matter. But Lowe clearly asserts that it is *not* 'the French sicknes,' and not surprisingly we discover why: Lowe may have been in service to the French King. In omitting the important detail found in earlier medical texts, that the disease originated in the French camp in Naples and thus is most closely associated with the French, Lowe rewrites medical history to posit the notion that the pox is the bane of England as a result of enmity with Spain, rather than France. Although Lowe claims that uncovering the origin and name of the disease is 'not greatly materiall' and that he 'will pass [these subjects] over,' the fact that he begins his tract with the absolution of France and the insistence of Spain's fault indicates the subtle ways even the most seemingly objective medical discourse might shape the way blame is assigned. The fact that almost all medical manuals follow the same pattern – a preliminary discussion of the origins and naming, a description of the symptoms, and then instructions for treatment – textually foregrounds the blame, allowing it to hover over the text as foreign spectre.[15]

---

15 We only have to look to the title of one tract to see how the way an author regards

Filthy Full of French

Travel to France was often seen in the literature as a dangerous activity, one that could lead to both physical and moral infection. The danger lay in the possibility that being in France will make the traveler like the French – i.e. lecherous and overly concerned with fashions – and that he will also carry home the French Disease.[16] In *The Hunting of the Pox*, for example, the author tells an allegorical tale of how the French Disease began. Superbus Publicus, a 'young Italian Gentleman, of birth decended well,' goes to France, 'The fashions there to know and learne' (B1v). There he meets a Neapolitan-born courtesan named Veneris who passes her malady on to him:

> She was the first that seazed upon Superbus in his sport,
> And made him poore and leane, God knowes, as men of him report;
> And altered all his body cleane, that strangers where he came
> Did call him Morbus Gallicus, or French diseased man. (B2r)

For the author, it does not matter that Superbus came originally from Italy; when he contracts the disease he must be called Morbus Gallicus. Significantly, the quest for French fashion is what leads to his ultimate demise. The desire 'to know and learn' modish apparel is what leads him down the slippery slope to Veneris, whose attendant 'hounds' 'fell on at length Superbus flesh, till that his life they ended' (B2r). The several different hounds that attack Morbus are distinct symptoms of the pox. One 'subtill hound' feeds on Morbus's 'glans,' while another 'curre' 'did raise up branny scales.' The dogs attack Morbus's 'gay and silken clothes,' revealing the primary reason he has contracted the disease: his persistent preoccupation with luxury apparel (B2v, B3v).

The immorality that infects the traveler is most apparent when he returns home. In Shakespeare's *Henry VIII*, three gentlemen discuss the courtiers who, returning to England after accompanying Henry to the Field

---

the disease prescribes the way it will be read: Προφυλακτικον *[Profulacticon]: Or Some Considerations of a Notable Expedient to root out the French Pox from the English Nation*. In naming the disease, it is very rare to see an association with England itself. We find two examples in satirical and dramatic literature. In a satirical prose dialog, Robert Greene's character Nan says that the pox is 'so surely now rooted in England' that 'it may better be called *A Morbus Anglicus* than *Gallicus*.' Greene, *A Disputation Between a Hee and Shee Conny-Catcher*, p. 232. In Thomas Middleton's *A Mad World, My Masters*, Sir Bounteous Progress asserts that 'the pox is as natural now as an ague in the springtime.' Middleton, *A Mad World*, IV.ii.23–24.

16See Williams, 'An Elizabethan Disease' for a catalogue of citations of pox as a side effect of French travel.

of the Cloth of Gold,[17] have lost all English decorum and replaced it with an overt concern for French fashion and loose morals:

> CHAMBERLAIN. Is't possible the spells of France should juggle
> Men into such mysteries?
> SANDS. New customs,
> Though they be never so ridiculous
> (Nay. Let 'em be unmanly), yet are followed. (I.iii.1–4)

Travel to France has enchanted the English courtiers to such an extent that they will follow 'ridiculous' fashions, both sartorial and behavioural, even if the 'customs' are considered effeminate. The English seem to be absolved of their new French obsessions as they are under the 'spells of France,' 'juggled' into confusion by their visit to the Continent. In describing the courtiers, Shakespeare alludes to Holinshed's account of English courtiers who were sent to France to negotiate the return of Touraine to the French several months before the events of the Field of the Cloth of Gold: 'when these yoong gentlemen came againe into England, they were all French in eating, drinking and apparel, yea, and in French vices and brags . . . so that nothing by them was praised but if it were after the French turne; which after turned them to displeasure.'[18] By imitating the manners and customs and fashions that they encountered at the meeting of the two kings, the English courtiers become 'all French.' What this ultimately means is that they, too, inherit the 'vices' of the French, which leads to a public chastisement and dismissal from court. Shakespeare suggests that by displaying their interest in French fashions, they are also suspected of carrying the French Disease. The 'reformation of our travell'd gallants' (I.iii.20) necessarily entails leaving all that is French behind:

> LOVELL. They must either
> (For so run the conditions). Leave those remnants
> Of fool and feather that they got in France,
> With all their honorable points of ignorance
> Pertaining thereunto, as fights and fireworks,
> . . . .
> renouncing clean
> The faith they have in tennis and tall stockings,

[17]The Field of the Cloth of Gold refers to the decadent display of wealth at the two-week long meeting in 1520 between Henry VIII and Francis I of France in the vale between a village in Calais and a village in Ardres. This meeting was designed to cement the tenuous friendship between the two countries. See Jocelyne G. Russell, *The Field of the Cloth of Gold*.

[18]Holinshed, *Chronicles*, vol. 3, p. 635.

> Short blist'red breeches, and those types of travel,
> And understand again like honest men,
> Or pack to their old playfellows.
> . . . .
> SANDS. 'Tis time to give 'em physic, their diseases
> Are grown so catching. (1.3.23–37)

The courtiers are in dire need of medical attention to rid themselves of the infectious diseases they have contracted by visiting France. Their French Disease, however, cannot be treated with mercury or guaiacum. The 'physic' they require is a renunciation of French customs such as 'fights,' whores ('fireworks'), and 'tennis.' To cure themselves they also need to give up French fashions such as 'feather,' 'tall stockings,' and puffed hose ('short-blistered breeches'). This, in turn, will allow them to 'understand again like honest men.' Here, the pox becomes a metaphor for the dangers of contracting French habits while traveling abroad, a malady that has entered England and has 'grown so catching.'[19]

Soldiers were perceived to be especially susceptible to immoral influence from abroad.[20] Mingling with soldiers of other nations was an invitation to amoral behaviour, opening the doors of the English nation to this suspect behaviour. In *The Ladies Looking Glass*, Barnabie Rich explains how this occurs, speaking specifically of the Dutch-Spanish conflict:

> And as the Armies of the Low countries are compounded of *English*, of *Scots*, of *French*, of *Spanish*, of *Italians*, of *Germans*, and of all the nations of Christiandome collected and gathered together: so the sinnes of all those countries and of all the world besides are everyday ingrossed and transported into England. We have stolne away the pride and ambition of the *Spaniard*, the fraud and falsehood of the *French* . . . (A4^{v})

By coming into contact with soldiers of other nations, the English are likely to acquire their sins. English soldiers, however, are given agency and thus are to be blamed for 'transporting' this behaviour back to England, evidence that 'sins' can be imported as a commodity. What is more, the vices can be 'stolen;' the English

---

[19]Sermonist William Walker cites the example of Lord Russell, who traveled abroad yet retained his Christian virtues, unlike the courtiers of England: 'O that our Gallants would imitate the example of this noble Lord, and would have care to keepe the *bit* of *Gods* grace, and the bridle of his *Feare*, to governe theire unbridled affections. Verely then they should not rush headlong, as now they doe, into all vice and irreligion.' Walker, *A Sermon*, sign. G2^{v}.

[20]See Hoenselaars for a discussion of English soldiers going abroad in early modern history plays. Hoenselaars, *Images of Englishmen*, p. 81.

soldiers have grown so covetous of European iniquities that they must rob these nations of their sins, including those that carry the pox.

Authors found especially fertile ground in the continual animosities with France for emphasizing the English soldier's fault for spreading the French Disease. As Gordon Williams observes, 'visits to France were humorously regarded as an extreme hazard' and 'for the soldiery fighting on the Continent, venereal infection appears more of a danger than the enemy.'[21] In 'Epigram 9' of *Humorous Ordinarie*, Samuel Rowlands cleverly shows how relations with France lead to contracting the French Disease:

> This Gentleman hath served long in *France*,
> And is returned filthy full of French,
> In single combat being hurt by chance,
> As he was closely foyling at a Wench:
> Yet hot alarm's he hath indur'd good store,
> But never in like pockie heate before. (B2ᵛ)

Hand to hand conflict is used as a metaphor to describe the soldier's relations with a prostitute and the resulting infection. Significantly, the 'pockie heat' is more debilitating to him than the many previous wounds he had received from the enemy. The main problem, though, is that he has '*returned*' to England, 'filthy full of French,' that is, both Frenchified and diseased. In Shakespeare's *Henry V* we have a similar scenario of the soldier infecting England with the pox as a result of his participation in the wars with France. After the battle of Agincourt, Pistol learns that his wife is 'dead i' th' spittle / Of a malady of France' (V.i.81–82). After participating in the unlikely defeat of the French forces, and receiving a beating from Fluellen, Pistol recognizes the fact that, since his wife died of the pox, it means his own 'Honor is cudgell'd.' This perhaps suggests that Pistol understands that he too has the disease and gave it to his wife, which is further emphasized by the plan he lays out for himself: 'To England will I steal . . . / And patches will I get unto these cudgell'd scars, / And [swear] I got them in the Gallia wars' (V.i.85, 87–89). As a result of the disease, Pistol has pock marks on his body that he will cover with 'patches,' only to claim that they are injuries received in combat.[22] The syphilitic sores are seen as more grievous than those

---

21Williams, 'An Elizabethan Disease,' p. 45.

22Velvet patches were used to cover scars as well as sores from pox. What the patches were covering was not always discernable. See, for instance, Shakespeare, *All's Well that Ends Well*, IV.iv.94–101. In some cases, it was entirely too obvious: Sir Pockhole in *The Knight of the Burning Pestle* claims that his nose has been cut away and 'in the place this velvet plaster stands.' Beaumont, *The Knight of the Burning Pestle*, III.429. See also Beaumont and Fletcher, *Cupid's Revenge*, IV.i.176–179.

wounds from combat, physically as well as morally. While wounds received in war were a sign of valour and commitment to the protection of one's nation, marks of the pox were symbolic of immorality and evidence of dalliance with the enemy, thereby calling into question the soldier's national fealty. Rather than serving as an elaborate metaphor, the French Disease is very real, causing pain and death. However, even in describing the 'pockie heat' and 'cudgell'd scars' that result from the pox, the symptoms must necessarily be seen as a 'malady' both contracted in and associated with France.

Luxury and Lechery/Vanity and Venery[23]

In the late sixteenth and early seventeenth century, the importation of silk, satin, and velvet from the Continent had reached an all time high. After wine, the primary imports were silks and velvets from Italy.[24] By the late years of that century, luxury cloth imports from Spain, as well as from France and Italy, had increased six-fold and were the most prominent class of imports.[25] By the turn of the century, there was a growing complaint from those involved in the manufacture of English cloth: the increased consumption, both at home and abroad, of textiles from the Continent, contributed to a crisis for the English domestic wool industry – England's major source of employment and primary export trade.[26] As the depression in the cloth industry in the late sixteenth and early seventeenth century was in large part blamed on the craze for foreign fashions, grievances against the consumption of foreign goods were almost always also complaints about the decline of the wool trade at home. The proliferation of literature in the period that takes up the subject of foreign fabrics reveals the extent to which the disruption of the cloth trade had become a national concern. Indeed, popular writers of the time were in effect echoing the preoccupations of the authorities who were troubled by the precarious position in which the domestic industry had been placed by the burgeoning trade in foreign cloth. The assault in print on those who bought and wore foreign clothes, and the linkage of those clothes to disease, also indicated the damage these actions inflicted on England's nationhood.

In the hands of these writers, the obsession with luxury goods from France in particular, represented leisure, decadence, disease, and – most crucially – dissolution of the virtues associated with English textiles: charity,

---

23Portions of the following section appear in a recent article. Hentschell, 'Treasonous Textiles,' pp. 543–546 and pp. 549–551.

24Davis, *English Overseas Trade*, p. 27.

25Stone, 'Elizabethan Overseas Trade,' p. 49.

26Bowden, *The Wool Trade*, p. 186.

hospitality, and humility.[27] Foreign fabrics on English bodies were not only an affront to the cloth industry, but also blurred the line between English and foreign. Unabashed consumption of the fabrics from the Continent compelled writers of the period to associate those who wore foreign fashion with the scandalous qualities of the country of origin. Simply donning the fabrics and fashions from these countries invited the corruption into England. As Barnabe Rich laments, '*Sinne* hath her *Silkmen* and *Mercers*, that doth serve her of *lace, silke, sattin, velvet, cloath of silver, cloath of gold . . . Sinne* hath her *Merchants*, that will transport the commodities behooveful for the commonwealth, into forraine countries, and will return backe again *toies* and *trifles*' (A4^{v}–B1^{r}). Silkmen and Mercers, those who traffic in luxury goods, are seen as evil agents who peddle their vice-ridden fabrics in England. Woven into the clothing is the vice of pride, which carries with it the French Disease. Thus, avoiding French fabric, seen as 'toies and trifles,' served a dual purpose – one would uphold the integrity of the nation though rejecting vanity associated with the French as well the disease nominally assigned to them. By avoiding luxury textiles one could also avoid lechery – the two words were synonymous in the early modern period.

More disturbing than the soldiers and courtiers who contracted the French Disease while in France consorting with strangers and taking in their customs, are those who have shown symptoms of the disease never having left England. In *The Time's Whistle*, by R.C., the speaker describes a young gallant guilty of this very sin: 'Nothus . . . / hath been late in France, / Yet never crost the seas' (2513–2515). Although he has never left England, the speaker is 'sure hee's hugely Frenchifide, / Gallicus Morbus is his owne, I swear' (2518–2519). The 'Frenchifide' Nothus has received 'Gallicus Morbus' for his pains. Or, perhaps more accurately, contracting the disease Frenchifies the gallant, who is *not-us*. Which came first, significantly, is not clear. The desire to ape the French fashion, in particular, leads to the disease, especially among those who have not left England. Samuel Butler, in his 'Satire Upon Our Ridiculous Imitation of the French,' lambastes the English who have the desire to 'study all [France's] Tricks and Fashions / With epidemic Affectations' (7–8). The aping of French fashion, undertaken as a sort of academic exercise, is itself a disease. It is no wonder, then, that the epidemic of 'affectation' should lead to the spread of the other French disease. The Frenchified Englishman has received

27 For a discussion of the interplay between pathology and commerce, see Harris, *Sick Economies*, especially chap. 2, 'Syphilis and Trade: Thomas Starkey, Thomas Smith, *The Comedy of Errors*,' pp. 29–51.

More Tricks, than ever they were taught:
With sly Intrigues and Artifices
Usurp their Poxes, and their Vices;
With garnitures upon their Shoes,
Make good their Claim to gouty Toes;
By sudden Starts, and Shrugs, and Groans
Pretend to Aches in their Bones,
To Scabs and Botches, and lay Trains
To prove their Running of the Reins (37–46)[28]

The price for imitating the French in their apparel is the 'usurp[ation]' of their 'poxes and vices.' The diseases that the English contract are the 'tricks' that attend preoccupation with foreign styles. With the contraction of the French pox, the English lose their proper national identity. The speaker concludes that in the aping of the French, the English 'Be *Natives* wheresoe'er they come, / And only *Foreigners* at home' (59–60).

The trope of the Frenchified English person, who has lost his or her own national identity in his obsession with French fashion, is common. In his eighty-eighth epigram, 'On English Monsieur,' for example, Ben Jonson ridicules the vainglorious pride in apparel of his subject and specifically the Englishman's obsession with clothes and accessories from France. Attired head to toe in French clothing, the Englishman becomes unrecognizable as such: he mutates into a 'Monsieur' through his very apparel. Jonson, however, does much more than simply deride the man's vanity. By asking his reader to marvel at the Englishman whose clothing belies his nationality, he puts into question the very identity of the English subject: 'Would you believe, when you this Monsieur see, / That his whole body should speak French, not he?' (1–2) Could the reader imagine, continues the speaker,

That so much scarf of France, and hat, and feather,
And shoe, and tie, and garter should come hither
And land on one whose face durst never be
Toward the sea, farther than half-way tree?

---

[28]Gout and gonorrhea (the 'running of the reins') were often seen as symptoms of the pox. As Margaret Pelling observes, 'By the early seventeenth century venereal disease had become another example of a condition identified differently according to the social class of the person affected. Among the upper or aspirant classes, syphilis – the "bone-ache" – was euphemistically called gout, rheumatism, or even sciatica.' Pelling, 'Appearance and Reality,' p. 98. This is echoed in Barnabie Rich's estimation of the French Disease in *The Honestie of this Age*: 'in poore men we use plaine dealing, & call it the *Poxe*, but in great personages, a little to gilde over the loathsomness, wee must call it the *Gowt*, or the *Sciatica*.' Rich, *Honestie*, sign. F4^r.

> That he, untravelled, should be French so much,
> As Frenchmen in his company should seem Dutch? (3–8)

The Englishman, though never having ventured beyond his homeland, has forsaken any signs that reveal his proper national identity by wearing the various French garments. He has invited foreign fashion 'hither,' thus becoming a foreigner in his own land. The body of the English subject, covered over with 'so much' that is French, not only obscures his Englishness, but also welcomes the unsavory qualities stereotypically associated with the French: vanity and moral laxity. The speaker then wonders if the monsieur's father, 'when he did him beget' had 'the French disease, with which he labours yet' (9, 10). The 'disease' with which the monsieur 'labours' is both his overt concern for fashion and also clearly the pox, which is evidenced through this concern. The disease is written on his body, not in scabs, but in scarves, silks, and feathers imported from France.

The young man of fashion was the primary target for the satirists who linked the pox with luxury clothing. To be sure, members of all social groups were susceptible to and concerned with the disease.[29] In the literature of the period, however, the writers seem to be focused on the affliction of the gentry – or those who had class aspirations. Perhaps this is because more privileged men, the very people who should be behaving according to their rank, were outwardly displaying their venery through a display of their vanity. John Marston's 'A Cynick Satyre,' from *The Scourge of Villanie* (1598), suggests that the gentleman donning foreign attire invites both physical infection and evil into England:

> Seest thou yon gallant in the sumptuous clothes,
> How brisk, how spruce, how gorgiously he showes,
> Note his French-herring bones, but note no more,
> Unlesse thou spy his fayre appendant whore
> . . . .
> Is this a *Man*? Nay, an incarnate devill,
> That struts in vice, and glorieth in evill.[30]

The gallant in fancy fabrics, as Marston tells us, 'struts in vice,' suggesting that the clothes in which he parades around London represent evil itself. At the same time, these words indicate that by wearing these clothes he 'struts' 'vice' 'in;' he brings it, and evil, into the city. The foppish man's choice of clothes and his accompanying prostitute also suggest the pox. The fabric

---

29For a discussion of the pox in relation to class concerns, see Boehrer, 'Early Modern Syphilis,' p. 212 and Anselment, 'Seventeenth-Century Pox,' pp. 193–194.

30Marston, 'A Cynick Satyre,' verse 17–20, 26–27.

from which his suit is made, herring-bone, is a silk or velvet from Lyon having a herring-bone pattern. The proximity of the words 'bone' and 'French' would have been an obvious joke to Marston's audience as an ache in the bone was a well-known symptom of the pox.

In *The Hunting of the Pox* we see one of the best examples of how gallants' concern with fashion and manners collapses into the disease itself. The poem begins with the author's encounter with Pild-Garlicke, who appears to have symptoms of the pox: 'He had of Spanish buttons store upon his forehead mixt; / And where that they were falne away, there stooles in place were fixt' ($A4^r$). While the scabs and scars on Pild-Garlicke's forehead indicate that he is suffering from the symptoms of cutaneous pox, it is the description of Pild-Garlicke's attire that clearly reveals that he has the French Disease. The author sees him as

> a man that's male-content, His hat without a band:
> A sattin dublet somewhat torne, with bootes and breeches sutable,
> He seemd a gentleman, whose mind to fashion was not mutable.
> A falling band, God dambe me call'd, a rapier by his side,
> He ware no cloke; for comlinesse a cloke doeth often hide. ($A4^r$)

The purposeful disorder of his dress signals the affected persona of a malcontent; his disheveled clothing is an outward expression of his inward melancholia. Despite the seeming lack of attention to his clothes, Pild-Garlicke has a steadfast 'mind to fashion,' seen perhaps most clearly in his lack of cloak, which would hide the 'comliness' of his slightly – but deliberately – tattered 'sattin doublet.' Pild-Garlicke's luxury clothes, though, reveal the lechery that lurks beneath them. Both the scabs on his forehead and the clothes on his back give evidence for his affliction. Excess in apparel – or, as here, excessive attention to apparel – was a sign of one's pride that marked him as an outsider within his own land. His close affiliation with Morbus Gallicus renders Pild-Garlicke a Frenchified Englishman who cannot uphold English values so long as his desire for French clothing is 'immutable.' As Anselment asserts, 'the sense of otherness implicit in this dismissal of the English Monsieur or the man of mode invokes a standard of communal values: those outside are the dissolute and depraved who would sap the energies of the nation's vigor.'[31] Again, we see the concern with French fashions as a marker of the French Disease that has infiltrated the pure space of England. There is a recognition of the Englishmen's moral questionability. Insisting that the Englishman is an outsider also deflects blame from England. He is perceived as a foreigner in his own land and the physical signs of his disease as well as his clothes register this foreignness.

---

[31] Anselment, 'Seventeenth-Century Pox,' p. 199.

Vanity and venery were seen as particular problems among the wealthier members of urban society. It is significant that Pild-Garlicke is identified as a 'gentleman.' This is certainly evident through his clothes, but also through the symptoms of his venereal disease. The author at one point indicates the contemporaneous collocation of class and the disease: 'he the pox hath not three times, is not a gentleman' (B1^{r}). Pild-Garlicke himself says that he does not need to read the author's book because 'thrice have I read it all my selfe' (A4^{v}). His 'reading' of the book indicates that he has been afflicted with the disease three separate times and also that – according to the conventional wisdom – he can now be counted a gentleman. In *The Irish Hubbub*, Barnabie Rich similarly asserts that 'He shall not be accounted a Gentleman if that he doth not carry this mark of the pox about him' (E1^{r}).

While satirical texts focus their attention on the wealthy gallant, fashionable women are not immune from the disease. In *Pleasant Quippes for Upstart Newfangled Gentlewomen*, the speaker reveals the communicable dangers that are related to French farthingales:

> These hoopes that hippes and haunch do hide,
> and heave aloft the gay hoyst-traine:
> As they are now in use for pride,
> so did they first beginne of paine.
> When whoores in stewes had gotten poxe,
> This French devise, keep coats from smocks. (151–156)

The author suggests that the ostentatious farthingales, the apparatus made from whalebone that puffed out the skirts of ladies' kirtles and also prevented the dress from dragging on the ground, were invented by the French as a result of symptoms of the pox. The women who contracted the 'poxe' in whore-houses ('stewes') wore the farthingale to keep their dresses ('coats') from the undergarments ('smocks'), which were thought to carry the disease. In criticizing English women for adopting this fashion, the speaker suggests that wearing French accessories is indicative not only of vanity, but also of the disease's entry into the social body of England.

While there was concern that imported fashions and fabrics introduced venereal disease when they crossed national borders, once in the country, these fabrics were then capable of corrupting the *moral* fabric of England itself, exposing the land to the sins of the city. Just as 'pox was the reality that undermined many of the pretensions of urban life and symbolized its vice and falsity,'[32] so too did foreign luxury fabrics. In *Michaelmas Term*, Thomas Middleton links sexually transmitted disease specifically with the silks that

---

32 Pelling, 'Appearance and Reality,' p. 104.

country girls wear when they come to the city to be whores: 'So farewell wholesome weeds, where treasure pants, / And welcome silks, where lies disease and wants' (I.ii.49–50). In giving up modest country clothing in favour of the urban uniform of luxury goods, one must necessarily open oneself up to the lechery associated with the fabric. The French Disease, whether sartorial or physical, was regarded as a sin of the city, so it was mainly those in urban areas, or those susceptible to the lure of the city, that fell victim to the disease. As Sheldon Watts explains, 'Unlike urban folk or mercenary soldiers, rural people who spent their lives within a day or two's walking distance of their place of birth generally followed behavioral patterns which excluded casual sex, and with it the risk of syphilis.'[33]

The Link to Cloth

Although the texts that I have examined are satirical in their nature and metaphorical in their linking clothing to the disease, the question of whether early modern people believed that cloth could transmit the pox remains. In *Great Venus Unmasked*, Gideon Harvey reminded his readers that the French, with their 'entailed manginess,' 'are slovens in their linen' and thus could transmit their disease through cloth.[34] Despite the fact that the pox became increasingly identified as a venereal disease, in several texts we see an assumption that the disease may also be transmitted through non-sexual means. In *Medela Medicinae*, Marchamont Nedham details pervasive common notions of the transmission of the pox: 'they generally argue it may be done by *Kissing*, by the *same Bed*, the same *Close-stool*, by Meats and Drinks, by *Sweat*, by *Breathing*, by the same Hot-house, by Linen, by Clothes, by the same Cup, by putting on anothers Glove or Stockin, and indeed by all the ways of Conversation.'[35] While some individuals believed that one could contract the disease through direct contact with an infected individual, others believed that the disease could be picked up just as easily through food or clothing. All major medical writers on the subject during the period agreed that unclean underclothing and linens, or cloth that came into contact with a pock-ridden person, were particularly to be avoided.[36] In

---

33 Watts, *Epidemics and History*, pp. 128–129.

34 Harvey, *Great Venus Unmasked*, p. 12.

35 Nedham, *Medela Medicinae*, p. 136.

36 This fear of cloth as a transmitter of the disease may come from the same fear that developed with the plague. Thomas Cogan, in *The Haven of Health* (1584), advises individuals to take care in coming into contact with 'clothes of those persons or places where the plague hath beene. For these thinges retaine the infection longer than the ayre it selfe . . . The clothes, especially of wollen, except they be washed, fumed, ayred, and

1547, Andrew Boorde warns that 'the cause of these impedimentes or infyrmytes doth come many wayes, it maye come by lyenge in the shetes or bedde there where a pocky person hath the nyght before lyen in . . .'[37] William Clowes's revised treatise on the disease shows that the 'primitive' cause of the *lues venerea* 'is some bodily touching, either of some infected body, as by sheets, or wearing infected apparell' (U1^{r-v}). Peter Lowe acknowledges that the primary cause of the disease is 'the act of Venus,' but he claims that 'it proceeds also by lying in uncleane lynnen' and 'by wearing the garments of them which are infected' (B2^{r}). In the *Praxis Medicinae* (1632), Walter Bruele asserts that cutaneous pox was simply 'communicated to the mouth and skinne by clothes.'[38] Even in the later years of the seventeenth century we see that the belief in cloth as a source of transmission remained strong: Daniel Sennert posits 'that the contagious inquination [pollution], sent forth from the body infected with the venereal disease, may adhere to the garments.'[39]

To be sure, lesions did secrete onto clothes. Richard Wiseman describes one patient who was so replete with running sores that 'his shirt, drawers, and stockings [were] stiff with the matter that flowed from them.'[40] Despite the widespread dread of contact with 'infected' cloth, the medical community could not fully corroborate such a link. As we now know, it is highly unlikely that spirochetes from this venereal disease can be transmitted through non-biological means. Theodor Rosebury explains that 'compared with other microbes, which survive and multiply in many different environments, these VD microbes grow, in nature, only in man. Outside his tissues they not only fail to grow, but are quickly killed . . . The microbes' delicacy, their inability to survive outside human tissues, prevents them from being transmitted from one person to another by any sort of *indirect* means.'[41]

Despite the pervasive belief that cloth was a transmitter of the disease – and thus was to be avoided at all cost – it was curiously also often the very thing that was used in the treatment of the disease. For example, in order

---

layd foorth oftentimes in the winde and sunne, continue contagious by the space of three yeares and more.' Cogan, *Haven of Health*, sign. L1^{r}.

[37]Boorde, *The Breviary of Health*, sign. Bbiii^{v}.

[38]Bruele, *Praxis Medicinae,* p. 390.

[39]Sennert, *Two Treatises*, sign. B8^{r}.

[40]Wiseman, *Severall Chirurgicall Treatises*, p. 35.

[41]Rosebury, *Microbes and Morals*, p. 7. Fabricius claims that in the period 'a syphilitic barber, an infected cup or towel, or a kiss from a diseased person were enough to pass on the disease.' While there may have been remote chances of contracting the disease through indirect means, contact with infected human tissue is widely regarded as the only sure way to contract the disease. Fabricius, *Syphilis in Shakespeare's England*, p. 20.

to ease the inflammation of his own sores with a concoction of lyme and water, Hutten 'took a sponge or a linen cloth and dipped it in the water . . . and often time warmed and moistened my sores therewith washing and wiping away all the filthiness. Then I took a cloth so moistened and lapped it about my sores.' (B1^{r}). William Bullein, in his *Bulwark of Defence Against All Sickness*, explains that, when treating a patient, a caregiver should 'lay very many clothes on him, till he sweat, for the space of twoo houres, then ease some of the cloathes, and have warmed linnen cloathes, and rubbe all the bodie drie' (fol. 48). In his 1596 treatise, Clowes explains that some unctions should be applied on 'linnen cloth' (Cc1^{v}); some should be applied with a stick where 'a piece of linen cloth' will be tied 'like unto a painters pencill' (Dd4^{r}). The genitals were clearly the area of the body most associated with the disease, and in this area we see that cloth was important in the treatment process. Clowes details a particular case where a 'double hot cloth' was applied to the 'fundament' of a patient (X4^{r}), while the author of *The Rich Store-House of Treasury for the Diseased* suggests one liquid remedy for treating genital swelling: 'take a fine linnen cloth, and annoint the yarde [penis] under the skinne' (I3^{r-v}). Given that the expense of cloth in the period guaranteed that it would literally be used to pieces, it is very likely that the linen used to apply ointments and soothe and open sores on the genitals and elsewhere were rags derived from old bedclothes. Is it possible that medical experts believed that cloth was a transmitter of the disease at the same time they used it so often in treatments?

Conclusion

The intended audience and purpose of early modern medical manuals and satire concerning the pox were clearly different. As we have seen, however, one persistent, common element in these two types of text was that they deflected blame for the disease from the English to another nation, usually the French. Both medical manuals and satirical texts also linked the contraction of the French Disease to apparel. For the medical community, it was possible that this fiction provided a vehicle to exonerate upstanding infected individuals who refused to acknowledge that they might have consorted with prostitutes or other high-risk people.[42] Those who contracted the disease were not always or necessarily blamed for sexual iniquities

---

[42]John Graunt, an indexer of the mortality bills of seventeenth-century England, expressed frustration that deaths from the French Disease could never be accurately estimated since so many denied having the disease. Graunt, *Natural and Political Observations*, p. 22.

'because they could supposedly contract the disease in a variety of other ways as well.'[43] As Clowes (1585) makes clear, 'This sicknesse is sayd first to be engendred by the accompaning with unclene women, which although it be moste commonly true, yet it is not alwayes so, nor in all persons' (A2^{v}). The general perception, however, *was* that the pox was associated with immoral behavior – especially consorting with prostitutes – and authorities clearly had an interest in perpetuating the notion that it could be picked up in a variety of ways. As in the early years of AIDS in the western world, the myth of contraction through the clothes of the infected (and other non-biological means) served to create a panic befitting a disease so closely associated with sexual immorality.

As Kevin Siena has argued, 'medical authorities employed the frightening image of venereal disease to help create and enforce danger beliefs aimed at policing behavior – behavior that was usually, but not always, sexual.'[44] Spreading the belief that the pox could be passed on through cloth, an item that virtually everyone touched every day, engendered anxieties that *anyone* could contract the disease and thus be susceptible to the shame and fear associated with it. The disturbing image of the infected person, while pathologized in medical discourse, was made increasingly familiar though popular satire. In this literature, the commonplace association of the French Disease and the desire for French clothing served as a warning for those who would follow foreign fashions. The legitimate fear of the pox thus translated into a biting, inflated xenophobic rhetoric intent on vilifying the French, especially, and other Catholic countries, in order to distance the English from associations with the new disease.

In this deflection of blame onto the other we can see how the discourse around the pox contributed to early modern English nation formation. As we have seen, the insistence on locating the disease – and the sins of vanity and venery with which it is associated – *elsewhere* is a crucial aspect of the rhetoric of these authors. These narratives of the pox, whether fictional or medical, didactic or satiric, serve to consolidate an emerging nationalism in their insistence on an English detachment from the disease. It is in knowing the strangers and all their iniquities that we can identify and thus celebrate ourselves for not being *them*. Nations, and the sentiments of belief in nations, are necessarily constructed and performed; one important way in which this occurs is through printed texts.[45] As Benedict Anderson has famously

---

[43]Bentley, *Shakespeare and the New Disease*, p. 27.

[44]Siena, 'Pollution, Promiscuity, and the Pox,' p. 555.

[45]See Richard Helgerson's remarks in *Forms of Nationhood* on the 'four-way exchange' of texts, nations, authors, and discursive communities: 'All are both produced and

argued, printed language is a fundamental aspect of nascent nationalism because the readers, 'connected through print, formed . . . the embryo of the nationally imagined community.'[46] Particularly in times of crisis – as we see so clearly with the advent of the pox into England – the discourse of nationalism helps a community cope with unnerving and scandalous threats. In this sense, the language of nation 'fills the void left in the uprooting of communities and kin, and turns that loss into the language of metaphor.'[47] While the language in the fictive as well as medical literature on the pox is often metaphorical, usually hyperbolic, and always crafted, it is important that we regard the inflated rhetoric as more than just a cavalier chauvinism. Rather it is an integral contribution to the articulation of national identity in the early modern period.

Colorado State University
Fort Collins, Colorado

Cited Works

Anderson, Benedict. *Imagined Communities: Reflections on the Origins and Spread of Nationalism*. New York: Verso, 1983.

Anselment, Raymond. 'Seventeenth-Century Pox: The Medical and Literary Realities of Venereal Disease' *Seventeenth Century*, 4:2 (1989): 189–211.

Barrough, Philip. *The Method of Physick, Containing the Causes, Signs, and Cures of Inward Diseases in Man's Body From the Head to the Foote*. London: Richard Field, 1596.

Beaumont, Francis. *The Knight of the Burning Pestle*, pp. 390–431 in *Renaissance Drama: An Anthology of Plays and Entertainments*, ed. Arthur F. Kinney. Malden, Massachusetts and Oxford: Blackwell, 1999.

Beaumont, Francis and John Fletcher. *Cupid's Revenge*, pp. 315–448 in *The Dramatic Works in the Beaumont and Fletcher Canon*. Vol. 2. ed. Fredson Bowers. Cambridge: Cambridge University Press, 1970.

Bentley, Greg W. *Shakespeare and the New Disease: The Dramatic Function of Syphilis in Troilus and Cressida, Measure for Measure, and Timon of Athens*. New York: Peter Lang, 1989.

Bhabha, Homi K. 'DisseminNation: Time, Narrative, and the Margins of the Modern Nation' pp. 291–322 in *Nation and Narration*, ed. Homi K. Bhabha. New York: Routledge, 1990.

Boehrer, Bruce Thomas. 'Early Modern Syphilis' *Journal of the History of Sexuality*, 1:2 (1990): 197–214.

---

productive,' p. 13. For an excellent discussion of the relationship between the body and nationalism in early modern England, see Susanne Scholz, *Body Narratives*.

[46] Anderson, *Imagined Communities*, p. 47.

[47] Bhabha, 'DissemiNation,' p. 291.

Boorde, Andrew. *The Breviary of Health*. London: William Powell, 1557.

Bowden, Peter J. *The Wool Trade in Tudor and Stuart England*. London: Macmillan, 1962.

Bruele, Walter. *Praxis Medicinae*. London: John Norton for William Sheares, 1632.

Bullein, William. *Bullein's Bulwark of Defence against all Sickness, Sores, and Wounds that do Daily Assault Mankind*. London: John Kingston, 1562.

Butler, Samuel. 'Satyr Upon Our Ridiculous Imitation of the French' pp. 49–52 in *Satires and Miscellaneous Poetry and Prose*, ed. René Lamar. Cambridge: Cambridge University Press, 1978.

R. C. *The Times' Whistle*, ed. J. M. Cowper. London: Early English Text Society, 1871.

Clowes, William. *A Briefe and Necessarie Treatise Touching the Cure of the Disease Called Morbus Gallicus, or Lues Venerea, by Unctions and Other Approoued Waies of Curing*. London: Thomas East, 1585.

Clowes, William. *A Briefe and Necessary Treatise Touching the Disease Now Usually Called Lues Venerea, by Unctions and Other Approued Waies of Curing: Newly Corrected and Augmented*. London: Edm. Bollifant 1596.

Cogan, Thomas. *The Haven of Health*. London: Henrie Midleton, 1584.

Davis, Ralph. *English Overseas Trade, 1500–1700*. London: Macmillan, 1973.

Fabricius, Johannes. *Syphilis in Shakespeare's England*. London: Jessica Kingsley Publishers, 1994.

Foa, Anna. 'The New and the Old: The Spread of Syphilis (1494–1530)' pp. 26–45 in *Sex and Gender in Historical Perspective*, eds. Edward Muir and Guido Ruggiero. Baltimore: The Johns Hopkins University Press, 1990.

French, Roger and Jon Arrizabalaga. 'Coping with the French Disease. University Practitioners' Strategies and Tactics in the Transition from the Fifteenth to the Sixteenth Century' pp. 248–287 in *Medicine from the Black Death to the French Disease*, eds. Roger French, Jon Arrizabalaga, Andrew Cunningham and Luis Garcia-Ballester. Aldershot: Ashgate, 1998.

Gilman, Sander. *Disease and Representation: Images of Illness from Madness to AIDS*. Ithaca and London: Cornell University Press, 1988.

Graunt, John. *Natural and Political Observations Mentioned in a Following Index, and Made Upon the Bills of Mortality*. London: Thomas Roycroft, 1662.

Greene, Robert. *A Disputation Between a Hee and Shee Conny-Catcher*, pp. 196–278 in *The Life and Complete Works in Prose and Verse of Robert Greene*. Vol. 10. ed. Alexander B. Grosart. NewYork: Russell & Russell, 1964.

Harris, Jonathan Gil. *Foreign Bodies and the Body Politic: Discourses of Social Pathology in Early Modern England*. Cambridge: Cambridge University Press, 1998.

Harris, Jonathan Gil. *Sick Economies: Drama, Mercantilism, and Disease in Shakespeare's England*. Philadelphia: University of Pennsylvania Press, 2004.

Harvey, Gideon. *Great Venus Unmasked: Or a More Exact Discovery of the Venereal Evil or French Disease*. Second edition. London: Printed by B.G. for Nath. Brook, 1672.

Helgerson, Richard. *Forms of Nationhood: The Elizabethan Writing of England*. Chicago: University of Chicago Press, 1992.

Hentschell, Roze. 'Treasonous Textiles: Foreign Cloth and the Construction of Englishness' *Journal of Medieval and Early Modern Studies*, 32:3 (2002): 543–570.

Hoenselaars, A.J. *Images of Englishmen and Foreigners in the Drama of Shakespeare and His Contemporaries: A Study of Stage Characters and National Identity in English Renaissance Drama, 1558–1642*. Rutherford, N.J.: Fairleigh Dickinson University Press, 1992.

Holinshed, Raphael. *Chronicles of England, Scotland, and Ireland*. Vol. 3. New York: AMS Press Inc., 1976.

Hutten, Ulrich Von. *De medicina guaici, et morbo gallico*, trans. Thomas Paynell. London: Thomas Bertheleti, 1533.

Jonson, Ben. 'On English Monsieur' pp. 251–252 in *Ben Jonson: A Critical Edition of the Major Works*, ed. Ian Donaldson. Oxford: Oxford University Press, 1985.

Lowe, Peter. *An Easy, Certain, and Perfect Method to Cure and Prevent the Spanish Sickness*. London: J. Roberts, 1596.

Marston, John. *The Scourge of Villanie,* pp. 93–176 in *The Poems of John Marston*, ed. Arnold Davenport. Liverpool: Liverpool University Press, 1961.

Massinger, Philip. *The Emperor of the East,* pp. 401–488 in *The Plays and Poems of Philip Massinger,* Vol. 3. ed. Philip Edwards and Colin Gibson. Oxford: The Clarendon Press, 1976.

Middleton, Thomas. *A Mad World, My Masters,* ed. Standish Henning. Lincoln: University of Nebraska Press, 1965

Middleton, Thomas. *Michaelmas Term*, ed. Richard Levin. Lincoln: University of Nebraska Press, 1966.

Miller, John. *Popery and Politics in England, 1660–1680*. Cambridge: Cambridge University Press, 1973.

Nedham, Marchamont. *Medela Medicinae*. London: Richard Lownds, 1665.

A New Method of Curing the French Pox. Amsterdam: John Taylor and Thomas Newborough, 1690.

Pelling, Margaret. 'Appearance and Reality: Barber-Surgeons, the Body, and Disease' pp. 82–112 in *London 1500–1700: The Making of the Metropolis*, ed. A.L. Beier and Roger Finlay. London and New York: Longman, 1986.

Pleasant Quippes for Upstart Newfangled Gentlewomen, ed. Edwin Johnston Howard. Oxford, Ohio: The Anchor Press, 1942.

Rosebury, Theodor. *Microbes and Morals: The Strange Story of Venereal Disease*. New York: The Viking Press, 1971.

Rich, Barnabe. *The Honestie of this Age*. London: Thomas Dawson, 1614.

Rich, Barnabe. *The Irish Hubbub Or, The English Hue and Crie*. London: George Purslowe, 1617.

Rich, Barnabe. *My Ladies Looking Glasse*. London: John Legat, 1616.

Rowlands, Samuel. *Humors Ordinarie*. London: William Firebrand, 1605 (?).

Russell, Jocelyne G. *The Field of the Cloth of Gold: Men and Manners in 1520*. London: Routledge & Kegan Paul, 1969.

L. S. Προφυλακτικον*[Profulacticon]: Or Some Considerations of a Notable Expedient to root out the French Pox from the English Nation*. London, 1673.

Schleiner, Winfried. 'Infection and Cure Through Women: Renaissance Constructions of Syphilis' *Journal of Medieval and Renaissance Studies,* 24:3 (1994): 499–517.

Schleiner, Winfried. 'Moral Attitudes toward Syphilis and Its Prevention in the Renaissance' *Bulletin of the History of Medicine,* 68 (1994): 389–410.

Scholz, Susanne. *Body Narratives: Writing the Nation and Fashioning the Subject in Early Modern England.* New York: St. Martin's Press, 2000.

Sennert, Daniel. *Two Treatises,* trans. Nicholas Culpeper. London: John Streater, 1673.

Shakespeare, William. *All's Well That Ends Well,* pp. 538–575 in *The Riverside Shakespeare.* 2nd ed. Ed. G. Blakemore Evans. Boston: Houghton Mifflin, 1997.

Shakespeare, William. *Henry V,* pp. 979–1020 in *The Riverside Shakespeare.* 2nd ed. Ed. G. Blakemore Evans. Boston: Houghton Mifflin, 1997.

Shakespeare, William. *Henry VIII,* pp. 1026–1064 in *The Riverside Shakespeare.* 2nd ed. Ed. G. Blakemore Evans. Boston: Houghton Mifflin, 1997.

Siena, Kevin P. 'Pollution, Promiscuity, and the Pox: English Venereology and the Early Modern Medical Discourse on Social and Sexual Danger' *Journal of the History of Sexuality,* 8:4 (1998): 553–574.

Sontag, Susan. *AIDS and Its Metaphors.* New York: Farrar, Straus and Giroux, 1989.

Stone, Lawrence. 'Elizabethan Overseas Trade' *Economic History Review,* 2nd ser. 2. (1949): 30–58.

A. T. *A Rich Store-House of Treasury for the Diseased.* London: Thomas Purfoot, 1596.

J. T. of Westminster. *The Hunting of the Pox: A Pleasant Discourse Between the Author, and Pild-Garlicke.* London: J. White, 1619.

Walker, William. *A Sermon Preached at the Funerals of the Right Honourable, William Lord Russell.* London: Thomas Snodham, 1614.

Watts, Sheldon. *Epidemics and History: Disease, Power, and Imperialism.* New Haven: Yale University Press, 1997.

The Whore of Babylon's Pockey Priest. London: Thomas Fox, 1679/80.

Williams, Gordon. 'An Elizabethan Disease' *Trivium,* 6 (1971): 43–58.

Wiseman, Richard. *Several Chirurgicall Treatises.* London: E. Flesher and J. Macock, 1676.

Linguistic Dis-ease: *Foreign Language as Sexual Disease in Early Modern England*

Diane Cady

Language is a virus
William Burroughs

The pox first appeared in Europe at the end of the fifteenth century. In the decades that followed, the disease accumulated names almost as rapidly as it spread across the Continent. The Germans and the English called it the French Disease. The French, in turn, dubbed it the Italian disease. The Japanese thought the Chinese or, alternatively, the Portuguese spawned the illness. The Russians blamed the Poles, and the Persians blamed the Turks. Still others argued that contact with the indigenous people of the 'New World' brought the disease to Europe. By 1524, Ulrich von Hutten identified some 200 names for the pox, most of which linked the disease to various nationalities.[1] In 1530, Girolamo Fracastoro attempted to detach the pox from the nation and jettison it to a pastoral space. According to Fracastoro, the shepherd Syphilis was the first to contract the disease as punishment for insulting Apollo. Yet, as suggested by the very title of his treatise – *Syphilis, sive Morbus Gallicus* – the disease is not easily separated from nationality. It is as if the pox refuses the natural and chooses the nation.

Why is this disease so inextricably tied to the nation in the early modern period, as if nationality itself is a sign of infection? On the most basic level, labelling another country as the source of the pox releases an individual – and indeed an entire nation – from blame for a disease that was often seen as a sign of divine retribution. Projection also serves a nation's ideological needs in a more complex fashion. First, it helps a nation manage its anxiety about a mysterious disease for which there is no cure. By displacing illness onto a given group, the 'mainstream' can assure itself that it is impervious

[1]Nelkin and Gilman, 'Placing Blame for Devastating Disease,' p. 365.

to infection. Second, by making foreigners synonymous with disease, the nation wields a powerful tool for constructing national identity. As Susan Sontag explains in a discussion of syphilis,

> there is a link between imagining disease and imagining foreignness. It lies perhaps in the very concept of the wrong, which is archaically identical with the non-us, the alien. A polluting person is always wrong, as Mary Douglas has observed. The inverse is also true: a person judged to be wrong is regarded as, at least potentially, a source of pollution.[2]

Thus a pernicious dialectic develops: disease and its stigmatizing effects are projected onto certain groups and these groups in turn are stigmatized (or perhaps more correctly, pathologized) through their association with disease. Links established between certain groups and diseases become added proof that these groups are rightly ostracized and serve as a rallying cry for their continued marginalization and surveillance. By projecting disease onto others, a nation can consolidate national identity, differentiating citizens (the healthy) from aliens (the diseased).[3]

Once the connection between foreigners and disease enters the social imaginary it becomes available to describe other national ills, many of which are suspected of infiltrating England from the Continent. For example, in *A Treatise of the Canker of England's Commonwealth* (whose title makes reference to one of the most visible signs of the pox), Gerard de Malynes describes the imbalance between foreign and domestic commodities as 'the unknowne disease of the politicke body.'[4] And as Roze Hentschell demonstrates in her article in this volume, blaming foreign clothing for the transmission of disease converts an economic matter into an issue of public health. Certainly these metaphoric deployments of disease are not unique to the early modern period. As Sontag has shown, they pervade our own historical moment as well, an issue to which I will return at the end of this essay. However, at a time when another metaphor dominated early modern society – the idea of the nation as a body – these images of foreigners and foreign influences as disease had a particular power to horrify.[5]

---

[2]Sontag, *Aids and Its Metaphors*, p. 48.

[3]On the ideological motivations behind blaming others for disease, see Sontag, *Illness as Metaphor*; and Sontag, *AIDS and Its Metaphors*; Nelkin and Gilman, 'Placing Blame for Devastating Disease'; Foa, 'The New and the Old,' pp. 26–45; Gilman, 'Plague in Germany, 1939/1989,' pp. 175–200; and Gilman, *Picturing Health and Illness*.

[4]Malynes, *A Treatise of the Canker of Englands Commonwealth*, sign. B2^r. Unless otherwise indicated, early modern spellings are reproduced.

[5]See Harris, *Foreign Bodies and the Body Politic*, for an extended and fascinating discussion of how various foreign agents (including Jews, Catholics and witches) are

In this essay I focus on one specific social ill imagined to infect early modern England: foreign words. It is no coincidence that when England's anxiety about the influx of strangers reaches its zenith, writers begin to complain that foreigners are flooding the language, as well as the country. Associating foreign language with pollution and disease pathologizes the presence of foreign words. It also provides opponents of foreign immigration with additional 'proof' that anything that smacks of the alien is diseased and polluted and needs to be kept out of the country. We can see, then, why Fracastoro's fiction does not take hold. The connection between the alien and disease is itself a fiction that is too vital for the construction of national identity to be surrendered. The trope of foreign language as disease serves, however, another function. In this period polluted language is not only depicted as something foreign, but also as something feminine. The English language is likened to a male body continually besieged by this feminine and feminizing infection. Women, as much as foreigners, threaten its supposed masculinity. As we will see in plays such as *Jack Drum's Entertainment* and *Englishmen for my Money, or A Woman Will Have Her Will*, women's bodies are the sites where the domestic and the foreign, the healthy and the diseased, commingle promiscuously. The image of foreign language as disease and women as conduits through which this disease enters the body politic, reminds the nation that it must keep an eye on its women as well as its borders.

★ ★ ★

Oure language is so rustye
So cankered and so dull

Foreign words were not always imagined as a disease that infected the English language. Indeed, for much of the fifteenth and sixteenth centuries it was English that was thought to be, as *The Boke of Philype Sparowe* puts it, a 'cankered' language.[6] According to a number of writers, the problem with English was twofold. With its monosyllabic words and harsh sounds, English seemed ineloquent when compared to the more mellifluous classical lan-

imagined to be infiltrating the body politic. See also Healy, *Fictions of Disease*.

6Skelton, *Philip Sparrow*, p. 82. Also cited by Jones in *The Triumph of the English Language*, p. 27. Jones amasses a wealth of early modern opinions about English, and my discussion of the shifting attitudes toward English is indebted to his study, as well as Bailey, *Images of English*, pp. 17–57. On the development of a national language and literature in the sixteenth century and the role they play in the construction of England as a nation, see Helgerson, *Forms of Nationhood*. For a discussion of the role gender plays in the development of national English, see Fleming, 'Dictionary English and the Female Tongue,' pp. 290–325.

guages and continental vernaculars. For example, in a translation of *Xenophon*, Wylliam Barkar complains that compared to Greek 'oure tongue is a rude and a barren tong.'[7] Even in the nationalistic *First Boke of the Introduction of Knowledge*, Andrew Boorde concedes that 'the speche of Englande [is] a base speche to other noble speeches, as Italion, Castylion and French.'[8] Part of the difficulty with English was that it lacked the copious vocabularies of other languages. As Ralph Lever observes in *The Arte of Reason, Rightly Termed, Witcraft*, such a situation leaves the speaker of English feeling that there are 'moe things, than there are words to expresse things by.'[9]

To overcome English's deficiencies a number of sixteenth-century writers recommend importing foreign words. As Richard Eden explains in a letter to Sir William Cecil, by adopting words from 'Latine and other tongues' what was once an 'indigent and barbarous' language becomes an 'enriched and amplified one.'[10] Richard Carew also promotes linguistic borrowing in 'An Epistle Concerning the Excellencies of the English Tongue.' He notes that 'the long words that we borrow being intermingled with the short of our owne store, make up a perfect harmonie, by culling from out which mixture (with judgment) you may frame your speech.'[11] Many advocates of this policy imagine foreign words as a kind of linguistic citizen, taking up residency in the English language. In *The Boke Named the Governour*, for example, Thomas Elyot argues that 'wordes late comen out of Italy and France' have been 'made denizens amonge us.'[12] And in the *Remains Concerning Britain*, William Camden notes that

> the alteration and innovation in our tongue as in all others, hath beene brought in by the entrance of Strangers, as Danes, Normans, and others which have swarmed hither, by trafficke, for new words as well as for new wares, have always come in by the tyranne Time which altereth all under heaven...it hath beautified and enriched out of other good tongues, partly by enfranchising and endenizzing strange words...happily containing themselves within the bounds prescribed by Horace.[13]

While Camden imagines foreign words remaining 'happily contained' within English's linguistic boundaries, his description of foreigners 'swarm-

[7]Barkar, *The Bookes of Xenophon*, sign. A6.

[8]Boorde, *The Fyrst Boke of the Introduction of Knowledge*, p. 122.

[9]Lever, *The Arte of Reason, Rightly Termed, Witcraft*, fol. 5^v.

[10]Cit. in Moore, *Tudor-Stuart Views on the Growth, Status, and Destiny of the English Language*, p. 95.

[11]Carew, 'An Epistle Concerning the Excellencies of the English Tongue,' p. 43.

[12]Elyot, *The Boke Named the Governour*, 1.22.96.

[13]Camden, *Remains Concerning Britain*, p. 29.

ing' into England perhaps reflects the growing concern at the end of the sixteenth century that not only the language, but also the country, has been inundated with strangers. Although immigration into England is not unique to the end of the sixteenth century, a dramatic increase in the number of immigrants does occur during this period, in part because of religious persecution in Flanders.[14] Foreign craftsmen settling in England were expected to share their skills and methods with their English counterparts, laws forbidding alien apprentices, restricting the number of alien journeymen in a foreign shop, and criminalizing the separation of English and alien apprentices were enacted to ensure the transmission of these foreign skills.[15] Thus, just as the importation of foreign words might mitigate English's deficiencies, the influx of skilled foreign workers could have a salubrious effect on the English economy, which had suffered since the collapse of the wool industry in 1551. However, many English artisans believed that these laws were not adequately enforced. William Cunningham has illustrated that English craftsmen petitioned Tudor-Stuart monarchs incessantly about foreign commodities, which threatened to 'beggereth' domestic trade.[16]

Foreigners were imagined to be displacing Englishmen not only economically, but sexually as well. Indeed, the economic and the sexual often converge in complaints about strangers. For example, in a sermon that served as a catalyst for the May Day Riots of 1517 (in which some 2000 apprentices sacked French and Flemish craftsmen's homes and attacked Florentine and German merchants) a preacher warns that 'strangers not only deprived the English of their industry and profits arising therefrom but dishonoured their dwellings by taking their wives and daughters.'[17] Here, what begins as an economic threat quickly slips into a warning about sexual dispossession and disgrace. While economic worries may be paramount in the minds of the English crowd, the preacher seems to understand that painting a picture of a sexually rapacious group of strangers who threaten their wives and daughters may do more to enflame their anger. Such is the case in the opening scene of *Othello*. Iago and Roderigo begin with warnings about economic loss: 'thieves, thieves, thieves! / Look to your house, your daughter, and your bags' (1.1.79–80) and ''Swounds, sir, you're robbed'

---

[14]For example, perhaps as many as 10,000 Flemish lived in various parts of England in 1567. By 1573, the number had increased to 60,000. For a discussion of England's changing demographics, see Brennan, 'The Cheese and the Welsh,' pp. 40–64; and Cunningham, *Alien Immigrants to England*.

[15]Brennan, 'The Cheese and the Welsh,' p. 62.

[16]Cunningham, *Alien Immigrants to England*, p. 168.

[17]Cit. in Brennan, 'The Cheese and the Welsh,' p. 62.

(1.1.86). However, it is their graphic description of Desdemona's 'gross revolt' with the 'extravagant and wheeling stranger' (1.1.135–137) that spurs Brabanzio into action. Images of sexual dishonour and dispossession are effective weapons in anti-foreign rhetoric because women are not simple economic assets (the property of their husbands and fathers), but rather economic assets, which, if stolen, affect a man's personal honour as well as his economic livelihood.[18]

There may be more at stake in this equation than a man's personal honour. As a number of scholars have noted in recent years, early modern notions of the nation gravitate towards the somatic.[19] Such an orientation allows for more than just colourful and elaborate analogies. As Mary Douglas explains, the body 'is a model which can stand for any bounded system. Its boundaries can represent any boundaries which are threatened or precarious.'[20] Pollution is imagined to enter through the body's orifices, those places that are simultaneously within the boundaries of the body and are in contact with the potential pollution outside those boundaries.[21] If pollution is symbolic,[22] miscegenation serves as its perfect symbol. Literally the mixing of races (*miscere* + *genus*), miscegenation represents a boundary crossing wherein something from the outside enters the social body through a vulnerable orifice. Miscegenation becomes a way to translate immigration into bodily terms.

The xenophobic play *The Pedler's Prophecy* clearly presents miscegenation as a pollution that threatens the nation's supposed purity. The peddler criticizes the mariners for bringing into England 'Fortie thousand enemies to the Crowne, / The deadly poison of hell' in the form of 'Jewes, Ruffians, Moores, Turkes and Tartarians.' With these, he argues, they have 'mixed the virgins' (D^{r-v}), so that now

> Three parts of London are already Alians,
> Other mongrels, Alains children, mischieviously mixed,
> And that with the most detestable
> Which here for ever hath their dwellings fixed:
> Still you Mariners bring them in daily. ($D2^{r-v}$)

---

[18]On women as economic assets that reflect men's honour, see Stallybrass, 'Patriarchal Territories: The Body Enclosed,' pp. 123–144; and Woodbridge, 'Palisading the Elizabethan Body Politic,' pp. 327–353.

[19]The literature on this subject is extensive. See, for example, Hale, *The Body Politic*'; Stallybrass, 'Patriarchal Territories: The Body Enclosed'; Woodbridge, 'Palisading the Elizabethan Body Politic'; Paster, *The Body Embarrassed*; Harris, *Foreign Bodies*, especially pp. 1–47; and Scholz, *Body Narratives*.

[20]Douglas, *Purity and Danger*, p. 116.

[21]Douglas, *Purity and Danger*, p. 122.

[22]Douglas, *Purity and Danger*, p. 126.

These lines take to a hysterical and nightmarish extreme William Camden's depiction of foreigners swarming into England. The image of an ever-growing population of aliens suggests an epidemic. And indirectly, foreigners are presented as a sexual disease, one transmitted into the body politic through the sexual mixing of English virgins with this 'deadly poison,' (a phrase which, as we will see in a moment, physician Daniel Sennert will use to describe the pox). According to the *Pedlar's Prophecy*, miscegenation is an issue of national security because through interracial marriage foreigners become permanent residents in England where they breed a 'mischieviously mixed' race of children. In addition, much like the projection of disease onto others, describing interracial children as 'mongrels' is a way to differentiate Englishmen and foreigners from one another. These lines suggest that they are different species and any mixing between the races will produce nonhuman offspring. Iago and Roderigo draw on similar images of bestiality and monstrous offspring to agitate Brabanzio: they tell him that 'an old black ram / Is tupping your white ewe' (1.1.88–89); that 'your daughter and the / Moor are now making the beast with two backs' (1.1.117–118); and that if he fails to stop the marriage, 'you'll have your daughter / covered with a Barbary horse, you'll have your nephews neigh / to you, you'll have coursers for cousins and jennets for germans' (1.1.112–115). Since deformed offspring were one of the unfortunate side effects of the pox,[23] these images of bestial coupling and monstrous births further link foreigners with disease. If Englishwomen are 'mischieviously mixed' with foreigners, disease will be the result, a disease that will seep into the body politic.

The opening scene of the *Pedler's Prophecy* articulates more explicitly the national ramifications of interracial marriage. When the peddler asks the father why his daughter remains unmarried, the latter explains that he is loath to marry her to a stranger. The mother agrees that such marriages should be avoided:

> Yea either they be Alians, or Aliant sonnes indeed,
> Who through marriage of English women of late,
> Hath altered the true English blood and seed,
> And therewithal English plaine maners and good state,
> All the naughtie fashions in the world at this day,
> Are by some meanes brought into England. (B2ᵛ–B3ʳ)

In these few lines one finds a terse construction of the foreigner as potentially polluting other. Aliens and their children are grouped together in line one

---

[23]Healy, *Fictions of Disease*, pp. 126–128.

and placed in opposition to 'Englishness,' a notion that is developed through repetition: there is 'English blood and seed' and 'English plaine maners and good state,' and miscegenation threatens to alter all of these. Such dilution constitutes pollution since the 'naughtie fashions in the world' are brought into England through these marriages. Finally, reference to 'the good state' reminds the reader that interracial marriage is a matter of national security.

I will have more to say about the ways in which foreigners and miscegenation supposedly threaten the 'good state' in a moment. For now, however, I want to return to early modern attitudes towards English, and specifically changes taking place in those attitudes during the last quarter of the sixteenth century. In many ways these changes parallel the anxieties surrounding foreigners. As already noted, for most of the sixteenth century English writers found their tongue deficient because of its monosyllabic qualities and its dearth of words. As a curative, writers such as William Camden recommend enfranchising foreign words, provided they remain 'happily contained' within their linguistic boundaries. By the end of the sixteenth century, however, writers are no longer complaining that English is too barren a tongue. Rather, the concern now is that the language has become too fertile and that, much like the foreign population as imagined in *The Pedlar's Prophecy*, it is increasing exponentially. John Florio, for example, argues in his prefatory letter to *A Worlde of Wordes*, that there is a 'yearly increase' of words.[24] In 'Of English Verse,' Edmund Waller fears that on account of this lexical influx, works written today will be incomprehensible tomorrow: 'We write in sand, our language grows / And like our tide, / our work o'erflows' (l.15–16). A number of Waller's contemporaries blame this linguistic overflow on the practice of importing foreign words. For example, in his dedicatory letter to *The Shepheardes Calendar*, E.K complains that by filling English's deficiencies with 'peces and rags of other languages, borrowing here of French, there of the Italian, everywhere of the Latine...they have made our English tongue a gallimaufray or hodgepodge of al other speeches.'[25] In *The Arte of English Poesie*, George Puttenham states that a 'mingle mangle' occurs 'when we make our speech or writings of sundry languages using some Italian word, or French, or Spanish, or Dutch, or Scottish' (Ee4v). No longer are foreign words linguistic citizens harmoniously intermingling with native words; rather, their presence has 'mischeviously mixed' the language.

The image of foreign words as 'mingle-mangle,' a disorderly mess that refuses to stay within its prescribed borders, suggests the transgressivity and fungibility of the grotesque body as described by Mikhail Bakhtin. Like

---

[24]Florio, *A Worlde of Wordes*, sign. B1r.

[25]E.K., 'Dedicatory Epistle to *The Shepheardes Calendar*,' p. 503.

Douglas, Bakhtin sees the body as a place where larger social relations are configured. According to his now familiar formula, the grotesque body is organized around the lower stratum, particularly the belly, the anus, and the genital organs. It is unfinished and borderless and continually threatens to outgrow its limits, spilling over into the classical body, which seeks to remain separated and impermeable.[26] During the early modern period, one sometimes finds foreign language appearing, quite literally, as something grotesque. In Ben Jonson's *Poetaster*, for example, Crispinus has a penchant for using polysyllabic words, most of which are foreign in origin. Crispinus is not cured of the habit until the end of the play, when Virgil gives him an emetic and he expels a long series of polysyllabic words into a basin (5.3.456–553).

If foreign words represent the grotesque, English during this period can be understood in terms of the classical body which seeks to remain hermetically sealed and protected from this linguistic overflow. As Sir John Cheke notes in a letter to Thomas Hoby, 'I am of the opinion that our own tung shold be written cleane and pure, unmixt and unmangled with borrowing of other tunges's.'[27] Ruling the language is one way to keep English 'cleane and pure, unmixt and unmangled.' Ben Jonson observes that through Grammar 'wee free our Language from the opinion of Rudnesse, and Barbarisme, wherefore with it is mistaken to be diseased.' Jonson's description of unruled language as 'diseased' reflects the growing dis-ease during this period that a flood of words threatens English' s purity and must be stopped by creating a kind of grammatical moat around the language.[28]

Although Bakhtin is silent on the subject of gender, a number of scholars have observed that the grotesque body is far from gender neutral. Mary Russo, for example, is not surprised that the 'senile, pregnant hag' exemplifies the grotesque in *Rabelais and His World*. The word grotesque 'evokes the cave—grotto-esque. Low, hidden, earthly, dark, material, immanent, visceral.'[29] 'Grotto-esque' images of women's bodies pervade early modern discourse. For example, Hugh Chamberlein describes the womb as a dungeon in *The Accomplisht Midwife*.[30] While in his *Brievyary of Helthe* Andrew Boorde defines the female genitalia as inherently diseased:

26Bahktin, *Rabelais and his World*, pp. 21–30.

27Cheke, 'A Letter of Syr J. Cheekes to his loving frind Mayster Thomas Hobby,' p. 12.

28Puttenham's claim that the most 'naturall [and] pure' English is the 'usual speech of the Court and that of London and the shires lying about London within 1x. myles, and not much above,' might also be read as an attempt to draw boundaries around 'proper' English, an attempt that reflects the class biases that are also often involved in the construction of national language. See *Arte of English Poesie*, sign. Riij$^{r–v}$.

29Russo, *The Female Grotesque*, p. 1.

30Hobby, 'Secrets of the Female Sex,' p. 202.

> Vulva is the Latyn word. In greke it is named Hystira. In englishe it is named a womans secret member the which is the gate or dore of the matrix or belly, and there may brede many diseases as ulcers, skabbes, apostumes, fissures, fystles, festures, the Pockes and burnynge of an harlot.[31]

Like Chamberlein and Boorde, early modern physicians believe that women's bodies are more moist and humid than men's and that the production of liquids – blood, milk, tears – is their central task. These fluids slosh together in an undifferentiated liquidity. This liquidity, combined with a woman's extra orifice, leads to the theory that a woman's body is less hermetically sealed than a man's and, like the grotesque body, is in constant danger of overflowing its boundaries.[32] One finds a similar notion in the opening scene of *The Tempest*. Gonzalo observes that their sinking ship is 'as leaky as an unstaunched / wench' (1.1.42–43). Although the *Norton Shakespeare* glosses 'unstaunched wench' as 'a freely menstruating woman,' the word more generally means 'unsated,' 'unrestrained' and 'not watertight'.[33] Given the association of women's bodies with liquidity and fungibility, the analogy depends not on a comparison between the ship and a woman's body at a particular moment in her cycle, but rather on her permanent bodily state as constructed by early modern medicine. We can also see the various definitions of 'unstaunched' coming together in early modern discourse, as the unrestrained quality of women's bodies is offered as an explanation for why women cannot be sexually sated. Images of women's overflowing bodies are not only linked with a rapacious sexuality, but also a verbal excessiveness as women's open mouths and open bodies are continually coupled in early modern discourse. Master Morose, for example, compares Epicene to a 'conduit pipe,' which 'will gush out with more force when she opens again' (4.4.77–79). Juliet Fleming has demonstrated how such notions continued even into the Enlightenment, as when Samuel Johnson was asked how his dictionary will contain 'those words and phrases which hastily begot, owe their birth to the incontinence of female eloquence.'[34] The image of women's speech as both conduit and incontinent neatly conveys the links between the grotesque body, women's anatomy and women's language.[35]

---

[31]Boorde, *Brievyary of Helthe*, chap. 237.

[32]On early modern constructions of female anatomy, see Maclean, *The Renaissance Notion of Women*, especially pp. 28–46; Crawford, 'Attitudes on Menstruation in Seventeenth Century England,' pp. 47–73; Eccles, *Obstentrics and Gynaecology in Tudor and Stuart England*.

[33]See definitions 1a, 1b and 2, *OED*.

[34]Fleming, 'Dictionary English and the Female Tongue,' p. 294.

[35]A later example of this link between liquidity and loquaciousness appears in *Les*

Given the associations between women's bodies and their verbal incontinence, it should come as no surprise that the flood of foreign words imagined to be encroaching upon English is also depicted as something feminine. As discussed above, Richard Carew advocates importing foreign words. Nonetheless, his overall impression of foreign tongues is far from commendatory. For example, he describes the interjections in Italian and French as 'effeminate' and compares the latter to a 'nice...Woman, scarce daring to open her lippes for feare of marring her Countenance.' Italian, he concedes, is pleasant, 'but without Sinews, as a still fleeting Water.'[36] While initially Carew's description of Italian may seem more gender neutral than his description of French, to be 'without sinews' (that is, without strength) is often read as a sign of effeminacy in the early modern period. In addition, 'fleeting,' with its connotations of changeability and fluidity, evokes the image of bodily overflow described above.[37] Indeed, Carew may be referencing a specific body of water in this passage: the Fleeting Ditch, an open sewer that ran from Ludgate Hill and Fleet Street. Just like Chamberlein's horror at the close proximity between a woman's vagina and the body's 'sink,' Camden's depiction of Italian as 'fleeting water' unites the grotesque and the feminine.

More frequently, English writers presented foreign speech as something feminine by linking it with feminine rhetorical ornament. For example, in *The Flower of Fame*, Ulpian Fulwell states

> I have not the gifte of flowing eloquence, neyther can I enterlace my phrase with Italian termes nor powder my style with frenche Englishe or Inkhorne Rhetoricke, neyther cowche my matter under a cloake of curious inventions, to feede the daintie eares of delicate yonkers.[38]

To ensure that the connection between femininity and foreignness is not missed, foreign words are coupled with particularly feminine kinds of physical embellishment, such as powdering and donning feathers. Thomas Wilson makes the association between feminine ornament and foreign

---

Bas-bleus (1878): 'Ah! Quand les femmes écrivent, c'est comme quand elles parlent! Elles ont la faculté inondante; et comme l'eau, elles sont incompréhensibles.' Barbey d'Aurevilly, *Les Bas-Bleus*, p. 303. For discussions of the ways in which early modern discourse constructs women's bodies as 'naturally' grotesque, and their supposed links with sexual and linguistic excess, see Stallybrass, 'Patriarchal Territories'; Parker, *Literary Fat Ladies*, pp. 1–35; Woodbridge, 'Palisading the Body Politic,'; Boose, 'Scolding Brides and Bridling Scolds,' pp. 179–213; Paster, *The Body Embarrassed*, especially pp. 23–63; and Harris, 'This Is Not a Pipe,' pp. 203–228.

36 Carew, 'An Epistle Concerning the Excellencies of the English Tongue,' p. 43.

37 See definitions 2 and 3 under 'fleeting' in the *OED*.

38 Fulwell, *The Flower of Fame*, sign. Biii^{v}.

language more explicitly in *The Arte of Rhetorique* when he chastises those who 'seeke so far for outlandish English,' that 'like as they love to goe in forraine apparel, so thei wil powder their talke with oversea language.'[39] Wilson presents foreign language as a cosmetic or ornament used to adorn one's speech, suggesting that to be 'outlandish,' with its dual sense of foreign and inappropriate, is to be feminine.

The connection between femininity and excessive rhetorical ornament is not new to the early modern period. It has been viewed as the particular vice of women (or effeminate men) since at least the classical period. Granted, classical writers such as Quintilian recognize that rhetorical embellishment is a necessary device for effective writing and speaking, but they draw distinctions between the 'proper' use of rhetoric (a trope) and the 'improper' use of rhetoric (a solecism). However, as Quintilian himself admits in the *Institutio Oratoria*, it is not always an easy distinction to make since the gap between a trope and a solecism is notoriously small. Despite these difficulties, Quintilian does attempt to differentiate between the 'proper' and 'improper' use of rhetoric. Elegance, he notes, is the greatest gift, but only when 'natural and unaffected' ('cum sequitur non cum adfectatur'), a quality that he associates with a healthy, strong body.[40] Unnatural, affected rhetoric, however, he associates with excessive, feminine cosmetics:

> The man who attempts to enhance these physical graces by the effeminate use of depilatories, and cosmetics, succeeds merely in defacing them by the very one he bestows them on. Again, a tasteful and magnificent dress, as the Greek poet tells us, lends added dignity to its wearer: but effeminate and luxurious apparel fails to adorn the body and merely reveals the foulness of the mind. Similarly, a translucent and iridescent style merely serves to emasculate the subject which it arrays with such a pomp of words.[41]

Femininity, then, becomes the mark of improper rhetorical embellishment. By differentiating proper, masculine tropes from improper, feminine solecisms, writers such as Quintilian can claim mastery: they know what is excessive and feminine, even if others do not. Quintilian's use of gender to construct an otherwise nonexistent difference is similar to the way in which early modern nationalistic discourse makes use of the language of disease.

---

[39]Wilson, *The Arte of Rhetoric*, p. 118.

[40]Quintilian, *Institutio Oratoria*, 1 v.5.8.Pr. 19. Citations and translations are from Butler's edition of the text. See Parker, 'Virile Style,' pp. 201–222 for a discussion of Quintilian's analogy between proper rhetoric and a healthy body.

[41]On the gendering of rhetoric, see Brody, 'The Eunuch and Vicious Writing,' pp. 11–36; Lichtenstein, 'On Platonic Cosmetics,' pp. 37–54; Parker, 'Virile Style'; and Sharon-Zisser, '"*Illuster nôtre langue maternelle*",' pp. 393–414.

Labelling certain tropes masculine and proper and others feminine and improper becomes a way to construct mastery, just as labelling certain groups foreign and diseased and others domestic and healthy becomes a way to construct national identity.

At the same time that foreign words are being presented as a feminine pollution, there is a movement to assert English's supposedly inherent masculinity. In large part this project takes the form of tracing English's linguistic roots to the ancient Teutonic language. The Teutonic people were thought to be a particularly manly race, a masculinity reflected in their language, which contained harsh consonants and monosyllabic words. It is precisely through these characteristics that English's Teutonic roots were established. Thus, what had previously been thought to be one of English's flaws was transformed into important evidence of its linguistic origins and made a special virtue of the language. Indeed, rather than being the deficient language, English is now thought to be the cure for other languages' deficiencies. As James Howell suggests in his preface to the *Lexicon Tetraglotton*, it would be advantageous for French, Italian, and Spanish to include 'so male a speech' as English in their ranks because 'by her consonants and tougher strains / [it] will bring more arteries 'mong your soft veins.'[42] Much like Quintilian, Howell's depiction of English as 'so male a speech' serves as a way to oppose it to the feminine, foreign language that supposedly threatens to pollute it. The clean and pure speech that Cheke advocates is not only free from foreign words, but also decidedly male.

Thus, we see a shift occur in the late sixteenth and early seventeenth centuries: no longer are foreign words the panacea for English's maladies, but the disease that threatens the very masculinity of the English language. The threat to the masculinity of the English language not only comes from the outside, from the influx of potentially polluting foreign words, but also from the inside, from native female speakers of English. Given early modern anxieties that women's bodies are always in danger of breaching and the links made between women's leakiness, their open bodies, and their open mouths, it should not come as a surprise that women's language is thought to be as diseased and potentially polluting as that of foreigners. In *The Boke Named the Governour*, for example, Elyot urges Englishmen

> to speke none Englisshe but that which is clean, polite perfectly and articulately pronounced, omitting no letter or sillable as foolish women often times do of a wantonness, whereby diverse noble men and gentilmennes children (as I do at this day knowe) have attained corrupte and foule pronunciation.[43]

42Howell, *Lexicon Tetraglotton*, p. 1.

43Elyot, *The Boke Named the Governour*, 1.5.33.

Elyot's description of 'corrupte and foule pronunciation' echoes Puttneham, who equates barbarous pronunciation with those who say 'a dousand for a thousand, isterday for yesterday, as commonly the Dutch and French people do' (Ee3), once again suggesting a link between foreign and female speech. Elyot's observation that women often speak improperly out of 'wantoness' is particularly striking. While 'wanton' generally connotes carelessness and excessiveness, it of course also contains the sense of sexual accessibility and transgressivity. It is women's so-called nature – their fungibility and potential for transgression – that makes them such a threat to clean, pure pronunciation. Women are a conduit, not only in the sense of gushing forth words, but also in the sense of passing on polluted language to others.

This depiction of women as transmitters of polluted language parallels in many ways early modern theories about women as transmitters of the pox. In most stories about the origin of the disease, prostitutes play a central role. For example, one popular theory was that a Valencian prostitute contracted the pox by having sex with a leprous knight. She, in turn, slept with a number of King Charles VIII's soldiers, who were passing through Valencia on their way to Naples. In a hypothesis popularized by Paracelsus, a prostitute with an ulcerated vagina had sex with a leprous Frenchman. Gideon Harvey believed that 'the new pretty toy' was acquired by Columbus' Neapolitan sailors in the New World. When they returned home they infected the prostitutes of their city, who in turn infected the French soldiers who invaded Naples in 1494–1495. Harvey explains that the French soldiers were 'almost starved for want of women's flesh, which they found so well seasoned, and daubed with mustard, that in a few weeks it took 'em all by the nose.'[44] These stories share a similar and significant element: they present 'wanton' women and polluted foreigners as co-conspirators in the spread of dread disease, a mischievous mixing that affects the 'good state.'

However, if one looks closely at venerologists' theories about the pox, it becomes clear that prostitutes are not the only potential transmitters of this 'new pretty toy.' Like most physicians of the time, Pietro Rostino believes that humidity is one of the central causes of infectious disease. He speculates that the humidity necessary for the spawning of the pox comes from a woman's ulcerated vagina.[45] Yet, as discussed above, humidity supposedly is characteristic of all women's bodies. Thus, any woman has

---

[44]Harvey, *Great Venus Unmasked*, Book I, Article 2, p. 3. For a discussion of versions of these stories, see Schleiner, 'Infection and Cure Through Women,' pp. 503–504; Healy, *Fictions of Disease*, pp. 130–132. Hutten also discusses possible origins of the disease in *Of the Wood Called Guaiacum*, fols. 1^r–3^r.

[45]Schleiner, 'Infection and Cure Through Women,' p. 503.

the potential to pass on the disease. The anonymous author of *A New Method of Curing the French-Pox* goes even further. He suggests that women's bodies are not simply conduits for passing disease onto others, but are actually the vehicles by which the disease comes into being:

> when a Common Woman has kept company with many Men, that the Seeds (which are of different, and often times of opposite qualities) being mixed into that woman's Womb (which is *naturally fitted* to preserve the Seeds and all their Spirits) do forcibly justle against one another [emphasis added].[46]

Here, the womb is imagined as a caldron where the seeds of various men mingle promiscuously. While at first the author's target seems to be the behavior of the 'common woman,' the fact that the womb is 'naturally fitted' for the production of the disease suggests that it might be quite common for any woman to produce the disease and pass it on to others. According to Ulrich von Hutten the problem is that a man cannot tell if a woman is infected because 'this thing as touching women resteth in their secret places, having in those places little pretty sores ful of venom poison, being very dangerous, for those that unknowingly medle with them.'[47] In fact, Peter Lowe suggests that a man is *less likely* to contract the pox from a prostitute because women who have sex infrequently are in a greater state of heat and excitement and therefore more likely to pass sexual disease on to their lovers.[48] Thus all women's bodies must be approached with caution. Daniel Sennert perhaps articulates the early modern anxiety about women's bodies the most succinctly when he notes that 'the place from whence comes life, is also the breeder of the most deadly poison.'[49] Any woman's body, then, is a potential site and cause of contamination, a contamination that can be passed onto others in much the same way Elyot imagines noblemen and gentleman's children being infected by women's 'wanton' speech.

Much like the theories about the pox's origins, foreign language is imagined to infiltrate England through a sexual union between a foreigner and an Englishwoman. One particularly notable example is found in *Jack Drum's Entertainment*, which explicitly links foreign language and sexual

---

46 *A New Method of Curing the French Pox*, pp. 29–30. For discussion of this theory see Schleiner, 'Infection and Cure through Women,' pp. 505–506; and Siena, 'Pollution, Promiscuity and the Pox,' pp. 562–571.

47 Hutten, *Of the Wood Called Guaiacum*, fol. 6^{v}.

48 Lowe, *An Easie, Certaine, and Perfect Method, to Cure and Prevent the Spanish Sicknes*, sign. B2^{v}.

49 Sennert, *Practical Physick*, p. 114.

disease. The play's subplot features a pox-ridden French teacher, Monsieur John, who repeatedly tells his English companions that he 'burnes' (E^r) and 'burst[s] vor a vench' (C^v) and spends most of the play trying to procure a whore. Since an increased libido was thought to be one of the side effects of the disease, the Frenchman's comments serve as a way to inform the audience that he has the pox. (Pain while urinating was another symptom, lending added significance to Monsieur John's complaints that he is 'burning,' a term that would have called to mind the common slang for gonorrhea – 'the burning of a harlot' – invoked by Boorde earlier). Yet there might be a deeper anxiety conveyed here as well. Monsieur John finds Englishwomen particularly attractive:

> I by my trot, ang you helpe mee to a Vench
> now, mee teach you French...
> your Secke is hote, and make mee brule, and brule,
> and burne, for a (hee) by gor your Seck is hote. (E^r)

Much like the *Pedlar's Prophecy* and the preacher who agitated the crowd before the May Day riots, Monsieur John's comments evoke the anxiety of a sexually rapacious stranger who threatens to dispossess English husbands and fathers of their wives and daughters. In addition, his assertion that he will 'burst' if he does not have an Englishwoman calls to mind the incontinent stranger whose polluted body (here clearly marked through disease) threatens England's purity. Monsieur John's offer to pay for the Englishwoman through French lessons links the polluted foreigner's body, which threatens to 'burst' and contaminate the English nation through a sexual liaison with an Englishwoman with his polluting language which threatens the purity and masculinity of English.

This is not the only passage in the play where the pox and foreign language intersect. When the Englishmen thwart Monsieur John's efforts to woo Camellia's maid, Winifride, he mutters 'a grand poc on you all' and immediately threatens, 'me teach you much French vor dis' (C^v). Monsieur John's dual curse implies that both his diseased body and his diseased language can be used as weapons of revenge. Indeed, this is precisely what happens at the end of the play. One of the Englishmen decides to play a joke on Monsieur John by presenting his wife as the bawd the Frenchman is so desperate to find. Fully expecting she will spurn Monsieur John's advances, the English husband leaves the Frenchman and his wife alone. However, instead of rejecting the stranger, the wife, after very little prompting, has sex with him. When the Englishman discovers what has happened, he is upset not only because of the sexual betrayal, but also because of the sexual infection that makes it dangerous for him ever to sleep with his wife again. The Frenchman apologizes, pointing out that the Englishman did tell him that the woman was a whore. In the end, he offers to teach the Englishman French as compensation, replacing one kind of pollution with another.

Alongside the theories about polluting strangers, *Jack Drum's Entertainment* confirms what doctors like Ulrich von Hutten and Daniel Sennert suggest about polluting women. The transmission of the pox is not exclusive to the 'common woman;' the assumedly chaste wife is as likely to be the 'breeder of the most deadly poison' as is the prostitute. A similar point is made in *Pedler's Prophecy*. In the play's opening scene, the peddler offers to sell the father spectacles that will allow him to keep an eye on his supposedly virginal daughter,

> [these glasses] will cause you to see as well behind as before
> For in your house is plaid manie a knacke,
> Which of my mind you shall know more.
> Though my spectacles you intend to buy,
> You shall perceiue your owne negligence,
> You suffer your children to sweare and lye,
> And you laugh thereat and haue patience,
> Fathers and mothers, kinsfolkes and friends,
> So inordinately do their children love:
> That they are parents of bodies, but poysoners of mindes. (B3^{v})

The reference to 'poysoners of mindes' recalls the depiction of foreigners as 'deadly poison' earlier in the play and also echoes Sennert's description of women's bodies as the 'breeders of poison.' In these lines, lenient parents become co-conspirators in England's contamination. The peddler's panoptic spectacles will allow a vigilant parent always to keep an eye on his child, a necessity if, as *Jack Drum's Entertainment* suggests, turning your back for even a moment can have dangerous ramifications for the nation. Because women are 'unstaunched' in the sense of leaky, they are 'unstaunched' also in the sense that they are never sexually sated. Therefore, they must be watched constantly.[50] The same might be said of women's speech. According to Elyot, women speak improperly out of wantonness, an observation

---

50The play *Nice Wanton* (1560) makes a similar point. In it, a young man and woman go astray because of lenient parents. The son becomes a gambler and takes up a life of crime in order to pay his debts, while the daughter acquires lovers and dies of the pox. While the play notes several times that the children have both a mother and a father, the audience sees only the mother, who at the beginning of the play indulges the children and who by the end of the play attempts suicide out of guilt for her children's horrible ends. The daughter's death presents, in a predictable way, the sexual wandering that young women are imagined to indulge in if left to their own devices. The absent father may warn the men in the audience that a similar fate will befall their families if they do not play an active role in rearing their children, but leave it instead to their wives.

that links women's unstaunched speech with their supposedly unstaunched bodies. Much like foreigners' language, which is also imagined as overflowing and polluting, the 'incontinence of female eloquence,' threatens English's purity, cleanliness, and inherent masculinity. If England wants to keep itself 'cleane and pure, unmixt and unmangled,' it will need to keep both foreigners and Englishwomen under surveillance to protect the 'good state.' Thus what we see in the image of foreign language as feminine disease is an ideological one-two punch: negative associations surrounding femininity and pollution are marshaled as a way to stigmatize foreign language, an effort that serves to consolidate national identity. Pejorative depictions of feminine speech as a pollution that threatens the purity of the English nation further reinforce gender ideology.

Understanding how this dual ideology works gives us a slightly different lens for reading a play such as William Haughton's *Englishmen for my Money or A Woman Will Have her Will.* On the surface the play seems to be a simple, xenophobic diatribe. G.K. Hunter, for example, calls the text 'a run-of-the-mill comedy.'[51] I would argue, instead, that the play articulates rather thoughtfully the link between pollution, femininity, sexuality and foreignness discussed above.[52] In the play, Pisaro, a Portuguese Jew, decides to marry his half-English daughters to three foreign merchants. They, however, prefer marriage to three Englishmen in debt to their father. The main action thus centres on the Englishmen's and the daughters' attempts to thwart Pisaro's will and fulfill their own. The play ends, as one might expect, with the Englishmen's marriage to Pisaro's daughters. On the way to this eventual outcome, several jokes are made at the foreigners' expense. For example, on a foggy night, Delio (the Frenchman) and Alvaro (the Italian) get lost on their way to Pisaro's house. At one point in their blind wanderings around the city, they run into Frisco, Pisaro's servant. Although he offers to lead them back to Pisaro's house, he actually has other plans:

> I shall lead you such a jaunt that you shall scarece give me thankes for Come sirrs follow mee: now for a durtie Puddle, the pissing Condit or a great Post, that might turne these two from Asses to Oxen by knocking their Hornes to their Fore-heads. (G^{v})

According to John Stow, one of the original functions of the pissing conduit was as a jail for 'night walkers and suspicious persons,' as well as those

---

[51] Hunter, 'Elizabethans and Foreigners,' p. 44.

[52] In her essay 'So Much English by the Mother,' Emma Smith treats some of the same passages I discuss here, although with a slightly different focus: she reads Pisaro's half-foreign daughters as emblems of a hybridized and feminized London.

'suspected of Incontencie.'[53] Thus, we might read Frisco's desire to find a 'dirtie Puddle' or a 'pissing Condit' as an effort to locate a place where he can dispose of the incontinent strangers and the pollution they represent. Although the foreigners eventually return to Pisaro's home, Frisco first takes them to Shoreditch, on the outside of the city. At this moment in the play the foreigners and the threat they pose to the nation are literally expelled outside the city walls.[54]

Despite their mixed heritage, Pisaro's daughters seem to present a singularly English point-of view. They reject their Portuguese heritage, which they associate with wantonness. As Mathea notes, 'Though I am Portingale by the Fathers side, / And therfore should be lustfull, wanton, light, / Yet Goosecap, I will let you know, / That I have so much English by the Mother, / That no base slauering French shall make me stoope'(G4^{v}). It is primarily through their investment in the English language that the daughters articulate their English identity. They repeatedly reject the foreign suitors because they cannot speak English. Laurentia, the eldest daughter, perhaps puts it most succinctly (if somewhat cruelly) when she tells her Dutch suitor, 'if needs you marry with an English Lasse, / Woe her in English, or sheele call you Asse' (E2^{v}). Nor will the daughters speak any languages besides English. Their father employs a tutor to teach his daughters the languages of the foreign suitors (although unwittingly he rehires the girls' Latin teacher, Anthony, who is a friend of the Englishmen). The girls vehemently oppose the idea of learning the foreigners' tongues. When Walgrave, Mathea's English lover, asks her if she is 'so mad as to turne French?,' she answers, 'Yes, mary when two Sundayes come together; / Thinke you Ile learne to speake this gibberidge, / Or the Pigges language? Why, if I fall sick, / Theyle say, the French et-cetera infected mee' (D2^{v}). Mathea's description of the Frenchman's speech as 'the Pigges language' and 'the French et-cetera' recalls the images of bestiality and disease described above.

53Stow, *Survey of London,* I.188, p. 17. On the conduit pipe as prison, see Harris, 'This is Not a Pipe,' p. 211.

54During their excursion in the fog, one of the foreigners cracks his head on a stage-post. Lloyd Edward Kermode notes that stage-posts 'indicate the largely invisible border between stage space and audience space, so they represent ideological limits and the edges of the Englishmen's control.' In addition, stage-posts are, in a confused way, connected with the columns of ancient buildings, in which images of defeated enemies were carved. Such an association makes Haughton's decision to use the stage-posts as weapons particularly appropriate. See Kermode, 'After Shylock: The 'Judaiser' in England,' p. 14. On depictions of foreigners on the early modern stage, see Hoenselaars, A. J., *Images of Englishmen and Foreigners in the Drama of Shakespeare and his Contemporaries.*

The daughters are instrumental in bringing about the play's conclusion, both because they participate in the tricks played against the foreigners and because they adamantly refuse to 'stoop' to their father's and the foreigners' desires. Given the daughters' witty repartee and their refusal to submit to their father's will, it might be tempting to read their disobedience as a challenge to patriarchal norms. However, as Kim Hall notes in her discussion of *The Merchant of Venice*, the potential transgressivity of the unruly woman in early modern drama usually is limited. Disorderly women often serve as tools for oppressing racial and cultural Others and when this task has been completed are converted into pliable wives and reintegrated into patriarchal society.[55] The same phenomenon occurs in Haughton's play. The daughters' comments about the foreigners' inability to speak 'proper' English are the primary device for constructing what it means to be English in the play. It is precisely the play's investment in 'proper' English as a marker of English identity that limits the inversion of gender hierarchies, since *Englishmen for My Money*, like so many of the texts discussed above, presents foreigners and women as equivalent threats to 'cleane and pure' English.

For example, early in the play, Pisaro sends Frisco to St. Paul's to find a Frenchman who can teach his daughters foreign languages. Frisco does not speak French, but he has a clear idea what a French language teacher would be like: 'a Monster in the liknesse of a man…a clipper of the King's English: and to conclude, a eternall enemie to all good language' (B2^{v}). Shortly after this statement, the play shifts scenes. We find Pisaro at the Burse, where he learns that his ships have been sunk by Spanish Galleys. While he is digesting this misfortune, a messenger persistently asks him for money. Pisaro lashes out at him: 'And what fits yours? A prating wrangling toung, / A womans ceaselesse and incessant babling, / That sees the world turnd topsie turvie with me; / Yet hath not so much witte to stay a while, / Till I bemone my late excessive losse' (C^{v}). The action then returns to Frisco at St. Paul's. Shortly after arriving there, he is approached by Anthony, who is disguised as a Frenchman: 'Pardon, for mine unciuill and presumptuous intrusion, who indeauour nothing lesse, then to provoke or exasperat you against mee.' Frisco interprets Anthony's wordy speech as a sign of his foreignness, stating that 'They say, a word to the Wise is enough: so by this litle French that he speakes, I see hee is the very man I seeke for' (D3^{r}). Anthony's copious and incomprehensible speech, much like Crispinus' language in Jonson's *Poetaster*, is dotted with polysyllabic and 'outlandish' words. At one point in Jonson's play, Crispinus is described as having 'much of the mother' in him because of his

55Hall, 'Guess Who's Coming to Dinner ?,' p. 104.

verbosity (3.1.184). Similarly, the juxtaposition of these scenes in *Englishmen for my Money*, where we move from Frisco's description of 'a Monster in the liknesse of a man,' to a 'woman's ceaselesse and incessant babbling,' back to Anthony's wordy, 'outlandish' speech, links foreigners and women through excessive verbiage.

While the daughters reject the foreigners because of their inability to speak English, it is Pisaro's servant, Frisco, who most explicitly articulates the danger to the nation that the foreigners represent. At one point in the play he beseeches the Englishmen to stop the daughters' impending marriages to the foreigners: 'Ah Gentleman, doe not suffer a litter of Languages to spring up amongst us' (B2v). And later, after discussing the sexual prowess of the foreigners, he observes, 'Oh the generation of Languages that our House will bring foorth: why every Bedd will have a propper speech to himselfe' (I3v). In these lines Frisco imagines the spread of foreign tongues in reproductive terms, associating the transmission of foreign language with sexual liaisons in much the same way that economic and sexual anxieties converge during this period. Haughton's intent might be similar to that of the preacher who spurred on the crowd before the May Day Riots. As in *Jack Drum's Entertainment*, the image of foreign language as a sexually transmitted phenomenon not only plays upon anxieties about lascivious strangers, but also, much like the fears of miscegenation discussed above, presents pollution in somatic terms, thus evoking the image of a vulnerable body politic. Frisco's description of a 'litter of languages' suggests that every stranger has the potential to produce several mischieviously mixed languages at once, calling to mind the worries of Waller and his contemporaries that English will 'overflow' because of this influx of foreign words. In addition, the image of language reproducing in a litter recalls the images of bestiality, disease, and monstrosity associated with foreigners, foreign language, and miscegenation that I described above. Like the *Pedler's Prophecy* and advocates of pure English, Frisco believes that preventing interracial marriages and the linguistic mingle-mangle that will follow is an issue of national concern. A foreigner is not just a 'clipper of the King's English,' but also 'an eternall enemie of all Good Language,' and, by extension, an enemy of the nation.

But perhaps most striking is the way in which Frisco presents the daughters' bodies as the site where linguistic corruption takes place. It is within their wombs that these litters and generations of languages will 'spring up amongst us.' The play configures women as the vulnerable orifice in the body politic through which diseased language enters the nation. Yet women are not just a passive conduit. While the daughters may reject the foreigners, their languages, and the wantonness associated with their own Portuguese heritage, they cannot reject their biological sex, a biological sex that, as both Ulrich von Hutten and Elyot claim, makes women 'naturally fitted' for sexual and linguistic transgression. As noted above, the talkative woman and the sexually available woman were frequently collapsed in early modern England. As a result, the daughters' skillful use of their tongues against their father and the foreigners becomes evidence that the daughters' bodies are unstaunched and that the anxiety surrounding their bodies as potential sites for corruption is well founded. I would suggest that even the second half of the play's title, 'A Woman Will Have her Will,' can be read in the same way. On the one hand it seems affirmative: women cannot be oppressed and will have what they want. But 'will,' with its connotations of desire, and in particular sexual desire, speaks to the anxiety that a woman's libido is something that cannot be suppressed: women will have what they sexually and linguistically desire. It is this characteristic of women's 'natures' that makes them potential polluters of the social body. 'Women will have their will' is a mantra throughout the play. I would suggest that its repetition is intended as a warning. Women *will* have their will. Their transgressivity is dangerous to the nation and must be contained. Certainly it is by the end of Haughton's play. Having served as mouthpieces for the construction of Englishness (a construction that the women are themselves excluded from) the play ends with the women being converted from talkative and rebellious daughters to silent and pliant English wives. The final message of *Englishmen for my Money* is that just as foreigners must be expelled outside the city walls, Englishwomen must be carefully secured within them.

★ ★ ★

> I'm not anti-immigrant. But I'm thinking about the future of the country.... It's too much for the country to absorb.
>
> Minneapolis resident quoted in *USA Today* (9 April 2001)

In 'The Excellencies of the English Tongue,' Richard Carew observes that no matter how long a stranger has lived in England, he 'carrieth evermore a watch-word upon his tong to descrie him by.'[56] Carew's description of non-native pronunciation as a 'watch-word,' with its valances of warning, surveillance and discrimination, neatly encapsulates some of the larger issues surrounding language regulation discussed in this essay. It is no coincidence that at the very moment when England is watching its borders, it becomes increasingly interested in watching its language. In the early modern period tropes of disease and pollution, as well as of femininity, become potent tools for pathologizing foreigners and their language and for carving out a national

[56] Carew, 'An Epistle Concerning the Excellencies of the English Tongue,' p. 40.

identity that seeks to differentiate itself from the alien. And in turn, these metaphors remind the nation that it must keep an eye on its women, who are ostensibly foreigners themselves because of their fungible 'natures.'

As I suggested at the beginning of this essay, tropes of disease and pollution continue to be deployed today, their longevity a testament to their potency. As in the early modern period, they are deployed primarily in anti-immigration rhetoric and by proponents of the 'English-only' movement. For example, *The New York Times* reports that in a recent speech Jean-Marie Le Pen argued that 'French culture was at risk from American ideas, spawned by a "mongrel nation."'[57] In The *Shemayisrael*, Eliezer Rauchberger describes the 'plague of non-Jewish immigration.'[58] The Ku Klux Klan deplores the 'plague of immigration' as well, and the Aryan organization Christian Identity, describes immigration as 'a destroying virus that attacks our racial purity.'[59] A speech by the racist Richard Barrett before a crowd at the Colorado State Capital deserves quoting at length for its elaborate deployment of illness metaphors:

> This political plague of homosexuality seeks more than to ooze into the ranks of the armed forces or to contaminate teams of high school football players. It is linked in its penchant to seek favors to, oh, so many other nasty strains. Like the Yellow Fever called greed, by which savings and loan manipulators would set themselves above their fair share of taxes. Or the Black Plague called immigration by which those not even citizens would claim for themselves our educational opportunities. Or the Scarlet Fever called jealousy, by which anti-social climbers would wrest away any job from any critic who dared to challenge their usurpation.[60]

The Department of Transportation Maritime Administration calls illegal immigration a crime that 'plague[s] our ports,'[61] and a recent headline in the *Miami Herald* announces that 'Spanish is spreading,' a phrase that recalls the early modern fears about encroaching foreign language.[62]

57Cit. in Erlanger, 'The World: Europe's Identity Crisis,' p. 5.

58Eliezer Rauchberger, 'Barak and the Arab Vote' in *Dei'ah veDibur: Information and Insight*. 13 December 2000. http://chareidi.shemayisrael.com/archives5761/vayishlach/VYSopoli tica.htm.

59Anti-Defamation League, *Hate on the World Wide Web: A Brief Guide to Cyberspace Bigotry*. October 1998. http://www.adl.org/special_reports/hate_on_www/hate_on_www.asp.

60Richard Barrett, 'Favors for None Rally.' Colorado State Capital. Denver, Colorado. 6 January 1994.

61Carlton, 'Department of Transportation Maritime Administration Statement before the Committee on Commerce, Science and Transportation,' p. 3.

62Viglucci, 'Spanish is Spreading Northward,' p. 1A. For a discussion of the similari-

At the beginning of *Illness as Metaphor*, Susan Sontag notes that 'one cannot think without metaphors. But that does not mean there aren't some metaphors we might well abstain from or try to retire.'[63] The association of foreigners and foreign language with disease is certainly one of these. Even if used in a seemingly benign way, the trope's long history lingers in the shadows. Sontag's warning is sound. Girolamo Fracastoro's *Syphilis, sive Morbus Gallicus* eventually becomes a reality. It is the fiction that supplies the name of a very real disease. Similarly, these conflations of disease, pollution, foreigners and femininity are fictions that can produce very real oppression and violence – something which, in our own historical moment, we would do well to keep in mind.[64]

Mills College
Oakland, California

Cited Works

Allen, Peter Lewis. *The Wages of Sin: Sex and Disease, Past and Present.* Chicago: University of Chicago Press, 2000.

Bailey, Richard. *Images of English: A Cultural History of the Language.* Ann Arbor: University of Michigan Press, 1991.

Bakhtin, Mikhail. *Rabelais and his World*, trans. Hélène Iswolsky. Bloomington, IN: Indiana University Press, 1984.

Barbey d'Aurevilly, Jules. *Les Bas-bleus.* Geneva: Slatkine Reprints, 1968.

Barkar, Wylliam. *The Bookes of Xenophon Contayning the Discipline, Schole, and Education of Cyrus the Noble kyng of Persie. Translated out of Greeke into Englyshe.* London: Reynolde Wolfe, 1552.

Boorde, Andrew. *Brievyary of Helthe for all Manor of Sycknesses and Diseases.* London: T. East, 1547.

Boorde, Andrew. *The Fyrst Boke of the Introduction of Knowledge*, ed. F.J. Furnivall. London: N.T. Trüber & Co., 1870.

Boose, Lynda. 'Scolding Brides and Bridling Scolds: Taming the Woman's Unruly Member' *Shakespeare Quarterly* 42 (1991): 179–213.

Brennan, Gillian. 'The Cheese and the Welsh: Foreigners in Elizabethan Literature' *Renaissance Studies* 8:1 (1994): 40–64.

---

ties between early modern anxieties about foreign language and modern American anxieties about the 'spread' of Spanish, see Helgerson, 'Language Lessons,' pp. 289–299.

[63]Sontag, *Illness as Metaphor*, p. 1.

[64]Earlier versions of this paper were given at the Renaissance Studies Colloquium at Cornell University in March of 1999, The Archipelagic Identities Conference in Oxford, England in April of 1999, and at the Renaissance Society of America Conference in Scottsdale, Arizona in April of 2002. I would like to thank these audiences for their thoughtful suggestions and comments.

Brody, Miriam. *Manly Writing: Gender, Rhetoric and the Rise of Composition.* Carbondale; Edwardsville: Southern Illinois University Press, 1993.

Camden, William. *Remains Concerning Britain*, ed. R.D. Dunn. Toronto: University of Toronto Press, 1984.

Carew, Richard. 'An Epistle Concerning the Excellencies of the English Tongue' pp. 37–44 in *Remains Concerning Britain*, ed. R.D. Dunn. Toronto: University of Toronto Press, 1984.

Carlton, Bruce J. 'Department of Transportation Maritime Administration Statement.' United States Senate. 24 July 2001. pp. 1–7.

Cheke, Sir John. 'A Letter of Syr J. Cheekes to his loving frind, Mayster Thomas Hoby' pp. 12–13 in *The Book of the Courtier*, ed. Walter Raleigh. London: David Nutt, 1900.

Crawford, Patricia. 'Attitudes on Menstruation in Seventeenth Century England' *Past and Present* 91 (1981): 47–73.

Cunningham, William. *Alien Immigrants to England*. London: S. Sonnenschien & Co; New York: The Macmillan Co, 1987.

Douglas, Mary. *Purity and Danger: An Analysis of the Concepts of Pollution and Taboo.* London; New York: Routledge, 1966.

E.K. 'Dedicatory Epistle to *The Shepheardes Calender*' pp. 501–505 in *Edmund Spenser's Poetry*, eds. Hugh Maclean and Anne Lake Prescott. New York; London: W.W. Norton & Company, 1993.

Eccles, Audrey. *Obstentrics and Gynaecology in Tudor and Stuart England*. Kent: Kent State University Press, 1982.

Elyot, Thomas. *The Boke Named the Governour*, ed. Donald W. Rude. New York: Garland Press, 1992.

Erlanger, Steven. 'The World: Europe's Identity Crisis' *The New York Times*, 5 May 2002, section 4, p. 5.

Fleming, Juliet. 'Dictionary English and the Female Tongue' pp. 290–325 in *Enclosure Acts: Sexuality, Property, and Culture in Early Modern England*, eds. Richard Burt, and John Michael Archer. Ithaca; London: Cornell University Press, 1994.

Foa, Anna. 'The New and the Old: The Spread of Syphilis (1494–1530)' pp. 26–45 in *Sex and Gender in Historical Perspective,* eds. Edward Muir and Guido Ruggiero. Baltimore: The Johns Hopkins University Press, 1990.

Florio, John. *A Worlde of Wordes, or Most Copious, and Exact Dictionaire in Italian and English*. London: Arnold Hatfield, 1598.

Fulwell, Ulpian. *The Flower of Fame. Containing the Bright Renowne & Fortunate Raigne of King Henry the VIII. Wherein is Mentioned of Matters, by the Rest of our Cronographers Ouerpassed*. London: William Hoskins, 1575.

Gilman, Sander. *Picturing Health and Illness: Images of Identity and Difference.* Baltimore; London: The John Hopkins University Press, 1995.

Gilman, Sander. 'Plague in Germany, 1939/1989: Cultural Images of Race, Space and Disease' pp. 175–200 in *Nationalisms and Sexualities*, eds. Andrew Parker, Mary Russo, Doris Sommer, and Patricia Yaeger. New York; London: Routledge, 1992.

Hale, David George. *The Body Politic: A Political Metaphor in Renaissance English Literature*. The Hague and Paris: Mouton, 1971.

Hall, Kim. 'Guess Who's Coming to Dinner? Colonization and Miscegenation in *The Merchant of Venice*' *Renaissance Drama* 22 (1992): 87–111.

Harris, Jonathan Gil. *Foreign Bodies and the Body Politic: Discourses of Social Pathology in Early Modern England.* Cambridge University Press, 1998.

Harris, Jonathan Gil. 'This Is Not a Pipe: Water Supply, Incontinent Sources, and the Leaky Body Politic' pp. 204–228 in *Enclosure Acts: Sexuality, Property, and Culture in Early Modern England*, eds. Richard Burt, and John Michael Archer. Ithaca; London: Cornell University Press, 1994.

Harvey, Gideon. *Great Venus Unmasked: Or a More Exact Discovery of the Venereal Evil, or French Disease.* 2nd ed. London: B. G. for Nath Brook, 1672.

Haughton, William. *Englishmen for my Money or a Woman Will Have Her Will.* ed. H. Hart. London: Malone Society at the Oxford University Press, 1912.

Healy, Margaret. *Fictions of Disease in Early Modern England: Bodies, Plague and Politics.* New York: Palgrave, 2001.

Helgerson, Richard. *Forms of Nationhood: The Elizabethan Writing of England.* Chicago: University of Chicago Press, 1992.

Helgerson, Richard. 'Language Lessons: Linguistic Postcolonialism, and the Early Modern English Nation' *Yale Journal of Criticism: Interpretation in the Humanities* 11:1 (1998): 289–299.

Hobby, Elaine. '"Secrets of the Female Sex": Jane Sharp, the Reproductive Female Body, and Early Modern Midwifery Manuals' *Women's Writing* 8:2 (2001): 201–212.

Hoenselaars, A. J. *Images of Englishmen and Foreigners in the Drama of Shakespeare and his Contemporaries: A Study of Stage Characters and National Identity in English Renaissance Drama, 1558–1642.* Rutherford, NJ: Associated University Press, 1992.

Howell, James. *Lexicon Tetraglotton. An English-French-Italian-Spanish Dictionary.* London: Thomas Leach, 1660.

Hunter, G.K. 'Elizabethans and Foreigners' *Shakespeare Survey* 17 (1964): 37–52.

Hutten, Ulrich von. *Of the Wood Called Guaiacum that Healeth the Frenche Pockes, and also Healeth the Goute in the Feete, the Stoone, the Palsey, Lepree, Dropsy, Fallynge Euyll and Other Dyseases.* London: Thomas Bertheleti, 1536.

Jack Drum's Entertainment: Or the Comedie of Pasquill and Katerine. London: W. Stansby, for P. Knight, 1616.

Jonson, Ben. *Poetaster*, ed. Tom Cain. Manchester; New York: Manchester University Press, 1995.

Jonson, Ben. *Epicene*, pp. 775–860 in *English Renaissance Drama: An Anthology*, ed. David Bevington, et al. New York; London: W.W. Norton & Company, 2002.

Jones, R.F. *The Triumph of the English Language: A Survey of Opinions Concerning the Vernacular from the Introduction of Printing to the Restoration.* Stanford: Stanford University Press, 1953.

Kermode, Lloyd Edward. 'After Shylock: The 'Judaiser' in England' *Renaissance and Reformation* 20:4 (1996): 5–26.

Lever, Ralph. *The Arte of Reason, Rightly Termed, Witcraft Teaching a Perfect Way to Argue and Dispute.* London: H. Bynneman, 1573.

Lichtenstein, Jacqueline. *The Eloquence of Color: Rhetoric and Painting in the French Classical Age*, trans. Emily McVarish. Berkeley: University of California Press, 1993.

Lowe, Peter. *An Easie, Certaine, and Perfect Method, to Cure and Prevent the Spanish Sicknes*. London: James Roberts, 1596.

Maclean, Ian. *The Renaissance Notion of Women*. Cambridge: Cambridge University Press, 1980.

Malynes, Gerard. *A Treatise of the Canker of Englands Commonwealth*. London: Richard Field, 1601.

Moore, J.L. *Tudor-Stuart Views on the Growth, Status, and Destiny of the English Language*, trans. Loenz Morsbach. Halle: M. Nieymer, 1910.

Nelkin, Dorothy, and Sander L. Gilman. 'Placing Blame for Devastating Disease' *Social Research* 55:3 (1988): 361–378.

Parker, Patricia. *Literary Fat Ladies: Rhetoric, Gender and Property*. London; New York: Methuen, 1987.

Parker, Patricia. 'Virile Style' pp. 199–222 in *Premodern Sexualities*, ed. Louise Frandenburg and Carla Freccero. New York: Routledge, 1996.

Paster, Gail Kern. *The Body Embarrassed: Drama and the Disciplines of Shame in Early Modern England*. Ithaca, NY: Cornell University Press, 1993.

The Pedlar's Prophecy, ed. W. W. Greg. London: Malone Society at the Oxford University Press, 1914.

Puttenham, George. *The Arte of English Poesie: Contrived into Three Bookes: The First of Poets and Poesie, the Second of Proportion, the Third of Ornament*. London: Richard Field, 1589.

Quintilian, Marcus Fabius. *Institutio Oratoria*, ed. and trans. H. E. Butler. Cambridge: Harvard University Press; London: William Heinemann Ltd., 1921.

Russo, Mary. *The Female Grotesque: Risk, Excess and Modernity*. Routledge: New York, 1994.

Schleiner, Winfried. 'Infection and Cure through Women: Renaissance Constructions of Syphilis' *Journal of Medieval and Renaissance Studies* 24:3 (1994): 499–517.

Scholz, Susanne. *Body Narratives: Writing the Nation and the Subject in Early Modern England*. New York: St. Martin's Press, 2000.

Sennert, Daniel. *Practical Physick*. London: Peter Cole, 1664.

Shakespeare, William. *The Norton Anthology of Shakespeare*, ed Stephen Greenblatt, et al. New York; London: W.W. Norton & Company, 1997.

Sharon-Zisser, Shirley. '"*Illuster nôtre langue maternelle*": Illustrative Similes and Failed Phallic Economy in Early Modern Rhetoric' *Exemplaria* 9:2 (1997): 393–414.

Siena, Kevin. 'Pollution, Promiscuity, and the Pox: English Venereology and the Early Modern Discourse on Social and Sexual Danger' *Journal of the History of Sexuality* 8:4 (1998): 554–574.

Skelton, John. *Philip Sparrow*, pp. 60–100 in *The Complete Poems of John Skelton, Laureate*, ed. Philip Henderson. London: J.M. Dent and Sons Ltd., 1959.

Smith, Emma. '"So Much English by the Mother": Gender, Foreigners and the Mother Tongue in William Haughton's *Englishmen for my Money*' *Medieval and Renaissance Drama in England: An Annual Gathering of Research, Criticism and Reviews* 13 (2001): 165–181.

Sontag, Susan. *AIDS and Its Metaphors*. New York: Farrar, Straus and Giroux, 1988.

Sontag, Susan. *Illness as Metaphor*. New York: Farrar, Straus and Giroux, 1977.

Stallybrass, Peter. 'Patriarchal Territories: The Body Enclosed' pp. 123–142. *Rewriting the Renaissance: The Discourses of Sexual Difference in Early Modern Europe*, eds. Margaret W. Ferguson, Maureen Quilligan and Nancy J. Vickers. Chicago: Chicago University Press, 1986.

Stow, John. *A Survey of London: Written in the Year 1598*, ed. Antonia Fraser. Great Britain: Sutton Publishing Company, 1994.

Viglucci, Andres. 'Spanish Is Spreading Northward In Florida' *The Miami Herald*, 22 November 2001, Final Section, p. 1A.

Waller, Edmund. 'Of English Verse' pp. 197–198 in *The Poems of Edmund Waller*, ed. G. Thorn Drury. London: Lawrence & Bullen, 1983.

Wilson, Richard. 'Observations on English Bodies: Licensing Maternity Shakespeare's Late Plays' pp. 121–150 in *Enclosure Acts: Sexuality, Property, and Culture in Early Modern England*, eds. Richard Burt, and John Michael Archer. Ithaca; London: Cornell University Press, 1994.

Wilson, Thomas. *The Arte of Rhetoric*, ed. Peter E. Medine. University Park, PA: Pennsylvania State University Press, 1994.

Woodbridge, Linda. 'Palisading the Elizabethan Body Politic' *Texas Studies in Literature and Language* 33:3 (1991): 327–354.

French Diseases and Italian Responses: Representations of the mal francese in the Literature of Cinquecento Tuscany[1]

Domenico Zanrè

On 28 May 1496, the Florentine chronicler Luca Landucci wrote the following entry in his *Diario fiorentino*: 'ci cominciava una certa infermità, che le chiamavano bolle franciose [...] e non si trova medicine, ma andavano senpre [sic] peggiorando' (A certain illness developed, which they called the French boils [...] and no medical treatment can be found, and the people were becoming increasingly sick).[2] By the end of the year, 'c'era già pieno di bolle franciose Firenze e 'l contado, ed erane in ogni città per tutta Italia e duravano assai' (Florence and the surrounding countryside was already full of the French boils; they were also present in every city throughout Italy and they were particularly virulent) (Landucci, *Diario fiorentino,* p. 141). Landucci's statement was supported by the contemporary physician Antonio Benivieni, who described the symptoms of the contagion: 'Pustules of various kinds broke out first on the genitals (sometimes it might be on the head, but this rarely) and thence extended over the whole body [...] Such pustules were followed and sometimes even preceded by pains in the joints which racked the body with no less torment, and reached their maximum as the pustules abated' (Benivieni, *De abditis nonnullis*, pp. 9, 11).

The malady that Benivieni was referring to in this passage was a sexually transmitted disease that was first reported in Italy in the last decade of the fifteenth century. Within a frighteningly short period of time, the disease had spread not only through the length and breadth of the peninsula, but also throughout Europe. The disease subsequently came to be known as syphilis, thanks to Girolamo Fracastoro's Latin poem, published in 1530.[3]

---

[1]This essay is based on a paper given at the Renaissance Society of America annual meeting in Scottsdale, Arizona in March 2002. I would like to thank the British Academy for their award of an Overseas Conference Grant, which made the trip possible.

[2]Landucci, *Diario fiorentino,* p. 132. Unless specified, all translations are my own.

[3]For a modern edition, see Fracastoro, *Syphilis*, trans. Eatough.

At the time of the outbreak in the last decade of the Quattrocento, however, its most widespread name amongst contemporaries was the *mal francese*. Its name was derived from the fact that it initially appeared during the French army's occupation of Naples in February 1495. From that moment on, the disease was referred to as the French sickness.

The exact origin of the disease remains a matter of great dispute. It is not my intention in this essay to rehearse the theories advanced by the competing schools of thought.[4] Rather, my aim is to study contemporary responses to the *mal francese*, and in particular to examine how the disease was utilised as a distinct literary topos by certain writers connected with the cultural milieu of mid-Cinquecento Tuscany. I will take as my focus the poet Agnolo Firenzuola, the often scurrilous dramatist Antonfrancesco Grazzini, and the controversial and enigmatic author identified only as il Grappa. All of these men operated on the fringes of official cultural production in the early decades of the sixteenth century and all of them were at the very least associated with, if not actually members of, the leading literary academies of the day.

The *mal francese* was a popular subject in cultural institutions such as the Accademia della Vigna, a Roman academy operating in the 1530s.[5] The members of this academy, the so-called Vignaiuoli (or 'Vintners'), were mostly well-educated men, who organised Roman-style banquets, where they read out and discussed their literary compositions. The majority of their output was in the form of burlesque poetry. This was a lively and entertaining vernacular medium, noted for its colloquialisms, linguistic hybrids, and double entendres, which was diametrically opposed to more formal and conventional literary styles. It had been typified in the Quattrocento by the writings of the Florentine barber Domenico di Giovanni, known as Burchiello, and was then developed and perfected by Francesco Berni in the early decades of the sixteenth century. The theme of the French Disease fitted in perfectly with the bawdy subject matter of Berni's satirical, tongue-in-cheek poetry and was particularly evident in his two 'Capitoli della Peste' of 1532. This latter work was itself influenced by the 'Capitolo del mal francioso' (1531), written by his friend and fellow academician Giovan Francesco Bini.[6]

---

[4]A detailed discussion of the various theories can be found in: French and Arrizabalaga, 'Coping with the French Disease;' Arrizabalaga, Henderson and French, *The Great Pox*; and Quétel, *History of Syphilis*.

[5]For information on the Vignaiuoli, see Maylender, *Storia delle accademie d'Italia*, vol. 5, pp. 466–467.

[6]Berni's 'secondo capitolo della peste' contains the following verses: 'Piange un le

The use of the *mal francese* as a literary vehicle for burlesque satire is evident in the largely unknown work by il Grappa, entitled *I cicalamenti del Grappa intorno al sonetto 'Poi che mia speme è lunga a venir troppo.'*[7] This commentary, first printed in Mantua and dated 1545, purports to be a scholarly exegesis of poem 88 of Petrarch's *Canzoniere*. A clue as to the content and tone of the composition is provided in the subheading: 'Dove si ciarla allungo delle lodi delle donne et del mal francioso' (where one chats at length about women and the French Disease). The commentary is dedicated to a certain Signora Antea Arcifanfana of San Petronio Vecchio; clearly a fictitious name that sets the stage for the ludic pronouncements that are to follow. Signora Antea, il Grappa informs the reader, is an ideal dedicatee, since she herself is 'un cimitero di mal francioso' (a veritable graveyard of the French Disease) (*I Cicalamenti*, fol. 2ʳ). Like her Boccaccian counterparts in the Preface to the *Decameron*, Signora Antea is shut away at home, with only her needle, thread, and spindle for company. Similarly, just like Boccaccio's 'gentildonne fiorentine,' she is suffering from an illness – in her case, it is not love-sickness, but rather the *mal francese*. The reader is assured from the very beginning that il Grappa will offer 'una spositione tanto nuova' (an exposition so original) that it will not only surprise other commentators, but even Petrarch himself, the original author of the sonnet (*I Cicalamenti*, fol. 6ᵛ).

Il Grappa's commentary begins with a rhetorical question: would Petrarch have acquired so much learning and knowledge, evident in his elegant compositions, if he had not contracted the *mal francese* from his beloved Laura? (*I Cicalamenti*, fols 15ᵛ–16ʳ). The reason that Petrarch spoke so warmly of her in his *Canzoniere* was thus to express his gratitude to her for bestowing him with such a gift. Indeed, according to il Grappa, women in general are to be praised, since they are the 'cagione di tanti nostri beni' (the reason for such great riches bestowed upon us) (*I Cicalamenti*, fol. 16ʳ).

The characteristics of the disease, according to il Grappa, are akin to the behaviour of a pedant towards his pupils: as long as students follow the rules and are obedient, they will be given useful instruction; when they choose to transgress and become disobedient, the *mal francese*, just like the

---

doglie e le bolle franciose | perché gli è pazzo, e non ha ancor veduto | quel che già messer Bin di lor compose' (One guy complains of his pains and the French boils because he's crazy, and he hasn't yet seen what Mr. Bini wrote about them). See Berni, *Capitoli*, ed. Dusi, pp. 77–81 (p. 78, vv. 34–36). Bini's 'Capitolo del mal francese' is contained in the *Opere burlesche di M. F. Berni e di altri*, pp. 163–172.

[7] *I Cicalamenti del Grappa intorno al sonetto "Poi che mia speme è lunga a venir troppo"* (Mantua: Venturino Ruffinelli, 1545). A copy of this work is contained in the Biblioteca Nazionale Centrale di Firenze; its classmark is Erotici 115.

pedant, is forced to scourge them in order to teach them a lesson. Whoever does not abide by the rules suffers as a result – this, il Grappa intimates, was the case with Petrarch, who apparently gave little care to his affliction, a fact that is evident in poem 88:

> Poi che mia speme è lunga a venir troppo,
> et de la vita il trappassar sí corto,
> vorreimi a miglior tempo esser accorto,
> per fuggir dietro piú che di galoppo;
> et fuggo anchor cosí debile et zoppo
> da l'un de' lati, ove 'l desio m'à storto:
> securo omai, ma pur nel viso porto
> segni ch'i' ò presi a l'amoroso intoppo.
> Ond'io consiglio: Voi che siete in via,
> volgete i passi; et voi ch'Amore avampa,
> non v'indugiate su l'extremo ardore;
> ché perch'io viva de mille un no scampa;
> era ben forte la nemica mia,
> et lei vid'io ferita in mezzo 'l core.[8]

> Since what I hope for is too long in coming and what is left of life is so short, I wish I had been wise earlier, to flee to the rear at more than a gallop; and I do flee now, even if so weak and lame on one side where desire has twisted me, safe but still in my face bearing scars that I got in the battle of love. Wherefore I counsel: You who are in the way, turn back your steps, and you whom Love inflames, do not wait for the fiercest burning, for, though I am alive, of a thousand not even one escapes. My enemy was strong, and her I saw wounded in the very heart![9]

The mock commentary begins with a discussion on the structure of the sonnet, which, we are informed, is divided into three parts (*I Cicalamenti*, fols 18^{v}–19^{r}). The first section, composed of verses 1–8, describes how Petrarch would have liked to have been made aware of his disorder; if he had been cogniscent of this, he would not have succumbed to the unbridled desires of the flesh ('vorreimi a miglior tempo esser accorto, | per fuggir dietro piú che di galoppo'). The consequences of his uncontrolled sexual escapades are all too evident in verses 7–8 ('ma pur nel viso porto segni ch'i' ò presi a l'amoroso intoppo'). As far as il Grappa is concerned, this is a clear reference to the ulcerated pustules that were so characteristic of the disease.

---

[8]This sonnet is located amongst a number of similar poems in the *Canzoniere* in which the author, believing himself to be freed from the bonds of Love, advises others to escape its insidious snares.

[9]The translation is taken from *Petrarch's Lyric Poems*, ed. Durling, p. 190.

The second part of the poem is composed of the first tercet (verses 9–11). Here, the reader is apparently confronted by an exhortation from Petrarch: those people who already have the malady are encouraged to sublimate their sexual activities and to master their libido, whilst those who are healthy are encouraged not to wait until the last minute to contract it: 'Voi che siete in via, | volgete i passi; et voi ch'Amore avampa, | non v'indugiate su l'extremo ardore.' In the last tercet (verses 12–14), there is an apparent reference to Madonna Laura. The wound in the middle of her heart is not due to an amorous arrow fired from Cupid's bow, but rather is a sign of her own contagion. Il Grappa does state quite categorically in his commentary that Petrarch endeavoured to exhort those who had not yet contracted the disease to do so as soon as possible. This rather perverse advice is justified by il Grappa on the grounds that 'il mal francioso è quello che in pochissimo tempo [...] ci fa santi, dotti e perfetti nelle migliori et più lodate discipline'; in other words, it renders the afflicted 'saintly, wise and perfect in the best and most praiseworthy pursuits'. The disease, then, should not be considered a bad thing in itself. If it were, il Grappa argues, Madonna Laura, who was after all such a strong woman and who was so resistant to wicked things, would not have caught it in the first place.

It is tempting to try and unmask the elusive – and allusive – author of this work. The 1545 Mantua edition of the *Cicalamenti* also contains the 'Comento del Grappa nella canzone di Firenzuola in lode della salsiccia'.[10] Giovan Mario Crescimbeni (1663–1728), author of the vast *Istoria della volgar poesia*, maintained that Agnolo Firenzuola was not only the author of the erotically equivocal 'canzone in lode della salsiccia,' but of the 'Comento' itself; in other words, that he was the figure behind the mysterious il Grappa. This declaration was challenged by Antonio Magliabechi (1633–1714), who contended that the person responsible for the 'Comento' was neither Firenzuola, 'né altro Fiorentino.'[11] Firenzuola was indeed accustomed to various appellations; he was known as 'il Pennato' in the Accademia della Vigna, and he concealed himself behind the character 'Celso' in his *Dialogo delle bellezze delle donne* (1540). Nevertheless, Magliabechi's comment on Firenzuola's lack of involvement does seem a valid assertion, particularly

---

[10]This work had been ascribed by early commentators to Grazzini; no doubt the confusion arose due to his 'Capitolo in lode della salsiccia,' written to Gismondo Martelli, one of the original founding members of the Accademia degli Umidi. Gismondo died in 1548, helping us to establish a terminus ante quem for the composition. The *capitolo* is contained in Grazzini, *Rime burlesche*, pp. 459–463. See also pp. XC–XCVI of this edition for Verzone's discussion of the authorship of the work.

[11]BNCF, Magl. IX, 104, 'Notizie di Scrittori Fiorentini,' fol. 36^{v}. Magliabechi did not provide any evidence for these assertions.

when we bear in mind the date of Firenzuola's death (1543) – two years before the publication of il Grappa's *Cicalamenti*. The possibility of the work being published posthumously cannot be discounted, though it does seem unlikely. What is certain is the fact that il Grappa was an educated *letterato* who appears to have been acquainted with several of the most famous contemporary writers of satirical works.[12] References are made in the *Cicalamenti* to the mock-heroic poem *La Moscheide* (The Battle of the Flies) by Merlino Cocaio, the *nom de plume* of Teofilo Folengo, and there are allusions to compositions by Giovan Francesco Bini and Giovan Maria Molza. It is also clear that il Grappa was very conversant with the practice of lampooning contemporary learned treatises. Such examples of literary *jouissance* formed part of the tradition of learned erotica prevalent in many of the sixteenth-century literary academies.[13] There is an allusion to these cultural institutions in the body of the text, as the author claims to have read out this commentary in the (presumably fictitious) Accademia de' Balordi, or Academy of the Harebrained.

Much of the vocabulary and style of the *Cicalamenti del Grappa* is remarkably similar to that found in the burlesque commentaries of Antonfrancesco Grazzini, who, together with Firenzuola, was responsible for a series of tongue-in-cheek compositions written in the early 1540s that mocked certain linguistic debates held in the Accademia Fiorentina, or Florentine Academy.[14] Furthermore, some of the themes used by Grazzini in his poetry are also evident in the *Cicalamenti*. Il Grappa had stated in his commentary of poem 88 that Petrarch's apparent baldness – 'la pelatina' – was due to alopecia, itself a symptom of the *mal francese*; this very same side-effect was highlighted by Grazzini on several occasions. In one sonnet he described it as 'cosa da tenerla in pregio e cara' (something precious, to be held in high esteem).[15] There is a further reference to this visual trait in his collection of *novelle* known as *Le Cene*: 'e non sarebbe stato mai uomo che lo avesse riconosciuto, come interviene ora a coloro che hanno quella spezie pazza di mal franzese che si chiama pelatina' (And no man would

---

[12]Alessandro Luzio and Rodolfo Renier contributed to the debate over the identity of il Grappa by discounting the names of several likely contemporary contenders, such as Pietro Aretino, Francesco Berni, and Niccolò Franco. See Luzio and Renier, 'Contributo alla storia del malfrancese,' p. 427.

[13]For a detailed discussion of this topic, see Frantz, *Festum Voluptatis*, especially pp. 9–42.

[14]For further details, see Zanrè, '«Che K.^{zo} vuol dire?»'. See also Plaisance, 'Réécriture et écriture.'

[15]Grazzini, *Rime burlesche*, sonnet LXXXIX, pp. 73–74 (p. 73, v. 4); see also sonnet XLII, pp. 37–38.

ever have been able to recognise him, as is the case these days with those people who contract that mad kind of *mal francese* called 'la pelatina').[16] If Grazzini was indeed the figure behind il Grappa, then Magliabechi's contention regarding the provenance of the author is inaccurate; however, without any form of concrete evidence, the true identity of this enigmatic individual can never be conclusively established.

If we accept that Grazzini and il Grappa were in fact the same person, then it naturally begs the following question: why did Grazzini choose to lampoon Petrarch, and why did he do so using an alias? To a certain extent, this playful commentary was part of the Florentine burlesque tradition of ridiculing established writers and cultural institutions, and was epitomised by the likes of Francesco Berni and his adherents. In broader terms it was indicative of the non-conformist attitude displayed by some sixteenth-century literati who were on the margins of official cultural acceptability. Such was the case with Grazzini, who was one of the original founding members of the short-lived and informal Accademia degli Umidi, or Academy of the Damp, where he was known by the name of 'il Lasca' ('the roach'). Within the space of three months – from November 1540 to February 1541 – Grazzini was compelled to watch the transformation of the Umidi into the official, Medici-sponsored Accademia Fiorentina.[17] Grazzini became one of the most vociferous protesters of the changes that were being implemented in the Fiorentina. His numerous acts of dissent and infringement against the authorities in the academy eventually resulted in his expulsion from it, following the reforms of 1547. Grazzini was thereafter forced to endure 19 years in the cultural cold before his readmission to the Accademia Fiorentina at the beginning of 1566.

Grazzini frequently included direct references, as well as passing allusions, to Petrarch's *Rime sparse* in his own poetry. In 1542 (three years before the publication of the *Cicalamenti*), Grazzini wrote a burlesque *canzone* to Lionardo della Fonte on the subject of the *mal francese*.[18] He explained the occasion of its bizarre composition in a line that deliberately parodied the opening sonnet of the *Canzoniere*: 'quand'era in parte altr'uom di quel che io sono, e che io

---

[16]Grazzini, *Le Cene*, ed. Bruscagli, I, 9 (p. 121, n. 4).

[17]The bibliography relating to the Accademia Fiorentina and its short-lived predecessor, the Accademia degli Umidi, is extensive. The most recent articles are by Zanrè, '«Che K.[zo] vuol dire?»'; Plaisance, 'Les Leçons publiques et privées'; and Bryce, 'The Oral World of the Early Accademia Fiorentina.' Other obligatory studies include: Di Filippo Bareggi, 'In nota alla politica culturale di Cosimo I'; Vasoli, 'Considerazioni sull'Accademia Fiorentina'; and two seminal works by Plaisance, 'Une première affirmation'; and 'Culture et politique.'

[18]See Grazzini, *Rime burlesche*, *canzone* III, pp. 143–148 (p. 145, vv. 11–13).

andava giuocando e puttaneggiando per tutto...' (when I was in part another man from what I am now, and when I used to play about and whore around everywhere). It is interesting to note that Grazzini chose to link petrarchan poetry with the French sickness, just as il Grappa was to do three years later in the *Cicalamenti*.

Grazzini would certainly have had a good knowledge of Petrarch's works, since the *Canzoniere* was the subject of the private readings held every Thursday for members of the Accademia Fiorentina.[19] Indeed, one of Grazzini's many acts of protest in the academy centred around his refusal to give a *lezione privata* on a sonnet from the *Canzoniere*.[20] For writers such as Grazzini, whose literary allegiance was predominantly to the *stile burlesco*, the promotion and imitation of petrarchan poetry was seen as a dry, unoriginal academic exercise that typified the excesses of sixteenth-century pedantry. In a letter of 10 July 1548, addressed to Lorenzo Scala, Grazzini declared that the burlesque genre was esteemed and appreciated by a large section of the Florentine populace:

> oggidì è fatto tanto conto, avuto in tanta stima, e tenuto in tanta riputazione, e non mica da' plebei, ma da uomini nobili e da signori, avendo le Petrarcherie, le squisitezze e le Bemberie, anzi che no, mezzo ristucco e 'nfastidito il mondo, perciocchè ogni cosa è quasi ripieno di *fior, fronde, erbe, ombre, antri, onde, aure soavi*.[21]

19Details of the *lezioni private* can be found in Plaisance, 'Les Leçons publiques et privées.'

20At a meeting on 27 October 1542, Grazzini's name was included in the list of those due to give a *lezione privata*. When asked to fulfil the obligation on 9 November of that year, however, he categorically refused: 'Giovedì alli nove di novembre 1542 lesse in Accademia privata nello studio di firenze per commissione del consolo Michelagnolo Vivaldi et seguitò la lectione delle rime del Petrarcha nel luogo ove si lasciò innanzi le vacantie cioè la sestina che comincia _____ [sic] finito che hebbe sua letione si trassero della borsa de i lettori privati per le due letioni prossime Antonfrancesco detto il Lasca et Piero Covoni fecesi loro intendere che non volsero leggere'; the details can be found in BMF, 'Annali,' fols 10^{v}–11^{r}. (On Thursday 9 November 1542, he gave a private reading in the Florentine Studio at the request of the Consul Michelagnolo Vivaldi, and his reading of Petrarch's poetry came next, commencing at the place where it had been left before the vacation, i.e., at the sextet that begins _____ [sic]. When he had finished his reading, the names of the readers for the next two private lectures were drawn – Antonfrancesco Grazzini, known as 'the roach,' and Piero Covoni made it clear that they did not wish to read). Grazzini's failure to comply with the request directly contravened the academy's statutes of the previous year, which decreed that every member was obliged to give a public and private *lezione*.

21The letter, dated 10 July 1548, was originally written as a preface to the *Primo libro delle opere burlesche del Berni ... , della Casa, del Varchi, del Mauro di messer Bino, del Molza, del Dolce, e del Firenzuola* (Florence: Giunta, 1548). It is reproduced in Grazzini, *Scritti*

> today it is depended upon, held in such esteem, and has such a reputation, and not only by the common man in the street, but also by noblemen and *signori*, since the poetic 'delicacies' of Petrarch and Bembo have pretty much bored and sickened the world. This is because almost every single thing is filled with 'flowers, leaves, grass, shadows, caves, waves, gentle breezes'.[22]

Here we have an instance of Grazzini's literary virtuosity; not only does he criticise Petrarch, but he does so by employing some of the Trecento poet's own verses. The seven nouns listed at the end of the quotation are taken from the fifth line of poem 303, entitled 'Amor, che meco al buon tempo ti stavi' (Love, who in the happy time stayed with me along these banks). Though he may ostensibly have been declaring his contempt for contemporary imitators of petrarchan poetry, Grazzini's mode of criticism nevertheless reveals his familiarity with the *Canzoniere*. Indeed, Grazzini's desire to parody Petrarch did not preclude his own attempts at compositions written in the style of the *Rime sparse*. These compositions were intended to demonstrate his creative skill and his ability to compete with the leading versifiers of the day. The irony is that in so doing, Grazzini was in effect contributing to the second-rate slavish imitations of Petrarch that he himself mocked.

It is evident that Grazzini was a complex character, whose writing frequently expressed divergent and often opposing literary views. This same contradictory attitude is revealed in his treatment of the *mal francese* with regard to both elegant courtesans and more common prostitutes. Grazzini had quite a penchant for their company. His poetry reflects this, with a variety of sonnets and madrigals that catalogue his relationships with women such as Giulia Napoletana, and the exotic-sounding Nannina Zinzera and Milla Capraia.[23] It is unclear whether he actually contracted the *mal francese*, though he certainly described its symptoms in several works, most notably in his *canzone* to Lionardo della Fonte.[24] In this composition, the author recounts a nightmare. During the course of his terrible dream, he imagines that he has caught the disease and proceeds to describe its horrific effects

---

scelti, ed. Fornaciari, pp. 168–170 (pp. 168–169).

[22]The translation of this line is taken from *Petrarch's Lyric Poems*, ed. Durling, p. 482.

[23]Georgina Masson has referred to Nannina as Grazzini's 'favourite' *cortigiana*; see her book *Courtesans of the Italian Renaissance*, p. 117. Poems addressed or referring to the following women can be found in Grazzini, *Rime burlesche*: Giulia Napoletana (*madrigalessa* XVIII, pp. 274–276; XIX, pp. 276–277; XX, pp. 277–280), Nannina Zinzera (*madrigalone* III, pp. 244–245), and Milla Capraia (*sonetto* CXXXVII, p. 110).

[24]See above, n. 18.

upon his body, particularly with regard to his sexual organs: 'discourteous, barbaric, tyrannous French sickness, you have completely deprived me of them.' He then continues with the following ludic lament: 'ond'io vo per tutto gridando come pazzo: ohimè!, ohimè!, ohimè!, dov'è il mio cazzo?' (And so I wander around shrieking like a madman: 'Oh my! Oh my! Oh my! Wherever is my cock?).

In the main, however, Grazzini takes a much more serious attitude towards the disease. He appears to have used it chiefly as a metaphor of blame, and his general representation of it reflects the contemporary view of the *mal francese* as a sign of alterity. Its very name was a loaded term containing multiple meanings; not only did it provide the disease with a suitable title, but it also served to identify it with a particular external group (or groups):

> Each newly affected country lost no time naming the new disease after the neighbour which it suspected, usually with good reason, of having been the source of contamination. The following gives an idea of the variety of names: the Muscovites referred to it as the Polish sickness, the Poles as the German sickness, and the Germans as the French sickness – a term of which the English also approved (French pox) as did the Italians (which presented certain difficulties). The Flemish and the Dutch called it the 'Spanish sickness,' as did the inhabitants of North-west Africa. The Portuguese called it 'the Castilian sickness,' whilst the Japanese and the peoples of the East Indies came to call it 'the Portuguese sickness'. Only the Spanish, oddly, enough, did not call it anything. (Quétel, *History of Syphilis*, p. 16)

As is so often the case with a new and virulent disease, ignorance and fear predominate in equal measure. Sixteenth-century responses were no different in this respect. The illness – whatever the name ascribed to it – was rapidly adopted as a metaphor for blame. The very process of assigning guilt and responsibility for its origin helped people to try and come to terms with it. As William Eamon has indicated, 'placing blame for devastating new diseases is a means of taking the mystery out of the incomprehensible, and of controlling what is terrifying. Locating blame is in a sense a quest for order and certainty' (Eamon, 'Cannibalism and Contagion,' p. 21). For a modern parallel, we need look no further than the early days of the AIDS epidemic in the 1980s, and the demonisation by many of certain minority groups in society. As far as Cinquecento Italy was concerned, the perceived Other included political, religious, social, and sexual outsiders, represented by the foreigner, the Jew, the leper, and the prostitute respectively. On occasion, contemporary writers conflated the suspected involvement of various demonised groups in order to emphasise the point. In 1525, Pietro

Mainardi argued in his *Epistola II ad Michaelem Sanctannam* that the disease had originated as the result of the sexual relationship between a Spanish prostitute and a leper. Paracelsus expressed very similar sentiments in his *Chirurgia magna* (1536), in which he accredited the development of the disease to the union of a French leper and a prostitute afflicted with venereal sores.[25]

The members of this latter group were marginalised on account of their profession. Prostitutes were generally regarded as being morally corrupt and unclean. Antonfrancesco Grazzini shared this view. Like other contemporary writers, he invariably equated prostitution with pollution to create, in his mind, an institution that was simultaneously civic and syphilitic. Thus, whenever he chose to write in a derogatory manner about *puttane*, he invariably portrayed them as carriers of the *mal francese*. Such is the case in his 'Canto di giovani impoveriti per le meretrici,' or 'Carnival song of young men impoverished on account of whores.' The song ascribes the financial ruin of so many promising *giovani* to the insatiable greed of the *puttane* they frequent. Not only are their clients expected to ply them with rings, necklaces, and expensive clothes, but so too with sumptuous banquets for both themselves and their families. Men who were once young and wealthy have been reduced to financial ruin in their old age on account of these 'ribalde meretrici,' or 'shameless harlots.' The climax of Grazzini's catalogue of woes, however, comes with the announcement that these women are riddled with syphilis: 'dopo alle spese e alla roba perduta e l'onore, | han tanto malfranzese | e coperto e palese: | anzi di doglie e gomme e piaghe infetti, | non trovano spedal che gli raccetti' (After all the expenses, clothes and honour that they have cast aside, they are completely infected with the French sickness: indeed they are so covered in pustules and wounds, that they are unable to find a hospital that will attend to them). If they were lucky enough, sufferers of the illness were treated in the so-called *Ospedali degli incurabili*, or Hospitals for Incurables, which were established in the sixteenth century. The purpose of these institutions was to look after the poor, the incapable, and those people who had been denied treatment in more general hospitals.[26]

One might speculate why a writer who was so at ease in the company of prostitutes should be so vitriolic towards them in this carnival song? In order to understand this, we need to consider the cultural context. Attacks against *puttane* were something of a literary tradition. Grazzini's contempo-

---

25For a fuller discussion, see Foa, 'The New and the Old,' p. 39.

26The creation and development of the *Ospedali degli incurabili* is discussed by Arrizabalaga, Henderson and French in *The Great Pox*; see especially pp. 145–170.

rary Giovambattista dell'Ottonaio, a fellow poet and author of more than thirty *canti carnascialeschi*, had previously written a 'Canzona de' puttanieri'; Grazzini's later 'Canto di giovani impoveriti per le meretrici' is very similar to it in terms of both tone and content. Both works featured in the collection of Carnival songs edited by Grazzini entitled *Tutti i trionfi, carri, mascherate o canti carnascialeschi andati per Firenze dal tempo del magnifico Lorenzo de' Medici fino all' anno 1559.*[27] This collection was published at a time when Grazzini was out of favour with the city's cultural élite. Grazzini's composition and inclusion of the 'Canto di giovani impoveriti per le meretrici' may have been intended as a public act of penance – an indication to the Medici regime that he was attempting to dissociate himself with Florence's stigmatised community and to mend his ways and change his behaviour.

The animosity expressed by Grazzini in the 'Canto di giovani impoveriti per le meretrici' and in others like it epitomised the general love-hate relationship that existed between prostitutes and the literati. On the one hand the women provided a service for their clientele that was in great demand; on the other, the sheer frequency of their business transactions had an adverse effect on both their health and the health of their customers. The misogynistic attitude inherent in much of the *poesia puttanesca* of this period reflected its distinctly male credentials – it was written by men, and for men.[28] However, these same authors – and their readers – invariably failed to recognise (or to admit) that it was due to their own sexual appetites that women became afflicted with the disease in the first place. It is perhaps ironic that a writer such as Grazzini, who penned burlesque and at times transgressive works, should participate in the literary demonisation of a social group that was itself marginalised by the contemporary community.[29]

So far I have discussed how the *mal francese* served as a literary motif in order to parody contemporary learned treatises. In addition, I have also

---

[27]The collection was published by the ducal printer Lorenzo Torrentino, which was ironic since Duke Cosimo I was subsequently to suspend the sale of the edition in March of that year, following complaints from Paolo dell'Ottonaio, the Canon of the church of San Lorenzo. Paolo had accused Grazzini of including in his edition a number of inaccurate versions of his brother Giovambattista's carnival songs. In January 1560, all of Giovambattista dell'Ottonaio's songs were removed from the edition, and in the following year a censored version of *Tutti i trionfi, carri, mascherate o canti carnascialeschi* was permitted to be sold to the public. For details, see Rodini, *Antonfrancesco Grazzini*, p. 25.

[28]For a discussion of the disease from a gender perspective, see Schleiner, 'Infection and Cure Through Women.'

[29]For more information on efforts to link prostitutes with the disease see Laura McGough's essay in this volume.

alluded to its function as a metaphor for blame, used in compositions that criticise and attack certain sectors of society that were considered 'deviant.' A further literary response to the pox can be found in works that personalise and contextualise it. For a good example of this, we need look no further than the writings of Grazzini's friend and fellow *letterato* Agnolo Firenzuola, some of which highlight the socio-cultural effects of the disease. The French sickness was an eminently suitable topos for Firenzuola, given his somewhat colourful early life. Born in Florence in 1493, he had studied law in Siena at the request of his father, despite his own lack of vocation towards the legal profession. In 1518, Firenzuola travelled to Rome, where he became acquainted with a number of prominent literati, including Francesco Berni, Giovanni Della Casa, Giovan Maria Molza, and Giovan Francesco Bini. All of these men belonged to the Accademia della Vigna. As a member of this academy, Firenzuola would have been well acquainted with the use of the *mal francese* as a traditional theme in contemporary vernacular poetry.[30] Indeed, he was no stranger to sexual transgression.[31] He was reminded of his propensity for 'giovenili piacevolezze' (youthful pranks) in a letter by Pietro Aretino, which described a particularly memorable incident from their past:

> Certo che io ritorno spesso con la fantasia a i casi de le nostre giovenili piacevolezze. Né crediate che mi sia scordato la fuga di quella vecchia che isgomberò il paese, impaurita da la villania che di bel dì chiaro e di su la finestra voi gli diceste in camiscia e io ignudo. Ho anco in mente il conflitto ch'io feci in casa di Camilla Pisana a l'ora che mi lasciaste ad intertenerla.[32]

> Indeed, I often whimsically recall examples of our youthful pranks. Don't think I've forgotten about the time when that old woman created an uproar in the town, terrified by your rude words to her in broad daylight at the window – you in your shirt and me stark naked. I also remember the carry-on that I had in Camilla Pisana's house when you left me to entertain her.

The letter also makes reference to their associations with some of the leading courtesans of the day. Firenzuola was known to have been intimate with cultivated *cortigiane* such as Tullia d'Aragona and Camilla Pisana, and he

---

30Information on Firenzuola's association with the Accademia della Vigna can be found in Fatini, *Agnolo Firenzuola*, 15–17.

31For further details, see Zanrè, 'Alterity and Sexual Transgression.'

32The letter is dated Venice, 26 October 1541. See Aretino, *Lettere*, ed. Procaccioli, no. 176 (pp. 471–472).

frequently referred to his numerous female acquaintances in his writings.[33] He paid a heavy penalty for his amorous adventures when he fell victim to the *mal francese* at the beginning of 1526.

Firenzuola's own experiences of the disease form the subject of two separate and quite distinct compositions. The first of these is an ostensibly light hearted poem entitled 'In lode del legno santo,' or 'In praise of the Holy Wood' (Firenzuola, *Opere*, pp. 957–961). Despite its inherently relaxed, jocular style, 'In lode del legno santo' provides scholars with a great deal of information, particularly with regard to the treatment of the affliction, as well as to contemporary perceptions of it. The *legno santo* was the name given to guaiac, or guaiacum, a genus of tree native to the West Indies and to the more temperate parts of North America, brought to Europe as a result of seafaring expeditions. This hard and heavy greenish-brown wood was referred to as *lignum sanctum* or *lignum vitae* ('holy wood,' or 'the wood of life'), because its resin, boiled down and made into a concoction, was alleged to have certain curative properties, particularly in relation to sexually transmitted diseases.[34] It is these very properties that Firenzuola praises in the poem. As he declares, 'Io non vorrei a fatica sognare | Di scriver d'altro mai che di quel legno' (I would not wish to dream of ever writing about anything else but that wood) (Firenzuola, *Opere*, p. 957, vv. 10–11).

The first rumours of the medicinal virtues of the wood are thought to have originated in Spain and Portugal between 1506 and 1516. It was believed to be most efficacious when taken as part of a course of treatment. Normally, the patient, wrapped in blankets, would shut himself (or herself) in a small warm room without any ventilation, in order to try and sweat out the disease. A strict diet was maintained, and a concoction made from the guaiacum was administered orally at regular intervals. The treatment would typically last a month or more until the body was cleansed of its impurities and the *mal francese* was eradicated.[35] References to the diet undertaken by contemporary sufferers are contained in Firenzuola's poem; German princes 'fra lor fan diëta così spesso' (follow diets in private on a very regular basis) (Firenzuola, *Opere*, p. 958, vv. 25–26). The medicinal effects of the wood were widely known in Germany at this time. Ulrich

[33]For further details, see Murray, 'Agnolo Firenzuola on Female Sexuality.' Firenzuola wrote several sonnets to a woman identified only as 'Mona Maria,' who may have been the courtesan Maria da Prato. See Firenzuola, *Opere*, sonnets 71 (p. 897), 98 (p. 954), 99 (p. 955), 100 (pp. 955–956). A particularly virulent composition to Tullia d'Aragona is contained in Firenzuola, *Opere*, sonnet 126 (p. 1002).

[34]For a detailed discussion of the history and efficacy of the *legno santo*, see Munger's excellent if dated article 'Guaiacum.'

[35]The treatment is discussed in Munger, 'Guaiacum.' pp. 206–208.

von Hutten's volume on the subject entitled *De guaiaci medicina et morbo gallico* ('On the medicinal properties of guaiacum and the French sickness') was published in Mainz in 1519. In book one of the work, von Hutten dwelt at length on his own case of *mal francese* and his subsequent cure using guaiacum. Not only did he describe the physical properties of the wood, but he also offered one of the earliest and most detailed accounts of its preparation into a medicine.

The central section of Firenzuola's composition appears to echo von Hutten's treatise, since it contains a discussion of the healing power attributed to the 'holy wood.' The patient, covered in sores and boils, is invariably unable to sleep at night due to the extreme pain. As soon as the concoction is administered to him, however, 'ogni suo membro in modo gli dispone, | Che può tornare a dormir con la moglie' (every limb is made better, so that he can go back to sleeping with his wife) (Firenzuola, *Opere*, p. 959, vv. 44–45). The sheer efficacy of the *legno santo* prompts Firenzuola to sing its praises, declaring it to be worth its weight in gold: 'Ma per tornar del legno al buon lavoro | Che, se ben mi ricorda, vi avisava, | Ch'al mal franzese valeva un tesoro' (But to return to the good work done by the wood; if I remember correctly, I advised you that, as far as the *mal francese* was concerned, it was worth a fortune) (Firenzuola, *Opere*, p. 959, vv. 49–51).

The most interesting – and entertaining – part of the poem is the final section, in which Firenzuola chooses to discuss his own experience of the disease and to describe his numerous attempts to rid himself of it. He has spent considerable sums of money on various medicines, all in an effort to find a cure. Indeed, he has exhausted the entire supplies of an apothecary in the process. His efforts, however, have been to no avail, so he comes to the following conclusion: 'Quanti danari ho speso per guarire, | Che meglio era giucarsegli a primiera' (I've spent a lot of cash on various cures; it would have been better to lose it playing at cards) (Firenzuola, *Opere*, pp. 960–961, vv. 97–98). He has tried a whole series of different remedies:

> Ho mutato aria, ho mutato paesi,
> Or ho abbracciata la poltroneria,
> Or in far esercizio i giorni ho spesi.

> I've changed air, I've moved town, first I became lazy and inactive, then I spent my days exercising. (Firenzuola, *Opere*, p. 961, vv. 109–111)

The initiatives employed by Firenzuola, commendable as they are, have proved futile. It is thus little wonder that he unreservedly praises the curative effects of the *legno santo*, for, in his own words, it saved him from an early grave ('Da poi che m'ha cavato dell'avello') (Firenzuola, *Opere*, p. 961, v. 124).

Firenzuola had no shortage of source material relating to the *legno santo*. Ulrich von Hutten's *De guaiaci medicina* was not only printed in Latin, but also in numerous vernacular languages. An Italian translation was published by Hieronymus de Benedictis of Bologna in 1521, and Firenzuola may well have availed himself of this edition. Another, even more successful work was Girolamo Fracastoro's *Syphilis sive morbus gallicus* (1530), published in approximately one hundred different editions during the course of the sixteenth century. In Book III of this poem, Fracastoro focused on the merits of the wood, extolling its virtues as the 'spes hominum, externi decus, et nova gloria mundi' (hope of mankind, pride and new glory from a foreign world) (Fracastoro, *Syphilis*, p. 107). The *legno santo* gained a large number of contemporary supporters who advocated its use. The Florentine goldsmith Benvenuto Cellini described in his *Vita* how he contracted the *mal francese* in Rome during the 1530s – at more or less the same time as Firenzuola – and how, despite the advice of doctors, he followed a course of treatment based on the 'holy wood':

> La infirmità gli era il vero che io l'avevo, ma credo che io l'avessi guadagnata mediante quella bella giovane serva che io tenevo nel tempo che io fui rubato. Soprastette quel morbo gallico a scoprirmisi piú di quattro mesi interi, di poi mi coperse tutto tutto a un tratto: non era innel modo de l'altro che si vede, ma pareva che io fussi coperto di certe vescichette, grandi come quattrini, rosse. I medici non mel volson mai battezzare mal franzese: e io pure dicevo le cause che credevo che fussi. Continuavo di medicarmi a lor modo, e nulla mi giovava; pur poi a l'ultimo, risoltomi a pigliare il legno contra la voglia di quelli primi medici di Roma, questo legno io lo pigliavo con tutta la disciplina e astinenzia che immaginar si possa, e in brevi giorni senti' grandissimo miglioramento; a tale che in capo a cinquanta giorni io fui guarito e sano come un pesce.

> It was true that I had caught the disease, but I think it must have been from that pretty young servant girl I was keeping at the time I was robbed. The French pox kept its distance for more than four whole months, and then it suddenly broke out all over. It did not show itself in the usual way, but I was covered with a number of small blisters, red ones, about the size of farthings. The doctors refused to christen it the pox, though I told them why I thought it was that. Anyhow I carried on with their treatment, without the least result. In the end, against the advice of the best doctors in Rome, I decided to take the *lignum vitae*. I did so with the greatest imaginable care and abstinence, and within a few days began to feel very much better; to such an extent, in fact, that at the end of fifty days I was completely healed and as sound as a roach.[36]

---

[36] *La Vita di Benvenuto Cellini*, ed. Davico Bonino, I, p. 59. The English version is taken from the translation by Bull, p. 111.

The *legno santo* was not without its critics, however. The celebrated physician Paracelsus had declaimed it in favour of the more traditional remedy using ointments and lotions made from mercury.[37] The widespread promotion of guaiacum as a suitable cure for the *mal francese* suffered a setback with von Hutten's death as a result of the disease in 1523. In subsequent decades following the publication of Fracastoro's *Syphilis*, the reputation of the *legno santo* as an effective antidote began to diminish. By 1546, Fracastoro himself admitted in his *De Contagione* that the concoction of guaiacum could produce ill effects, especially when mixed with wine rather than water: 'vidimus enim multos e potu vini illius male affectos in insanabilem aegritudinem decidisse' (I have observed many cases where patients drank this wine and were made ill by it, and lapsed into a condition beyond care) (Fracastoro, *De Contagione*, trans. Cave Wright, III, p. 279).

Fracastoro and von Hutten may have provided Firenzuola with the necessary background information to the disease and its methods of treatment, but the most likely, and certainly most accessible, contemporary source on the subject was Niccolò Campani da Siena's work entitled *Il lamento dello Strascino* of 1510. Campani was a fellow Tuscan writer who was also residing in Rome at the beginning of the Cinquecento, and it was here that he became infected with the *mal francese* some time in the first decade of the century.[38] His *Lamento* consists of two parts: in the first half, the narrator describes his own suffering; he both invokes and curses God, whilst regretting the loss of his good health and underlining the apparent hopelessness of his present situation. The second part of the poem is much more spirited and cheerful. Evidently the author has been cured of his affliction thanks to the *legno santo* and even dares to joke about the disease. It is possible that this light hearted second section served as the inspiration for Firenzuola's 'In lode del legno santo.'

By contrast, the darker first half of Strascino's *Il lamento* is seemingly reflected in Firenzuola's other poem on the *mal francese*, entitled 'Intorno la sua malattia' (Regarding the author's illness) (Firenzuola, *Opere*, pp. 799–807). This latter work – composed of 278 verses, divided into 4 sections – is completely different in tone and content; the colloquial, burlesque verses of 'In lode del legno santo' are replaced here with an altogether more sombre

---

[37]Arab doctors such as Avicenna (*Canon Medicinae*) and Rhazes (*Regem Mansorem*) had already recognised the use of mercury as an effective cure for skin disorders. For details, see French and Arrizabalaga, 'Coping with the French Disease,' pp. 248–287 (see especially pp. 255, 282, n. 21).

[38]Details of Strascino da Siena can be found in Luzio and Renier, 'Contributo alla storia del malfrancese' (see pp. 420–424).

penitential quality. In the work, Firenzuola provides an account of an interior monologue with God, in which he, as author, implores the Almighty to bring an end to his suffering. His pain is of such intensity that he has considered taking his own life; the only things that prevent him from following this course of action are the possible consequences such actions may have on his soul.[39] Paradoxically, his present life is in effect a form of death; his body, which he describes as an 'albergo degli affanni' (hostel of grief), is deprived of every kind of goodness and tranquillity, and peace (Firenzuola, *Opere*, p. 801, v. 70). If God were to intervene and take him from this world, his 'animo afflitto,' or afflicted soul, would be led to a new life, free from his present pains. In the final section of the poem, Firenzuola tries to convince God to come to his aid by talking of his faith. He declares that he doesn't want his anger, frustration, or impatience attributed to any wickedness on his part, but to the extreme desperation in which he finds himself. His final comment serves as a suitable leitmotif for his state of mind throughout the composition: 'sia la morte | Fine e riposo di sì lunghi affanni' (May death be an end and a solace to such long-drawn-out sufferings) (Firenzuola, *Opere*, p. 807, vv. 277–278).

The value of this poem lies not only in its function as a testament to the sufferings of one man, for it also serves as a social document that charts the symptoms of the malady. Firenzuola is careful to record many of the outward manifestations of the illness: the alternating bouts of heat and cold, the nightmares, the prodigious sweats, and the pain and lethargy experienced in all of his joints. In addition, certain biographical details allow us to date with precision the composition of this work. In the initial section, Firenzuola makes the following declaration: 'Quanto questo sia in me tu 'l sai, Signore, | Ch'essendo omai nel quarantesimo anno, | Mi trovo vecchio, infermo' (You know, Lord, how long I have lived with this inside me, because now that I am in my fortieth year, I find myself old and infirm) (Firenzuola, *Opere*, p. 800, vv. 31–33). Firenzuola was born in September 1493; thus, if he was 40 years old at the time of composition (assuming that the information is accurate), then the work would have been written in 1533. A further detail reveals the duration of his illness: 'Che già sette anni afflitto ha questo corpo' (This body has already suffered for seven years)

---

[39]'Io vorrei volentier tormi la vita | Con le mie proprie man, se la paura | De l'estremo giudicio non facesse | Torcer la voglia forse a miglior voglia' (I would willingly take my life with my own hands, if it were not for the fear of the Last Judgement, which made me alter my desire to perhaps a better one); see Firenzuola, *Opere*, pp. 799–800, vv. 20–23.

(Firenzuola, *Opere*, p. 803, v. 146). The information thus confirms the date of his initial contraction of the disease in 1526.

Similar compositional clues can be found in the more frivolous 'In lode del legno santo.' Delmo Maestri has demonstrated that this is an earlier work by pointing to certain textual references.[40] For example, Britonio and Casio are two contemporary figures who are cited in the work; these men made their living as minor poets at the papal courts of Leo X and Clement VII (Firenzuola, *Opere*, p. 958, v. 30). The city of Rome is specifically mentioned as the place of action in the poem (Firenzuola, p. 961, v. 104). This would appear to indicate that the work was composed some time between 1518 (Firenzuola's arrival in the city) and 1534 (death of Clement VII). Firenzuola's passing comment on the curative practices adopted north of the Alps may help to validate this hypothesis. If he was familiar with von Hutten's *De guaiaci medicina*, as seems likely, then 'In lode del legno santo' must have been composed post-1519. There is, however, an inherent contradiction with such a theory: how can Firenzuola claim to have been cured of the *mal francese*, thanks to the holy wood, if he later writes at length of his syphilitic suffering in 'Intorno la sua malattia'? Either he had experienced a state of remission, before an even more acute attack later in his life, or else he had been cured before contracting a further case of the disease at a subsequent date. An additional point to note is that Firenzuola spent much of his life in holy orders. Between 1518 and 1526, Firenzuola was a member of the Vallombrosan order. His decision to enter this order may, however, have been due to convenience, rather than religious zeal; after all, his father was a notary in the order, and he would have been in a position to assist the career of his son Agnolo during his stay in Rome. Indeed, Firenzuola was to take full financial advantage of his clerical benefices, whilst enjoying the position of procurator of the Vallombrosans in the papal curia. Interestingly, he was released from his vows in 1526; one wonders if this was due to his contraction of the *mal francese* in that same year. He did not assume his clerical obligations again until 1538, when he was made abbot of the monastery of San Salvatore at Vaiano. Firenzuola's ecclesiastical hiatus thus corresponds precisely to the period of time during which he was struggling to find a cure for his illness. In this light, 'Intorno la sua malattia' can be interpreted as a heartfelt, penitential call to God by a contrite sinner, a kind of 'Apologia pro vita sua' for his earlier youthful excesses.

---

[40]See the Introduction to Firenzuola, *Opere*, especially p. 14.

Not only did different writers represent a wide range of responses to the French Disease, but – as is clear from Firenzuola's poetry – even individual writers put the disease to a wide range of metaphorical uses, for different purposes and with different effects. Given his involvement in the Accademia della Vigna, one would expect Firenzuola to compose bawdy, humorous satire on the *mal francese*. Yet when he discusses the disease in his own works, he produces a much more sober and self-reflective discourse than one might have imagined. Even his poem on the *legno santo* seems rather void of critical satire, focusing on the very real issue of treatment. His own infection may have had a lot to do with this. In 1526, when he thought that he had been cured, he had room for some (relatively) lighter prose about the disease. Seven years later, though, when it became evident that the disease had not disappeared, his writing was characterised by much darker personal reflections.

It should be evident from this essay that the *mal francese* functioned as a very fertile and effective topos, whether it be in a ludic manner that was intended to parody contemporary genres, as a literary vehicle of attack directed against a particular group in society, or in personal accounts of the sufferings endured by the afflicted, and in objective descriptions of the symptoms. It proved to be an extremely popular and durable theme amongst writers of burlesque works in the Cinquecento, and it is perhaps little wonder that il Grappa chose to describe it as 'così buona e perfetta cosa' (Such a good and perfect thing).

University of Glasgow
Glasgow, Scotland

Cited Works

Manuscript Sources

Firenze. Biblioteca Marucelliana di Firenze (BMF) B.III.52–54, 'Annali degli Umidi, poi Fiorentina'.

Firenze. Biblioteca Nazionale Centrale di Firenze (BNCF) MS. Magl. IX, 104 'Notizie di Scrittori Fiorentini'.

Published Sources

Aretino, Pietro. *Lettere*, ed. Paolo Procaccioli. Milan: Rizzoli, 1990.

Arrizabalaga, Jon, John Henderson, and Roger French. *The Great Pox: The French Disease in Renaissance Europe*. New Haven: Yale University Press, 1997.

Benivieni, Antonio. *De abditis nonnullis ac mirandis morborum et sanationum causis*, trans. Charles Singer. Springfield, IL: Thomas, 1954.

Berni, Francesco. *Capitoli*. ed. Riccardo Dusi. Turin: UTET, 1926.

Bryce, Judith. 'The Oral World of the Early Accademia Fiorentina' *Renaissance Studies,* 9 (1995): 77–103.

Cellini, Benvenuto. *La Vita di Benvenuto Cellini.* ed. Guido Davico Bonino. Turin: Einaudi, 1973.

Cellini, Benvenuto. *The Life of Benvenuto Cellini,* trans. George Bull. London: Penguin, 1956.

Di Filippo Bareggi, Claudia. 'In nota alla politica culturale di Cosimo I: l'Accademia Fiorentina' *Quaderni Storici,* 23 (1973): 527–574.

Eamon, William. 'Cannibalism and Contagion: Framing Syphilis in Counter-Reformation Italy' *Early Science and Medicine,* 3:1 (1998): 1–31.

Fatini, Giuseppe. *Agnolo Firenzuola e la borghesia letterata del Rinascimento.* Cortona: Prem. Tipografia Sociale, 1907.

Firenzuola, Agnolo. *Opere.* ed. Delmo Maestri. Turin: UTET, 1977.

Foa, Anna. 'The New and the Old: The Spread of Syphilis (1494–1530)' pp. 26–45 in *Sex and Gender in Historical Perspective,* eds. Edward Muir and Guido Ruggiero. Baltimore: The Johns Hopkins University Press, 1990.

Fracastoro, Girolamo. *De Contagione,* trans. Wilmer Cave Wright. New York: The Knickerbocker Press, 1930.

Fracastoro, Girolamo. *Syphilis sive morbus gallicus,* trans. Geoffrey Eatough. Liverpool: Francis Cairns, 1984.

Frantz, David. *Festum Voluptatis: A Study of Renaissance Erotica.* Columbus, OH: Ohio State University Press, 1989.

French, Roger, and Jon Arrizabalaga, 'Coping with the French Disease: University Practitioners' Strategies and Tactics in the Transition from the Fifteenth to the Sixteenth Century' pp. 248–287 in *Medicine from the Black Death to the French Disease,* eds. Roger French, Jon Arrizabalaga, Andrew Cunningham and Luis Garcia-Ballester. Aldershot: Ashgate, 1998.

Grappa. *I Cicalamenti del Grappa intorno al sonetto 'Poi che mia speme è lunga a venir troppo.'* Mantua: Venturino Ruffinelli, 1545.

Grazzini, Antonfrancesco. *Le Cene,* ed. Riccardo Bruscagli. Rome: Salerno Editrice, 1976.

Grazzini, Antonfrancesco. *Rime burlesche edite e inedite,* ed. Carlo Verzone Florence: Sansoni, 1882.

Grazzini, Antonfrancesco. *Scritti scelti in prosa e poesia,* ed. Raffaele Fornaciari. Florence: Sansoni, 1911; repr. 1957.

Landucci, Luca. *Diario fiorentino, dal 1450 al 1516: continuato da un anonimo fino al 1542.* Florence: Sansoni, 1985.

Luzio, Alessandro, and Rodolfo Renier, 'Contributo alla storia del malfrancese ne' costumi e nella letteratura italiana del secolo XVI' *Giornale storico della letteratura italiana,* 5:3 (1885): 408–432.

Masson, Georgina. *Courtesans of the Italian Renaissance.* London: Secker and Warburg, 1975.

Maylender, Michele. *Storia delle accademie d'Italia,* 5 vols. Bologna: Cappelli, 1926–1930.

Medicine from the Black Death to the French Disease, ed. Roger French, Jon Arrizabalaga, Andrew Cunningham and Luis Garcia-Ballester. Aldershot: Ashgate, 1998.

Munger, Robert. 'Guaiacum, the Holy Wood from the New World' *Journal of the History of Medicine and Allied Sciences,* 4 (1949): 196–229.

Murray, Jacqueline. 'Agnolo Firenzuola on Female Sexuality and Women's Equality' *Sixteenth Century Journal*, 22:2 (1991): 199–213.

Opere burlesche di M. F. Berni e di altri, ed. Francesco Berni et al. Leiden: Van der Bet, 1823–1824.

Petrarch, Francesco. *Petrarch's Lyric Poems: The 'Rime sparse' and Other Lyrics*, ed. Robert Durling. Cambridge, MA, and London: Harvard University Press, 1976.

Plaisance, Michel. 'Culture et politique à Florence de 1542 à 1551: Lasca et les Humidis aux prises avec l'Académie Florentine' pp. 149–242 in *Les Écrivains et le pouvoir en Italie à l'époque de la Renaissance*. Second series, ed. André Rochon. Paris: Université Nouvelle de la Sorbonne, 1974.

Plaisance, Michel. 'Les Leçons publiques et privées de l'Académie florentine (1541–1552)' pp. 113–121 in *Les Commentaires et la naissance de la critique littéraire*. Paris: Aux Amateurs de Livres, 1990.

Plaisance, Michel. 'Réécriture et écriture dans les deux commentaires burlesques d'Antonfrancesco Grazzini' pp. 185–223 in *Réécritures 1: commentaires, parodies, variations dans la littérature italienne de la Renaissance*, ed. Jean Toscan. Paris: Université Nouvelle de la Sorbonne, 1983.

Plaisance, Michel. 'Une première affirmation de la politique culturelle de Côme Ier: la transformation de l'Académie des "Humidi" en Académie Florentine (1540–42)' pp. 361–438 in *Les Écrivains et le pouvoir en Italie à l'époque de la Renaissance*. First series, ed. André Rochon. Paris: Université Nouvelle de la Sorbonne, 1973.

Primo libro delle opere burlesche del Berni, della Casa, del Varchi, del Mauro di messer Bino, del Molza, del Dolce, e del Firenzuola, ed. Francesco Berni et al. Florence: Giunta, 1548.

Quétel, Claude. *History of Syphilis*, trans. Judith Braddock and Brian Pike. London: Polity Press, 1990.

Rodini, Robert. *Antonfrancesco Grazzini: Poet, Dramatist, and Novelliere, 1503–1584*. Madison, WI: University of Wisconsin Press, 1970.

Schleiner, Winfried. 'Infection and Cure Through Women: Renaissance Constructions of Syphilis' *Journal of Medieval and Renaissance Studies*, 24:3 (1994): 499–517.

Vasoli, Cesare. 'Considerazioni sull'Accademia Fiorentina' *Revue des Études Italiennes*, 25 (1979): 41–73.

Zanrè, Domenico. '«Che K.zo vuol dire?» A Re-Reading of Mid-Sixteenth-Century Linguistic Debates in the Accademia Fiorentina' *Italian Studies*, 53 (1998): 20–37.

Zanrè, Domenico. 'Alterity and Sexual Transgression in the Sixteenth-Century Tuscan Novella' pp. 159–178 in *The Italian Novella: A Book of Essays*, ed. Gloria Allaire. New York: Routledge, 2003.

Institutional and Policing Responses

Quarantining Beauty: The French Disease in Early Modern Venice[1]

Laura J. McGough

In 1556, Pietro Rostinio recounted his theory of the origins of the French Disease (commonly but problematically translated as syphilis). Little is known about Rostinio's life, other than that he translated, expanded upon and popularized earlier Latin medical treatises on the French Disease, especially the work of Antonio Brasavola (1500–1555).[2] Rostinio's popular medical book apparently reached a wide audience, with reprints in 1559 and 1565. After the French invasion of Italy in 1494, he explained, a most beautiful prostitute served the French troops. At the opening of her womb was a putrefying sore; the combination of the humidity and putrefaction of that 'place,' along with the rubbing of the male member against it, caused the male member to break out in ulcers. 'And this illness began to stain one man, then two, and three, & one hundred, because this woman was a prostitute and most beautiful, and since human nature is desirous of coitus, many women had sexual relations with these men (and became) infected with this illness.'[3] This beautiful prostitute was responsible for starting the epidemic of the French Disease that was dispersed through not only 'all of Italy, France, and throughout all of Europe,' but also Asia and Africa.[4] The only region that escaped the beautiful prostitute's influence

---

[1]This article is a revision of an earlier paper, 'Purifying the Body Politic: Venice's Response to Syphilis,' at The Body in Early Modern Italy Conference, Johns Hopkins University, Baltimore, MD, on 17 October 2002.

[2]On Brasavola's theory, see Foa, 'The New and the Old,' p. 39.

[3]Rostinio, *Trattato del Mal Francese*, fols. 21^{r-v}. The 1559 edition is a reprint of the 1556 edition. 'Nel campo de Francesi del mille quattrocento era una meretrice bellissima, la quale nella bocca della matrice haveva una apostema putrefatta, et gli huomini che usavano con lei fregolando il collo della matrice, per la humidità & putredine del loco, nel membro virile cõtrahevano una dispositione, che ulcerava.' fol. 21^{r}. 'Et questo male cominciò a macular prima un'huomo, poscia due, et tre, &cẽto, perche quella era publica meretrice & bellissima. & si come la natura humana è appetitosa del coito, molte donne usando con questi huomini, infettate si trovavano di tal male. Et queste l'han participato con altri huomini, tal che il detto male si è sparso per tutta la Italia, Francia, & per tutta l'Europa.' fol. 21^{v}.

was India, where the disease was, according to Rostinio, already well known, thereby making this woman the epidemiological equivalent of the 'shot heard round the world.'

Rostinio had constructed a 'Patient Zero,' a beautiful and promiscuous original patient, in much the same way that, centuries later, several epidemiologists and writer Randy Shilts would portray Gaetan Dugas, the Canadian airline steward, as responsible for the transmission of AIDS to dozens of North Americans on account of his physical attractiveness and promiscuity.[5] The beautiful Italian prostitute, however, was blamed not only for spreading disease, but also for having created the disease within her own body. She was never identified by name and could not have been alive (if she had ever existed) when Rostinio's book was published, whereas Gaetan Dugas was very much alive when he was identified as 'Patient Zero.' While Dugas was a living individual who became enveloped in myth, the beautiful prostitute was generic and nameless, always enshrouded in mythology.

Given the notoriety of historical figures such as Typhoid Mary,[6] modern readers are probably not surprised to learn that a sixteenth-century medical writer traced the origins of the epidemic to a single person. Nor would modern readers be surprised to read about prostitutes in connection with sexually transmitted diseases, since they are frequently described as a 'risk category.' But the association between the French Disease and sinful female sexuality was relatively new in the mid sixteenth century, as was the idea of tracing an epidemic to a single person. Whereas earlier theories of the French Disease's origins implicated bad air and shifts in the planets, this theory focused on the dangers of a woman's body, as well as on the dangers of temptation that women's beauty brought.[7]

Rostinio's reconstruction of the events of the late fifteenth century built on the long, slow development and acceptance of theories of contagion. Meanwhile, early modern Italians were responding to the threat of the French Disease by building institutions to enclose beautiful young women, separated from men who might find them sexually tempting. This

---

[4]'...Il detto male si è sparso per tutta la Italia, Francia, & per tutta l'Europa. Ho anco udito, che è in gran vigore nell'Asia, & che anco ne machiata l'Africa. Niente ragiono dell'India, che egli ivi è famigliarissimo.' fol. 21^{v}.

[5]Shilts, *And the Band Played On*. For commentary on Gaetan Dugas as 'Patient Zero,' see Griffin, *Representations of HIV and AIDS,* and Treichler, 'AIDS, Gender, and Biomedical Discourse,' p. 217.

[6]On how Mary Mallon became Typhoid Mary, see Leavitt, *Typhoid Mary*.

[7]On early theories of the French Disease's origins, see Foa, 'The New and the Old,' and Arrizabalaga, Henderson and French, *The Great Pox,* especially pp. 56-87.

article examines the construction of the myth of the 'most beautiful' prostitute as the originator of the first European epidemic of the French Disease and the dynamic relationship between this myth and the creation of institutions to enclose beautiful, promiscuous women to prevent the spread of disease. The myth of the beautiful prostitute as originator of disease enjoyed a degree of popularity in early modern Venice because it incorporated and expressed Venetian anxieties about a variety of fears: vulnerability to military conquest, which was still a threat, especially from the Turks, and the disruptive powers of beautiful women. This myth developed through the interaction of several overlapping discourses: medicine and the idea of contagion, military advice manuals, treatises on beauty, and Counter Reformation writings. Equally important were the interactions between writers and their social context, specifically the hospitals dedicated primarily to the care of French Disease patients and institutions for repentant or potential prostitutes.

Cultural, political, and military anxieties informed Venetian response to the French Disease and partially shaped the institutions created to prevent and cure the disease. As Paul Farmer has shown in the case of AIDS, origin myths about epidemics do far more than explain the biological origins of a pathogen. Origin myths locate blame for the epidemic within a wider geopolitical and moral framework.[8] Myths about the French Disease became commentaries on why the Italian city-states did not recover from the French invasion of 1494 and from subsequent Italian Wars (1494-1530).

The theory that a beautiful prostitute who had served the invading French army accounted for the late-fifteenth-century epidemic of the French Disease resonated with popular perceptions and reinforced efforts to control disease by placing certain types of women in institutions. In Venice, lay reformers in cooperation with the Church built three different institutions for women in response to the threat of the French Disease – the *Convertite* and the *Zitelle* in the sixteenth century, and the *Penitenti* in the eighteenth century. All of these institutions focused on female bodies as the location of disease, isolated women perceived to be fallen or vulnerable from the rest of the city, and promoted repentance in order to combat both moral and physical contagion. Although protection from disease was not the only motive for founding these institutions, these institutions' origins as part of the response to the French Disease has too often been overlooked.[9] Even after Venetian authorities judged the six-

[8]Farmer, *AIDS and Accusation*.

[9]On the *Zitelle*, see Chojnacka, 'Women, Charity, and Community in Early Modern

teenth-century institutions to have been a failure, they continued to be influenced by the image of the beautiful prostitute as responsible for the spread of disease and built a new institution for repentant prostitutes in the eighteenth century. Venice was not alone in responding to the French Disease by focusing on female bodies and urging permanent repentance for female sinners; in Genoa, Naples, and Rome, convents for repentant female sinners developed within hospitals built for those suffering from the French Disease.[10]

At the core of the idea of the beautiful prostitute is, of course, the prostitute: consequently it is important to define this word in its early modern context. During the sixteenth century, the problem of prostitution was defined primarily as a problem of sin. Monetary exchange was not part of the definition. The term prostitute, or *meretrice,* was a moral category that referred to a woman's sexual activities outside of marriage rather than an occupation or commercial transaction. In 1543, the Venetian Senate defined the word *meretrici* as those women who 'not being married have commerce, and practice with one, or more men' (commerce or *commercio* being used in the sense of intercourse, as in 'carnal commerce'). *Meretrici* were also defined as 'those who being married do not live with their husbands but stay separately, and have commerce with one or more men.'[11] Because the French Disease was closely identified with female sexual sin, response to the disease focused on the ultimate symbol of female sexual sin – the 'prostitute,' or, more accurately, the loose woman – rather than on the disease itself.

Prostitution and Disease: Humanist and Medical Discourse

The connection between prostitution and the French Disease was not immediately apparent to the earliest observers. Of the earliest chronicles written by non-medical observers of the 1490s epidemic, gathered and

Venice.' On all of the female communities, see Chojnacka, *Working Women of Early Modern Venice*, pp. 121-137, and Pullan, *Rich and Poor in Renaissance Venice.* On the *Convertite*, see McGough, 'Raised from the Devil's Jaws.' On these institutions in other Italian cities, see Cohen, *The Evolution of Women's Asylums since 1500.* In Bologna, see Ferrante, 'Honor Regained,' and Ciammitti, 'Conservatori femminili a Bologna e organizzazione del lavoro,'; in Rome, see Groppi, *I Conservatori della Virtù*, and Camerano, 'Assistenza richiesta ed assistenza imposta.'

10 Arrizabalaga, Henderson and French, *The Great Pox,* p. 168.

11 *Parte presa nell'Eccellentissimo Conseglio di Pregadi*, 21 February 1542 m.v. (21 February 1543).

published by the nineteenth-century historian Alfonso Corradi, none makes mention of a prostitute as the origin of disease.[12] Most blamed the invading French army for the disease, such as the Florentine chronicler Parenti, for example, who described the disease as new in 1496 and yet already extended through all parts of the world.[13] Although the hardships created by the war diverted most authors' attentions from speculating about the disease's origins in favour of descriptions about the myriad problems each city-state faced during the Italian Wars (1494-1530), occasionally a writer would offer his theory about where the disease came from. The Sienese historian Sigismondo Tizio argued that the disease was not new at all: it had been periodically plaguing humanity since the time of the Pharaohs, whenever God wished to punish humanity for their sins.[14] It took nearly a generation to resolve the issue of whether the disease was new or not, as described below. As Jon Arrizabalaga's contribution to this volume suggests, prostitutes were curiously absent from most early accounts. When early writers discussed the disease's origins, most usually ignored how the disease itself originated and focused their blame on the French army and its leader, Charles VIII.

Only two of Corradi's early commentators mentioned prostitutes or loose women in association with the French Disease, but they did not construct a theory of the disease's origins as lying within a particular woman's body. A chronicler from Bologna, Fileno dalle Tuate, remarked about the French Disease that 'there is no real remedy, except to let it run its course and it is found that women have it in their private parts (*in la natura*) and because of this many prostitutes were banished from Bologna and from Ferrara and other places.'[15] Fileno held women accountable for this disease, and punished prostitutes by expelling them from the city. Similarly, a writer from Ferrara explained that the disease arose from men having had sexual relations with 'dirty women.'[16] The two writers were building on a longstanding association between women's bodies and disease

---

12Corradi, 'Nuovi Documenti.'

13Pietro Parenti, cit. in Corradi, 'Nuovi Documenti,' pp. 15-16. 'Settembre 1496. Non sarà inconueniente far memoria della nuoua malattia uenuta in Italia a questi tempi, chiamata rogna franciosa, la quale in tutte parti del mondo si distese. Faua doglia intensissima; durava 8 in 10 mesi...'

14Sigismondo Tizio cit. in Corradi, 'Nuovi Documenti,' p. 16.

15Corradi, p. 19. 'Et non vera rimedio se non lasarla fare suo corso et se trovava che le feminine lo avevano in la natura e per questo ne funo chazate molte meretrize da bologna e da ferara e altri luoghi.'

16Corradi, p. 19. 'e questo provene per li homini hanno a fare con donne immonde....'

that could be found in Galen's writings and was expanded through centuries of medieval commentaries. The association between femininity and disease was already present in Western medical literature: the notion that an individual could cause an epidemic that would affect most of the known world was, as Arrizabalaga suggests above, relatively new.

Initial Venetian reports about the French Disease were war reports that focused on the soldiers and commanders infected, not on the origins of the epidemic. The Venetian diarist Marin Sanuto duly noted any reports of illness; noteworthy names were powerful men, with no mention of who had infected them. In 1498 and 1499, for example, Sanuto reported the French Disease as he did any other illness, with no sense of stigma or moral opprobrium. '*Item*, that Paulo Vitelli has a lot of the French Disease.' And

> Dom. Alvosio Valaresso has the French Disease; he wants money to give to the company, saying that he has had no pay and is becoming desperate.[17]

In 1499, when a Venetian galley was at Corfu, it was unable to set sail because the crew was infected with the French Disease.[18] Concerned about the availability of manpower and the need for resources, Sanuto focused on the immediate concerns: who was sick and what impact that had on Venice's military strength. Although Sanuto already believed that the French Disease was spread from person to person via sexual intercourse, his belief in the cosmic origins of the disease (much like his contemporaries outlined by Arrizabalaga and Hayton above) prevented him from speculating about a single individual, soldier or prostitute ultimately responsible for the epidemic.[19]

Critical to such a shift was the development of theories of contagion, which presented diseases as entities capable of transmission from person to person and from thing to thing. The idea of a 'Patient Zero' for the French Disease depended on such a notion of contagion, which, although implicitly present in the works of Aristotle, was more fully expounded and elaborated during the sixteenth century. Sexual transmission of the French Disease had been discussed since the late fifteenth century, but until the idea of contagion was more widely accepted physicians could challenge the idea of sexual transmission. Physician Antonio Scanaroli of Modena,

---

[17] *I Diarii di Marin Sanuto*, p. 47; pp. 288-289. 'Item, che Paulo Vitelli ha mal franzoso assai.... Et come dominio Alvosio Valaresso havia mal franzoso; voria danari per dar a la compagnia, dicendo non havia auto niuna paga et si vedea disperato.'

[18] Cited by Corradi, pp. 22-23.

[19] On his idea of celestial origins and the sexual transmission, see *I Diarii di Marin Sanuto*, Vol. I, 9 July 1496, pp. 233-234.

for example, argued in 1498 that sexual intercourse was not the means of transmission, but the disease instead arose spontaneously in the sexual organs.[20]

First published in Venice in 1546, Fracastoro's work on contagion was chiefly important, as Richard Palmer has argued, because it provided a language and image for the spread of disease that was more useful than previous images. The Greek philosophers had articulated the idea of contagion, which Fracastoro revitalized with new metaphors.[21] Living things, called *seminaria* or seeds, could reproduce themselves and cause disease by spreading directly from person-to-person, by attaching themselves to an object such as clothing which enabled their spread over a small distance, or by traveling through the air and infecting a wider geographical area. Although Fracastoro clung to the idea that changes in air and in the alignment of planets could produce new diseases, such as the French Disease, his ideas on contagion nevertheless provided fruitful metaphors for different ways of thinking about the origins of the French Disease. The emphasis on seeds themselves, which shares the same root as the word for semen, is important. This particular seed, which Fracastoro described as cold and sluggish, needed heat and activity before it could become an active disease. As he explained,

> This contagion was not very readily taken in by the body, because of the viscosity in which its germs (*seminaria*) had been buried; hence there was needed a sort of reciprocal heat in two bodies; thus somehow the germs (*seminaria*) became active, and were able to adhere to something else and to propagate themselves on nourishment analogous with themselves, but this, being as it were coagulated, they could not have done unless they had been heated.[22]

Fracastoro had thereby offered a mechanism through which this seed could become active and cause disease: reciprocal heat between two bodies.

It did not take a great leap of imagination for Rostinio to build on Fracastoro's theory of the mechanisms of contagion and link it to ideas about a prostitute who served French soldiers. The focus on a prostitute as originator of disease had already been articulated in 1536 with Paracelsus's *Chirurgia magna*, in which he argued that syphilis arose from the sexual

---

[20]Sudhoff, *The Earliest Printed Literature on Syphilis*, p. XLV.

[21]Palmer, 'The Control of Plague in Venice and Northern Italy,' pp. 91-93, and Nutton, 'Seeds of Disease.' In practice, public health officials recognized the possibility of contagion by imposing quarantine not only on sick individuals, but also on those who had been in contact with the sick. Carmichael, 'Contagion Theory and Contagion Practice in Fifteenth-Century Milan.'

[22]Fracastoro, *De Contagione*, p. 153.

union between 'a leprous Frenchman and a prostitute with uterine sores.'[23] Although Paracelsus's writings reached print only a few times before his death in 1542, he enjoyed enormous posthumous popularity in the 1550s.[24] Paracelsus was not the only physician to associate the French Disease with prostitution by the mid-sixteenth century. Those physicians who had argued since the early sixteenth century that this disease was transmitted primarily through sexual intercourse had warned against the dangers of prostitutes, although their advice was primarily preventive rather than a reconstruction of the origins of the disease. Indeed, as Arrizabalaga shows, Gaspar Torrella of Valencia argued that the only definitive way to prevent the spread of disease was to round up and treat all infected prostitutes.[25] Closer to Rostinio in time and space was the popular lecturer in anatomy at the University of Padua, Gabriele Fallopio, who also linked the problem of prostitution to the French Disease. Falloppio's enormous popularity as a lecturer during the 1550s ensured that his medical theories would receive a wide audience among practicing physicians throughout Venice and the Veneto.[26] Falloppio made an explicit link to the problems that 'beautiful prostitutes' presented because of their ability to transmit the French Disease to contemporaries, including his medical students. One pupil who kept careful notes of Falloppio's lectures described Falloppio's advice on how to avoid infection should the students succumb to the charms of a beautiful prostitute. Significantly, the prostitute was described as being not merely beautiful, but 'most beautiful,' the same description that Rostinio used in describing his Patient Zero (in Falloppio's Latin, *pulcherrimam*; in Rostinio's Italian, *bellissima*).[27] Charles Estienne's anatomical representations of women's bodies depicted women in erotic poses, displaying their genitalia as a form of foreplay, designed to titillate a male readership.[28]

---

[23]Schleiner, 'Infection and Cure through Women,' p. 504.

[24]Porter, *Greatest Benefit to Mankind*, p. 205.

[25]Arrizabalaga, Henderson and French, *The Great Pox*, p. 129. See also Arrizabalaga, above.

[26]Porter, *Greatest Benefit to Mankind,* p. 182.

[27]Schleiner, 'Moral Attitudes toward Syphilis and Its Prevention in the Renaissance,' p. 399.

[28]A good example of the overlap between anatomy and the erotic is Charles Estienne's work, published in Paris in the 1540s. It is unclear how widely available this text was in Venice, although the fact Estienne based his drawings on erotic images drawn by Italian artists suggests that French and Italian intellectuals borrowed from each other. See Estienne, *La Dissection des parties du corps,* pp. 294, 300, 310, 312. In the last image, the woman is lying on her back on the bed. On the association between Estienne and Italian erotic images, see Carlino, *Paper Bodies*, pp. 23-26.

The symbolic association between prostitution and the French Disease was thus already available for Rostinio; what was missing were the mechanics, about which Rostinio drew on both Fracastoro and the physician Antonio Brasavola for inspiration. In the first two editions of his book, Rostinio acknowledged his debt in the book's foreword to Antonio Brasavola, who attributed the French Disease to a prostitute suffering from a uterine abscess. By the third reprinting in 1565, however, Brasavola's name did not appear, as Rostinio situated the book within more recent scholarship about the French Disease.[29]

For Rostinio, the development of the French Disease as a contagious disease within the body of a prostitute depended on three crucial mechanisms: the friction generated through sexual intercourse with multiple partners, the ulceration of the prostitute's uterus, and the softness and therefore penetrability of the French soldiers' penises after coitus. The French Disease was a new disease, created by a change in the quality of the air; about the ability of new diseases to be created through poor air quality there could be no doubt, he argued.[30] But how this new disease, created through climate change, could become a contagious disease, transmitted from individual to individual through coitus, demanded explanation. The French invasion of Italy had occurred during a period of great humidity and flooding, so this poisonous air was already present when the most beautiful prostitute arrived to serve the invading army. The friction of intercourse, along with the humidity of the vagina and putridity produced by ulcerations within the woman's body, were essential in transforming this poison into a contagion. As Fracastoro had already explained, once the seeds of disease were present, all that was needed to make the germs active was heat. Apparently size and the dark, hidden quality of the vagina mattered as well, as the woman's 'cavernous place' enabled a sufficient quantity of bad air to enter.[31]

---

[29]The 1559 edition, for example, states that Rostinio has translated parts of Brasavola's work and added his own work. The 1565 edition makes no mention of Brasavola, but makes references to the popular empiric Leonardo Fioravanti's book *Capriccio Medicinale* (fol. 9^{v}), a reference that did not appear in the 1559 edition.

[30]'Non si deve dubitare, che li mali nuovi nascono per la mala qualità dell'aere, & quella qualità dell'aere è peggiore, quanto alla corruttione, quando egli seguita la humidità & calidità, che quando la siccità.' Rostinio, *Trattato del Mal Francese*, fol. 20^{r}.

[31]'Se dimãdi in questo male, che cosa sia questa venenosita, dicemo, che è una mala dispositione senza nome, ne da niuno è definita dico ma la dispositione di questo male qual è nasciuto, & dalla mala qualita dell'aere, & dalla frictione nel cavernoso loco della donna, dove èmala dispositione il male è da numerar tra li contagiosi.' fol. 21^{v}.

Equally troubling were penises gone flaccid after intercourse. The softness of the French penis after intercourse enabled the disease to penetrate the male member, ascend upwards through a man's body, enter his liver and infect the blood.[32] The object of sexual penetration, the penis, itself became penetrable, subject to infection. Through this vulnerability of the penis in its flaccid state, the male body became vulnerable to systemic infection. Anxieties about the military vulnerability of Italy, invaded by no less than four foreign armies during the Italian Wars, were projected onto this description of the mechanics of the French Disease's evolution.

Rostinio's theory was popular enough to be published three times within a decade, always in the vernacular, hence accessible to a wider audience than Latin treatises. But his theory never edged out all other theories of the French Disease's origins. The popular empiric Leonardo Fioravanti, for example, entered the debate in 1561 with his own theory of the disease's origins: cannibalism practiced by the desperate French army spawned the disease.[33] The French Disease continued to inspire speculation about its origins, partly because it originated in recent, historical time, but more importantly because the late fifteenth century epidemic represented a turning point in Italy's history. Once a collection of independent city-states that supported an interdependent commercial life, the Italian peninsula had fallen permanently under the sway of foreign nation-states, with the precarious exception of Venice, still independent but no longer as powerful. During the mid-sixteenth century, as intellectuals tried to make sense of Italy's military decline, they focused on the French invasion of Italy and the disease named after this event.

This preoccupation with military decline helps explain the Italian reading public's continued fascination with the origins of this disease as late as the 1560s, when the French invasion was no longer a living memory but an historical event. Contagion theory provided the medical reasoning to explain how a single individual could be responsible for a pandemic of the French Disease, but medical theories alone do not explain why doctors and the reading public were so captivated by the idea of a most beautiful

---

[32]Rostinio's complete explanation of these mechanisms is the following: 'Nel campo de Francesi del mille quattrocento era una meretrice bellissima, la quale nella bocca della matrice haveva una apostema putrefatta, et gli huomini che usavano con lei fregolando il collo della matrice, per la humidità & putredine del loco, nel mẽbro virile cõtrahevano una dispositione, che ulcerava, & per il mẽbro qual'è mollissimo ascẽdeva una mala qualita fino alle vie emũtorie, & alle parti del l'inguini. Et la natura per scacciar fuori la mala qualita venenosa ivi facea tumori, et ivi trasmettera la materia. Poi quella mala qualita fino al figato ascẽdeva, & maculava il sangue.' fol. 21^{r}.

[33]Eamon, 'Cannibalism and Contagion.'

prostitute as Patient Zero. Why a prostitute and not a soldier? And why a most beautiful prostitute? Medical ideas developed in dynamic relationship with other ideas, and were also influenced by the rich visual imagery of late Renaissance Venice, which, especially in the work of Titian, produced numerous representations of female beauty.

EXTREME BEAUTY: VULNERABILITY AND TEMPTATION

The potential danger of beauty was a common theme in Renaissance literature and art. This idea had its roots in the Jewish and Christian traditions, with stories about temptresses – Eve, Delilah, and even the heroine Judith – who brought about the downfall of men. Renaissance writers and artists built on these traditions and incorporated their own anxieties about beauty. As Brian Steele has argued, women's physical beauty could lead a viewer to think only of passing, sensual pleasures, whereas the representation of female beauty in art could serve the more ennobling goal of reminding viewers of the timelessness and moral value of art. Titian, for example, painted representations of ideal female beauty, such as the golden-haired woman reminiscent of Petrarch's Laura in his painting *La Bella,* rather than lifelike portraits of identifiable women.[34] For neoplatonists, art could resolve the problem of 'the ambiguity of beauty,' to borrow a phrase from Naomi Yavneh.[35] In Tasso's epic poem *Gerusalemme liberata* (1575), for example, the beautiful, evil temptress Armida, who distracts Christian soldiers from their goal of conquering Jerusalem during the Crusades, is converted to Christianity, thereby chastening her destructive sexuality.[36] Beautiful temptresses were generic in form, all possessing the same combination of long, golden hair, black eyes, and fair skin that Renaissance treatises described. An ideal beautiful woman was virtually never found in nature; she had to be constructed from many different women, each of whom might possess beautiful parts. One woman might have beautiful hair, another beautiful shoulders or neck, and so forth, but ideal beauty seldom existed in nature.[37]

---

[34]Steele, 'In the Flower of Their Youth,' pp. 491-502.

[35]Yavneh, 'The Ambiguity of Beauty.'

[36]Yavneh, 'The Ambiguity of Beauty,' pp. 133-134.

[37]Yavneh, 'The Ambiguity of Beauty,' 138-139; Cropper, 'On Beautiful Women, Parmigianino, *Petrarchismo,* and the Vernacular Style.' The best-known Renaissance treatise on women's beauty is by Agnolo Firenzuola. He constructed an ideal woman made of the various parts of women who attended a fictional party in his dialogue *On the Beauty of Women*. On Firenzuola's life, see Eisenbichler and Murray's introduction to Firenzuola, *On The Beauty of Women*, pp. xiii-xviii.

The idea that extreme beauty seldom existed in nature and was, therefore, almost a deformity explains the sixteenth-century association between excessive beauty and vice. Renaissance aesthetics emphasized the importance of harmony, balance, and moderation. The humanist Agnolo Firenzuola (whose own bout with the French Disease Domenic Zanrè describes in this volume) described ideal female beauty as 'ordered concord, akin to a harmony that arises mysteriously from the composition, union, and conjunction of several diverse and different parts.'[38] Beauty and virtue were therefore linked in the minds of Renaissance Italians.[39] Beauty and good health were linked as well, especially since sixteenth-century doctors published books that combined advice for healthy living with advice on cosmetics, hair dye, and skin ointments. Giovanni Marinello, who practiced medicine in Venice, dedicated his *Gli ornamenti delle donne* (1562) to 'chaste and young women,' with advice on how to cure leprosy, heal scabies, and colour the hair to appear more blonde.[40] The boundary between medicine and cosmetics, if it existed at all, was extremely fluid: beauty belonged to the realm of medicine as well as art.

Extreme beauty could upset the careful balance of symmetry and proportions. As the humanist and scientist Giambattista Della Porta explained, beauty was a sign of God's favour; extreme beauty, however, was often accompanied by vice. Because nature gave gifts in proportion, extremes of beauty were joined by a proportionate extreme of virtue as well as extreme of vice. An extremely beautiful male might be vainglorious and lead an army on an ill-advised expedition, such as the ancient Athenian general Alcibiades, held responsible for Athens' defeat in the Peloponnesian war. Extremely beautiful women all suffered from the same vice: sexual excess. The *bellissima* Helen of Troy was unfaithful to her husband, Della Porta explained, while Laïs was a courtesan and Faustina the allegedly unfaithful wife of Marcus Aurelius.[41]

As the Counter Reformation became a more important cultural force during the late sixteenth century, a moral discourse on beauty overlapped with the earlier discourse on beauty and harmony. Beauty was not only useless to a woman, it was potentially damaging for a wife. Vain, spoiled, and easily led into adultery, the beautiful wife brought more damage than

---

[38]Firenzuola, *On The Beauty of Women*, p. 14.

[39]Ames-Lewis and Rogers, *Concepts of Beauty in Renaissance Art*; Steele, 'In the Flower of Their Youth, pp. 481-502.

[40]Marinello, *Gli ornamenti delle donne*.

[41]Della Porta, *Della fisonomia dell'huomo*, p. 86. On Della Porta, see Eamon, *Science and the Secrets of Nature*, pp. 194-233.

pleasure.[42] Popular proverbs from the early modern period also suggested a certain mistrust of beauty, such as 'Beauty does not put food on the table' and 'Every beautiful new slipper becomes a worn-out old shoe.'[43]

The dangerously beautiful woman, who could defeat an army by distracting generals and soldiers, became a common theme, easily adapted to explain the origin and spread of the French Disease. Military discourse, especially treatises written during the Counter Reformation, reinforced the association between danger and extreme beauty. Ascanio Centorio's 1567 *Discorsi di guerra* praised chastity as a virtue for the soldier, giving the example of Scipio Africanus, general of the Roman army who brought Carthage to defeat during the Second Punic War. 'A most beautiful young woman being presented to Scipio Africanus while he was in Spain, not only did he abstain from her, but he did not even turn to admire her, and ordered that she be returned to her relatives.'[44] Scipio Africanus was therefore able to do what the French and Italian soldiers of 1494 had failed to do: resist the temptation of extreme beauty. Scipio Africanus saved the Roman republic from conquest by Hannibal's legendary military brilliance, while the republics of Venice and Florence all but crumbled.

Writers like Centorio lamented that contemporary Italian soldiers lacked the discipline of their ancient predecessors. Because of greedy leaders, the military had become an 'ignominious market,' 'no longer worthy of that past glory,' with soldiers weighted down in combat by carrying baggage filled with their own personal items. Here he underscored the prostitute's role in contributing to this moral and military decay, noting that armies were accompanied by 'an infinity of whores:' most soldiers even insisted on having their own prostitute at their very side as they fought.[45] His contemporaries needed to follow the example of the Turks and the Moors, whose soldiers he portrayed as more chaste. In mentioning the Turks and Moors as examples to follow, Centorio identified the principal

---

[42]Pancino, *'Soffrire per ben comparire,'* pp. 5, 32-34. This moralistic discourse was still evident in the early eighteenth century, when writers such as Francesco Beretta wrote advice manuals for noblemen choosing a spouse.

[43]Literally, 'Con le bellezze non si mangia,' and 'Ogni bela scarpa deventa bruta ciabata.' I have translated 'scarpa' as slipper to reflect the word's positive association in English (such as Cinderella's glass slippers) and translated 'ciabata' as shoe to reflect the negative connotations in English of old shoe. Cited by Pancino, 'Soffrire per ben comparire,' pp. 36-37.

[44]Centorio, *Discorsi di guerra*, fol. 12^{v}. 'Scipio Africano in Ispagna, essendogli presentata una bellissima giovane avanti, non solo da quella si astenne, ma non volse pur mirarla, et commesse che fosse restituita à suoi parenti.'

[45]Centorio, *Discorsi di guerra*, fols. 57^{v}, 39^{v}.

threats to European, especially Italian, security during the mid-sixteenth century. Of course, by contrasting the chaste Turks with the incontinent European armies, Centorio and other military commentators played on Venetian fears of their vulnerability to the powerful Turkish army. Beautiful prostitutes not only brought disease, but they destroyed armies, navies, and, by extension, entire empires. Although Counter Reformation discourse emphasized the importance of the male soldier's virtue and continence, no physician ever located the origins of the French Disease within the male body. Regarded as humid, containing a mysterious womb, the female body carried the symbolic burden of disease from which the virtuous male soldier should protect himself. Furthermore, religious imagery often reinforced the association between female beauty, prostitution, and danger, especially in the imagery of Mary Magdalene.

MARY MAGDALENES: THE BEAUTIFUL PROSTITUTE, REPENTANT

Sensual, even erotic, portraits of Mary Magdalene as a beautiful sinner linked feminine beauty with prostitution. A twelfth-century hagiography of Mary Magdalene described her temptation to promiscuity on account of her own beauty, which increased her vanity and made men almost blameless in their inability to resist her.[46] The sixteenth century witnessed a veritable explosion of paintings of the Magdalene, notably Titian's titillating paintings, which presented her with clothing barely clinging to her breast, almost inviting viewers to imagine touching her.[47] As Paula Findlen has noted, contemporary viewers responded to Titian's paintings with feelings of sexual arousal. During the 1550s, Ludovico Dolce described his response to seeing Titian's *Venus and Adonis* as a 'warming, a softening, a stirring of the blood...

> If a marble statue could by the stimuli of its beauty so penetrate to the marrow of a young man, that he stained himself, then, what must she do who is of flesh, who is beauty personified and appears to be breathing?[48]

Although sensual images of the Magdalene competed with religious images that depicted the penitent saint with hair covered and sombre visage, the erotic image of the Magdalene never disappeared.

46Rollo-Koster, 'From Prostitutes to Brides of Christ,' pp. 129-130.

47On the iconography of Mary Magdalene, see Mosco, *La Maddalena tra sacro e profano*; Haskins, *Mary Magdalene*; and Malvern, *Venus in Sackcloth*. On the sexualization of touch represented visually in Renaissance art, see Gilman, 'Touch, Sexuality and Disease.'

48Quotation from Findlen, 'Humanism, Politics, and Pornography in Renaissance Italy,' pp. 64-65.

The image of the repentant prostitute Magdalene became one of the central images of Counter Reformation Catholicism, partly a response to Protestant polemics against the sexual degeneracy of the Catholic Church.[49] Although repentance had long been one of the central themes of Christian thought, even greater emphasis was placed upon penitential practice during the late fifteenth and early sixteenth-century religious revival.[50] Ignatius Loyola, who would later found the Jesuit order, spent time in Venice, where his followers worked at the *Incurabili* hospital, established in 1537. By that time, a group of 'converted women' had gathered within the hospital, but had not yet moved to their own building (which would happen in 1542). Loyola's contacts with these Venetian patients may have inspired his ministry to former prostitutes, since the Society of Jesus supported the establishment of institutions for repentant prostitutes throughout their missions, including the New World.[51] An emphasis on repentance also became a key weapon against encroachments by Protestants into Catholic territory, as Catholics sought to maintain control over their faithful through appeals to conscience.[52]

Venice's health board (the *Sanità)* first responded to the problem of the French Disease in 1521. Noting that many gentlemen and gentlewomen were sick from the disease, not to mention others who were covered in sores and reduced to begging for survival on the streets near the crowded areas of San Marco and the Rialto, the health board ordered that the sick be taken to the newly-founded *Incurabili* hospital for a period of convalescence.[53] Although the hospital treated both male and female patients, only female patients were encouraged to repent by taking permanent monastic vows and entering a convent. As in Rome, Naples, and Genoa, Venice's convent for repentant prostitutes, the *Convertite*, developed as an extension of the city's *Incurabili* hospital (primarily for French Disease patients), making the convent an important arm in the city's fight to control disease.[54] Venice's institutional responses to the French Disease

---

49Lewis Wager's 1566 play about Mary Magdalene, for example, can be seen as a critique of Catholic mores. See Badir, '"To allure vntu their loue".'

50Cameron, *The European Reformation*, pp. 79-81; Fitzgerald, *Conversion through Penance in the Italian Church*; Lualdi and Thayer, *Penitence in the Age of Reformations*.

51O'Malley, *The First Jesuits*, pp. 32-33, 178-188.

52Luria, 'Rituals of Conversion,' pp. 72-73.

53ASV, Prov. alla Sanità, Busta 2, fol. 31^{r}, 12 February 1521 m. v. (12 February 1522) On the origin of the *Incurabili* hospital in Venice, see Nordio, 'L'Ospedale degli Incurabili nell'assistenza veneziana del '500.'

54Arrizabalaga, Henderson and French, *The Great Pox*, p. 168.

thereby both reflected and reinforced medical anxieties about the dangers of women's bodies and female beauty in particular.

Particularly prominent in both the *Convertite* and the hospital for the Incurables was iconography depicting the penitent Mary Magdalene, to whom the *Convertite* was dedicated. The *Convertite* contained several representations of the Magdalene, including a *Noli me tangere* by Luigi Benfatto as well as one by Alvise del Friso, in addition to Palma Giovane's painting on the church's ceiling of the Magdalene being lifted by angels.[55] The *Noli me tangere* scene refers to the text from the Gospel of John in which Mary Magdalene recognizes Christ after his crucifixion and resurrection who tells her not to touch him, since he has not yet ascended into heaven.[56] This scene delineates the boundary between the sacred and profane, represented by Mary Magadelen's corporality. This text also gives her a critically important role, since she was first among all to recognize the risen Christ. In late medieval accounts of her life, after Christ's ascension she took up preaching in the city of Marseilles, where she was renowned not only for her beauty but also for her eloquence.[57] Reformers hoped that the story of a beautiful, penitent woman who converted from a life of sin to become one of the central figures in Christ's life would inspire women in the *Convertite* to follow her example. Not only did medical, military, and visual images reinforce the associations between female beauty, danger, and disease, so too did the institutional life of sixteenth-century Venice.

THE *CONVERTITE* AND THE *ZITELLE*: ISOLATION OF BEAUTIFUL GIRLS AND WOMEN

Between 1525 and 1542, a group of 'converted women' remained with the hospital until they were able to move to a building of their own. In

---

[55]Boschini, *Le Minere della Pittura*, p. 404; these paintings were still found at the convent at the time of its suppression under French rule, see ASV, Edwards, Busta 2, 6 July 1807. On Benfatto and Palma Giovane, see Haskins, *Mary Magdalen*, p. 288; on del Friso, see Pallucchini, *La Pittura Veneziana del Seicento*, p. 22. Art within the church rather than the hallways and refectory would have been seen less often by the nuns, since they spent most of their time outside of the church and were confined to certain areas within the church. Minor artwork, such as small paintings of the Magdalene by an unknown artist, would likely have escaped the attention of contemporary observers; a few of these items appear in wills left by nuns, who bequeathed their portraits of Mary Magdalene to other nuns. See Laura McGough, 'Raised from the Devil's Jaws,' p. 127.

[56]Malvern, *Venus in Sackcloth*, p. 19.

[57]Jansen, 'Mary Magdalene and the Mendicants,' p. 22.

1551, they received permission to follow the Augustinian rule.[58] Although the only requirement for entry into the convent (besides the willingness to follow the religious life) was having led a 'licentious life' and therefore being a fallen woman, the nuns nonetheless quickly earned a reputation for beauty. The convent's governors, as well as the church hierarchy, regarded beautiful women as more vulnerable to sin than ugly ones. In making the case for why Isabetta Arrigona should be allowed to enter the *Convertite* in 1606, for example, the petition on her behalf explained that she was 'both young and beautiful,' and therefore not safe outside of matrimony or an institution. In fact, youth and beauty constituted the most important qualities that made Isabetta eligible for entry into the *Convertite*. She was not a prostitute, nor even an adulteress; her brief marriage to her husband, Michel, to whom she had been faithful, had foundered, leaving her few options to 'live honestly' outside of convent life.[59] Beauty thus gave an added edge to candidates who sought admission to the *Convertite*. This admissions process likely contributed to the institution's reputation for beautiful women. For example, in 1581 the popular writer Francesco Sansovino claimed that the convent housed a great number of penitent sinners, all most beautiful ('*gran numero di donne & tutte bellissime*').[60] By the 1580s, the convent enclosed more than 350 women, a number which remained fairly steady for the rest of the convent's history.[61]

The nuns' beauty was apparently what attracted the first rector in charge of the convent, Pietro Lion from Valcamonica, to seduce approximately 20 of the nuns and induce abortions in those he had impregnated. The apostolic nunzio Ippolito Capilupi reported in a letter of November 1561 that Lion confessed to asking the most beautiful among the nuns to undress and bathe in front of him '*che le più belle si spogliassero e andassero a bagnarsi nella cavana.*' Those who were unwilling to submit to his advances were sent to the convent's internal prison.[62] Prior to his public execution in Piazzetta San Marco in 1561, he wrote a confession, explaining that he had committed these acts because 'we are all subject to fragility... also I saw and knew about greater faults committed by others than what I was doing, it seemed to me that my faults were much inferior to those.'[63]

---

58 *Capitoli et Ordini per il buon Governo della Congregatione del Monastero di S. Maria Maddalena delle Convertite della Giudecca*, pp. 8-11.

59 ASVatican, SC, E & R, Positiones, 1606 Lett. T-V, undated letter from the *Convertite* in Venice.

60 Sansovino, *Venetia Cittá Nobilissima et Singolare*, p. 91b.

61 Pullan, *Rich and Poor in Renaissance Venice*, p. 378.

62 Molmenti, *La Storia di Venezia nella Vita Privata*, Vol. II, pp. 589-590.

63 MCC Codice Cicogna 3239, 10 November 1561.

Hinting that he was powerless to control himself, Lion played to contemporary prejudices about the power of feminine beauty.

By concentrating on beautiful women, the *Convertite* invited significant attention (and some trouble) from Venice's men. In November 1624, for example, the priest Francesco Montenegro was forbidden from saying the Mass at the *Convertite* after he was caught having sent a portrait of a nude man to one of the nuns inside; just four years earlier, the priest Giacomo Zenoni was denounced for having sent love letters to nuns in the *Convertite*, as well as to nuns in two other convents.[64] Priests were not the only men who found the nuns at the *Convertite* tempting. Men stopped by frequently to try to talk to them or just catch a glimpse of them, which was difficult to do once strict closure was imposed in 1563. It is clear that some Venetian men viewed women at the *Convertite* as unique from other nuns and thus open to their sexual advances. Piero, a musician, defended himself on charges of unlawfully trying to talk to the nuns by claiming that he thought they were 'women of the world,' not like other convents.[65] The attention that the nuns at the *Convertite* garnered must have only confirmed the authorities' initial suspicions about the effects of beauty on public order and public health. Extreme beauty was best corralled. A subsequent institution, the *Zitelle*, actually made beauty an official requirement for entry.

The statutes of the *Zitelle* explicitly required that girls who entered the institution be beautiful, thereby reflecting and reinforcing contemporary anxieties about the dangers of beauty and its association with disease. Like the *Convertite*, the *Zitelle* owed its origins to the hospital of the Incurables. After he came face-to-face with the French Disease while preaching in the hospital's church, Benedetto Palmio wrote that he felt inspired in 1558 to found an institution to protect young girls from the eternal damnation that could be their fate should they fall into sin on account of their beauty. A house of refuge would 'liberate from the danger of eternal damnation a certain type of virgin, who being very beautiful, and graceful' was at risk of losing her virginity due to the malice of others acting 'contrary to the health and to the purity of the Christian religion.'[66] The statutes of the *Zitelle* tried to ensure that only girls who were truly at risk of being deflowered – defined

---

[64]ASV, PS M, Busta 267, 28 November 1624; Busta 260, 2 July 1619.

[65]ASV, PSM, Busta 267, 1 August 1626.

[66]Archivio IRE, ZIT A1, 'Costituzione e Regole della Casa delle Citelle di Venezia,' Venice, 1738. Benedetto Palmio described himself as solely responsible for the selection of the *Zitelle*'s site, but several noblewomen were also involved. See Chase, 'The Casa delle Zitelle,' p. 73.

as 'at risk' on account of their beauty – were accepted into the *Zitelle*. New entrants had to be at least 12 years old but not older than 18, healthy, and beautiful; the governors should be particularly attentive to cases of impoverished, very beautiful girls, whose own parents or guardians might be tempted to let the girl be led astray in order to alleviate the family's extreme poverty. Two male governors interviewed each prospective entrant to determine whether she fit the institution's requirement. Detailed notes were not taken on a girl's appearance, but simply the judgment of *'bella'* or *'brutta'* (ugly).[67]

The requirement that girls be beautiful existed in similar institutions in other Italian city-states: Bologna's conservatory of S. Maria del Baraccano (founded in 1528), for example, required that the orphaned girls they accepted be at risk of losing their virginity on account of their beauty. Detailed descriptions of the girls' beauty (or lack of it) survive for the eighteenth century, for example the case of 13-year-old Caterina Felice Guastuzzi, whom the governors described as not so much beautiful as mediocre in appearance, on account of the shortness of her neck and her protruding shoulders.[68] The conservatory's governors could have been reading from Renaissance treatises on female beauty, which praised long, slender necks and 'graceful shoulders,' as Parmigianino depicted in his painting, *Madonna of the Long Neck*.[69]

Unlike the *Convertite*, which sought to save women who had already fallen into a life of vice and disease, the *Zitelle* made its mission to protect Venice's beautiful young girls before they ever reached that fate. The *Zitelle's* founders were aware that, as at the *Convertite*, these beautiful young girls could provide a temptation to those placed in charge of them. Once inside the institution, girls came under the care of a female hierarchy who taught the girls to read and to master a particular skill which would eventually make them suitable marriage partners or, if they chose, nuns in a cloistered convent.[70] Only virgins were allowed to enter the institution, where they were supposed to spend five or six years prior to marriage or entry into a convent.[71] A multi-layered hierarchy ensured that the girls, as well as their superiors, were well supervised. At the lowest level, the female

---

67 Archivio IRE, ZIT A1, 'Costituzione e Regole della Casa delle Citelle di Venezia,' Parte IV, Cap. III; on interviewing the girls, see Chojnacka, 'Charity and Poverty in Counter-Reformation Venice.'

68 Ciammitti, 'Fanciulle monache madri,' p. 469.

69 Firenzuola, *On the Beauty of Women*, pp. 63-65.

70 Chojnacka, 'Women, Charity, and Community,' pp. 73-79.

71 Archivio IRE, ZIT A1, *Costituzioni e Regole della Casa delle Citelle di Venezia*, Parte Quarta, Cap. III and Cap. XV.

teachers were elected among the *Zitelle* themselves; they were responsible for teaching the girls to read, to learn specific skills such as embroidery, and to make sure they prayed and dressed modestly. At the highest level, noblewomen and noblemen filled the roles of *protettrici* and *protettori* who performed the roles of trustees. Day-to-day contact with their girls was restricted to the female hierarchy; even physicians could not visit one of the girls alone, but had to be accompanied by a female administrator (confessors, however, were exempt from this requirement).[72]

Isolating these beautiful women was central to the Venetian public health strategy. By placing the *Convertite* and the *Zitelle* on the islands of the Giudecca, Venetians ensured that the institutions' inhabitants were physically removed from the mainstream of Venetian life. Cost played an important role in influencing decisions to locate these institutions on islands outside central Venice, but it was not the only factor. The idea of quarantine also influenced decision-making – especially the desire to isolate these girls and women from the rest of the city, ostensibly for their own protection, as well as for the benefit of the rest of the city. The practice of quarantine had become routine by the sixteenth century. First instituted in response to the plague in 1377 in Ragusa (modern day Dubrovnik, Croatia), quarantine became a regular practice throughout central and northern Italian city-states during the fifteenth century. Venice first imposed quarantine in 1423. By the mid-sixteenth century, Venice's health board (the *Sanità*) routinely isolated the sick and the potentially infected on islands, the Lazzaretto Vecchio and Nuovo.[73]

Significantly, Renaissance contagion theory did not focus on biological contagion alone: morals, people, and ideas were all potentially contagious, that is, capable of spreading from person to person. Church authorities repeatedly referred to heresy as a contagious disease; Pope Paul III had even complained to the Venetian ambassador that heresy had reached epidemic levels in Venice and therefore posed a threat of contagion to the rest of Italy.[74] 'Loose women' posed a similar threat to heresy: even casual contact with them could infect others and transform them into sinners. Venetian law tried to maintain a strict segregation between 'loose' and respectable women by insisting that disreputable women not attend

---

[72]Chojnacka, 'Women, Charity, and Community,' pp. 73-79.

[73]Richard Palmer, 'The Control of Plague in Venice and Northern Italy,' and Preto, *Peste e società a Venezia nel 1576*. On responses to plague throughout Italy, see Cipolla, *Fighting the Plague in Seventeenth-Century Italy* and *Public Health and the Medical Profession in the Renaissance*.

[74]Martin, *Venice's Hidden Enemies*, p. ix.

mass at certain hours and not speak to respectable women.[75] The health department warned that prostitutes could bring a variety of diseases, including plague. City health authorities specifically targeted immigrant prostitutes; in 1539 prostitutes of 'foreign origin' (usually from different Italian city-states) were ordered to leave the city on account of the 'disorder' they brought, and therefore the risk of plague.[76] The construction of a permanent institution for the *Convertite* marked an even more dramatic effort to segregate loose women from respectable women: enclosed within the convent's high walls, where iron bars prohibited physical contact between the nuns inside and the world outside, on the relatively uninhabited, far southwestern corner of the Giudecca, these nuns remained permanently quarantined from the rest of society. Described as a 'place of security' by the institution's founders, the nuns' permanent enclosure was also supposed to benefit other Venetians by 'placating... the wrath of God with the diminishment of sin.'[77] To be sure, all convents were walled in and enclosed during the late sixteenth century, as the Council of Trent's regulations requiring strict cloister for all nuns were imposed. But other convents were typically located in the heart of the city: residents wanted proximity to the sacred space of cloistered nuns. By contrast, the 'loose women' and vulnerable girls of the *Convertite* and *Zitelle* respectively inhabited corners of an island a safe distance from the political, symbolic, and residential centres of Venice.

Easily visible from the Piazzetta San Marco and the southern part of the city, the islands of the Giudecca are a short boat ride across a canal from Venice. Administratively, the Giudecca was part of the city of Venice. In the imagination of city inhabitants, however, the Giudecca was nonetheless regarded as separate and distinct from Venice itself. The sense of separateness derived from its history as well as its location, having served since the tenth century as a refuge for groups of Jews, exiled Venetians, and Eastern Orthodox communities.[78] As Vanessa Chase has argued, the decision to locate the institutions of the *Zitelle* and the *Convertite* on the islands of the

---

75All of the following compilations of laws regarding 'prostitutes' (*meretrici*) are available at the Biblioteca Marciana, Venice. *Parte presa nell'Eccellentissimo Conseglio di Pregadi sopra il vestire, & ornamenti di casa delle Meretrici* 21 February 1542; *Parte Prese nell'Eccel.mo Conseglio di Dieci in material delle Publiche Meretrici, con l'obbligo de Barcaruoli, e Carrozzieri* 30 June and 8 July 1615; *Terminatione Degl'Illustrissimi Sig. Provveditori alla Sanità in material de Meretrici* 20 December 1628.

76ASV, Provveditori alla Sanità, Busta 2, 12 and 16 September, 1539.

77ASV Convertite, Busta 50, *Capitoli et Ordini per il Buon Governo della Congregatione del Monastero di S. Maria Maddalena delle Convertite*, pp. 7-8.

78On the history of the Giudecca, see Basaldella, *Giudecca*.

Giudecca marked a shift in Venetian practice from the tradition of integrating charitable institutions into the fabric of neighbourhood life to the isolation and removal of these institutions to the outskirts of Venice.[79]

The idea of quarantine at least implicitly influenced the placement of these institutions on the outskirts of Venice.[80] The sixteenth century was the period when the idea and practice of quarantine enjoyed popularity among the Health Board magistrates as well as many learned physicians. It was during the early sixteenth century that the Jewish ghetto was first physically segregated and isolated, another practice of 'quarantine' applied to a marginalized people, suspected of contagion both moral and physical. Some important differences exist between the practice of quarantine during epidemics of plague and the enclosure and isolation of these sub-populations of young girls, promiscuous women, and Jews: foremost among the differences was that plague victims were subject to temporary, not permanent, quarantine. Another difference was that plague victims had no defining characteristic as a sub-population, being of either sex, any age, neighbourhood or religion.

Penitence Reaffirmed

By the late seventeenth century both the *Zitelle* and the *Convertite* came to be regarded as failures.[81] Despite this, state and ecclesiastical authorities continued to define the French Disease as a problem of women's bodies and women's unregulated sexuality; the solutions they proposed for these problems were more of the same – a new house of penitence for fallen women, but one that would specifically benefit the poor. In 1701, a new asylum began accepting penitent women, this one called the Pious Place for the Poor Penitent Sinners of Saint Job, or the *Penitenti*. Since the penitent women who entered did not adopt the religious life, they were not required to observe strict cloister; their expenses were therefore lower

---

[79]Chase, 'The Casa delle Zitelle,' p. 77.

[80]This idea is further developed in my forthcoming book, *Sex, Repentance, and Venereal Disease: A Tragedy Set in Late Renaissance Venice*.

[81]Because of the costs of entering the *Convertite*, the women who entered were seldom prostitutes, but either the former lover of a nobleman or, surprisingly, a virgin from an artisan family who could not afford to enter a traditional convent. Similarly, competition to enter the *Zitelle* was tough, so that ultimately the daughters of respectable artisan families entered the institution, edging out the more vulnerable girls. See McGough, 'Women, Private Property, and the Limitations of State Authority,' p. 34, and for a more detailed discussion McGough, 'Raised from the Devil's Jaws,' pp. 59-99.

than the *Convertite*'s.[82] Beauty was dropped as a requirement for entrance, signalling a shift in emphasis from beauty to poverty as the principal cause of prostitution and disease. [83]

What remained the same was the emphasis on women's bodies and women's need for moral reform. As Kevin Siena has shown in the case of the eighteenth-century Lock Asylum for the Reception of Penitent Women in London, cure for women was a two-stage process: first the body, then the soul. Men underwent only the first stage of this process.[84] Venice's policy was similar. Female patients being treated for the French Disease were transferred directly from the *Incurabili* hospital to the *Penitenti*, while male patients were merely released from the hospital. On 31 October 1793, for example, the physician-in-charge noted that five women were 'completely cured' and ready to go the following day to the *Penitenti*. Between 1793 and 1795, the hospital for the Incurables treated and 'cured' between 116 and 137 French Disease patients each year, fairly equally divided between men and women. When space was available, former female patients were sent to the *Penitenti*, but men were free to go where they pleased.[85]

What young girls and women faced was a state and ecclesiastical system that placed them behind walls in order to protect society from the threat of contagion, biological and moral. Medical and ecclesiastical discourse each reinforced the perception that women were responsible for the spread of the French Disease. Their beauty demanded that they be enclosed, in some cases permanently, for their own good and the benefit of the city as a whole. Women's repentance benefited not only the souls of the sinners, but the city as whole. By purging themselves of sin through repentance, the body politic's excess vice was reduced; furthermore, by becoming nuns, the amount of piety in the city was increased. The net effect was a dramatic change in Venice's moral ledger, thereby protecting the city as a whole from God's anger at sin, potentially enacted through epidemic disease. Despite the development of theories that focused on the culpability of the individual in the spread of disease, Venice responded to the threat of the French Disease by focusing on certain sub-populations deemed vulnerable or at risk. The symbolic weight these women bore

---

[82]Archivio IRE, PEN A1, *Capitoli per il buon governo del pio loco in ovvegno delle povere peccatrici penitentidi San Job* (Venice, 1731).

[83]For an explanation of this transition, see my forthcoming book, *Sex, Repentance, and Venereal Disease: A Tragedy Set in Late Renaissance Venice.*

[84]Siena, *Venereal Disease, Hospitals, and the Urban Poor*, p. 214.

[85]ASV PSO, Busta 76, fasc. 'Ammalati,' 31 October 1793 and fasc. 19.

permitted the rest of Venetian society to remain at ease, free of culpability for the disease's origins or transmission.

Johns Hopkins University
Baltimore, Maryland

Cited Works

Manuscript Sources

Vatican, Archivio Segreto Vaticano (ASVatican)
  Sacra Congregatione (SC), Episcoporum et Regularium (E & R), Positiones
Venice, Archivio di Stato di Venezia (ASV)
  Convertite
  Provveditori alla Sanità
  Provveditori sopra Monasteri (PSM)
  Provveditori sopra Ospitali (PSO)
Venice, Archivio Storico dell'Istituto di Ricovero e di Educazione (Archivio IRE)
  Zitelle (ZIT)
  Penitenti (PEN)
Venice, Museo Civico Correr (MCC)
  Codice Cicogna 3239

Published Sources

Ames-Lewis, Francis and Mary Rogers. *Concepts of Beauty in Renaissance Art*. Brookfield, VT: Ashgate, 1998.

Arrizabalaga, Jon, John Henderson, and Roger French. *The Great Pox: The French Disease in Renaissance Europe*. New Haven: Yale University Press, 1997.

Badir, Patricia. '"To allure vntu their loue": Iconoclasm and Striptease in Lewis Wager's *The Life and Repentaunce of Marie Magdalene*' *Theatre Journal* 51(1999): 1-20.

Basaldella, Francesco. *Giudecca: Storia e testimonianze*. Venice: [s.n.], 1986.

Boschini, Marco. *Le Minere della Pittura*. Venice: F. Nicolini, 1664.

Camerano, Alessandra. 'Assistenza richiesta ed assistenza imposta: il conservatorio di S. Caterina della Rosa di Roma' *Quaderni Storici* 82 (April 1993): 227-260.

Cameron, Euan. *The European Reformation*. Oxford: Clarendon Press, 1991.

Capitoli et ordini per il buon governo della congregatione del monastero di S. Maria Maddalena delle Convertite della Giudecca. Venice: Lovisa, 1719.

Carlino, Andrea. *Paper Bodies: A Catalogue of Anatomical Fugitive Sheets 1538-1687*. *Medical History* Supplement No. 19. London: Wellcome Institute for the History of Medicine, 1999.

Carmichael, Ann G. 'Contagion Theory and Contagion Practice in Fifteenth-Century Milan' *Renaissance Quarterly* 44 (1991): 213-256.

Centorio, Ascanio. *Discorsi di guerra*. Venice: Gabriel Giolito de' Ferrari, 1567.

Chase, Vanessa. 'The Casa delle Zitelle: Gender and Architecture in Renaissance Venice.' Ph.D. Diss. Columbia University, 2002.

Chojnacka, Monica. 'Charity and Poverty in Counter-Reformation Venice,' paper presented at Circolo Britannico, Venice, December 1995.

Chojnacka, Monica. 'Women, Charity, and Community in Early Modern Venice: The Casa delle Zitelle' *Renaissance Quarterly* 51:1 (1998): 68-91.

Chojnacka, Monica. *Working Women of Early Modern Venice*. Baltimore: The Johns Hopkins University Press, 1991.

Ciammitti, Luisa. 'Conservatori femminili a Bologna e organizzazione del lavoro.' *Quaderni Storici* 41 (August 1979): 760-4.

Ciammitti, Luisa. 'Fanciulle monache madri: Povertà femminile e previdenze a Bologna nei secoli XVI-VXIII' pp. 461-496 in *Arte e Pietà: i patrimoni culturali delle opere pie*. Bologna: Istituto per i beni culturali della Regione Emilia-Romagna: CLUEB, 1980.

Cipolla, Carlo M. *Public Health and the Medical Profession in the Renaissance*. Cambridge: Cambridge University Press, 1976.

Cipolla, Carlo M. *Fighting the Plague in Seventeenth-Century Italy*. Madison, WI: University of Wisconsin Press, 1981.

Cohen, Sherrill. *The Evolution of Women's Asylums since 1500: From Refuges of Ex-Prostitutes to Shelters for Battered Women*. New York: Oxford University Press, 1992.

Corradi, Alfonso. 'Nuovi documenti per la storia delle malattie veneree in Italia della fine del '400 alla metà del '500' *Rendiconti* 4:14-15 (Milan, 1871): 1-32.

Cropper, Elizabeth. 'On Beautiful Women, Parmigianino, *Petrarchismo*, and the Vernacular Style' *Art Bulletin* 58 (1976): 374-394.

Della Porta, Giambattista. *Della fisonomia dell'huomo*. Naples: Tarquinio Longo, 1598.

Eamon, William. *Science and the Secrets of Nature: Books of Secrets in Medieval and Early Modern Culture*. Princeton: Princeton University Press, 1994.

Eamon, William. 'Cannibalism and Contagion: Framing Syphilis in Counter-Reformation Italy' *Early Science and Medicine* 3:1 (1998): 1-31.

Estienne, Charles. *La dissection des parties du corps*. Paris: Simon de Colines, 1546.

Farmer, Paul. *AIDS and Accusation: Haiti and the Geography of Blame*. Berkeley: University of California Press, 1992.

Ferrante, Lucia. 'Honor Regained: Women in the Casa del Soccorso di San Polo in Sixteenth-Century Bologna' pp. 46-72 in *Sex and Gender in Historical Perspective*, ed. Edward Muir and Guido Ruggiero. Baltimore: The Johns Hopkins University Press, 1990.

Findlen, Paula. 'Humanism, Politics, and Pornography in Renaissance Italy' pp. 49-108 in *The Invention of Pornography: Obscenity and the Origins of Modernity, 1500-1800*, ed. Lynn Hunt. New York: Zone Books, 1993.

Firenzuola, Agnolo. *On The Beauty of Women*. Translated by Konrad Eisenbichler and Jacqueline Murray. Philadelphia: University of Pennsylvania Press, 1992.

Fitzgerald, Allan. *Conversion through Penance in the Italian Church of the Fourth and Fifth Centuries: New Approaches to the Experience of Conversion from Sin*. Studies in the Bible and Early Christianity, 15. Lewiston, NY: The Edwin Mellen Press, 1988.

Foa Anna. 'The New and the Old: The Spread of Syphilis (1494–1530)' pp. 26–45 in *Sex and Gender in Historical Perspective,* eds. Edward Muir and Guido Ruggiero. Baltimore: The Johns Hopkins University Press, 1990.

Fracastoro, Girolamo. *De contagione et contagiosis morbis et eorum curatione.* Translated by Wilmer Cave Wright. New York, London: Putnam, 1930.

Gilman, Sander. 'Touch, Sexuality and Disease' pp. 198–224 in *Medicine and the Five Senses,* eds. W. F. Bynum and Roy Porter. Cambridge: Cambridge University Press, 1993.

Griffin, Gabriele. *Representations of HIV and AIDS: Visibility Blue/s.* Manchester: Manchester University Press, 2000.

Groppi, Angela. *I conservatori della virtù: donne recluse nella Roma dei papi.* Bari: Laterza, 1994.

Haskins, Susan. *Mary Magdalene: Myth and Metaphor.* New York: Harcourt Brace, 1993.

Jansen, Katherine L. 'Mary Magdalene and the Mendicants: The Preaching of Penance in the Late Middle Ages' *Journal of Medieval History* 21 (1995): 1-25.

Leavitt, Judith Walzer. *Typhoid Mary: Captive to the Public's Health.* Boston: Beacon Press, 1996.

Penitence in the Age of Reformations, ed. Katharine Jackson Lualdi and Anne T. Thayer. Burlington, VT: Ashgate, 2000.

Luria, Keith. 'Rituals of Conversion: Catholics and Protestants in Seventeenth-Century Poitou' pp. 65-81 in *Culture and Identity in Early Modern Europe (1500-1800): Essays in Honor of Natalie Zemon Davis,* eds. Barbara Diefendorf and Carla Hesse. Ann Arbor: The University of Michigan Press, 1993.

Malvern, Marjorie M. *Venus in Sackcloth: The Magdalen's Origins and Metamorphoses.* Carbondale: Southern Illinois University Press, 1975.

Marinello, Giovanni. *Gli ornamenti delle donne.* Venice: Francesco de' Franceschi Senese, 1562.

Martin, John. *Venice's Hidden Enemies: Italian Heretics in a Renaissance City.* Berkeley: University of California Press, 1993.

McGough, Laura J. 'Women, Private Property, and the Limitations of State Authority in Early Modern Venice' *Journal of Women's History* 14 (Autumn 2002): 32–52.

McGough, Laura J. '"Raised from the Devil's Jaws": A Convent for Repentant Prostitutes in Venice, 1530–1670.' Ph.D. Diss. Northwestern University, 1997.

Molmenti, Pompeo. *La storia di Venezia nella vita privata.* Bergamo: Istituto Italiano d'arti grafiche, 1906.

Mosco, Marilena. *La Maddalena tra sacro e profano: da Giotto a De Chirico.* Florence: Casa Usher, 1986.

Nordio, Andrea. 'L'Ospedale degli Incurabili nell'assistenza veneziana del '500' *Studi veneziani* N. S. 32 (1996): 165–184.

Nutton, Vivian. 'The Seeds of Disease: An Explanation of Contagion and Infection from the Greeks to the Renaissance' *Medical History* 27 (1983): 1–34.

O'Malley, John W. *The First Jesuits.* Cambridge, MA: Harvard University Press, 1993.

Pallucchini, Rodolfo. *La pittura veneziana del Seicento*. Milan: Electa, 1981.

Palmer, Richard. 'The Control of Plague in Venice and Northern Italy, 1348-1600.' Ph.D. Thesis, University of Kent, 1978.

Pancino, Claudia. *'Soffrire per ben comparire. Corpo e bellezza, natura e cura'* pp. 5–42 in *Storia d'Italia,* Annali 19 *La moda*, ed. Carlo Marco Belfanti e Fabio Giusberti. Turin: Einaudi, 2003.

Parte presa nell'Eccellentissimo Conseglio di Pregadi. 21 February 1542 m.v. Venice: Pietro Pinelli, 1543.

Porter, Roy. *The Greatest Benefit to Mankind: A Medical History of Humanity*. New York: Norton, 1997.

Preto, Paolo. *Peste e società a Venezia nel 1576*. Vicenza: Pozzi, 1978.

Pullan, Brian. *Rich and Poor in Renaissance Venice: The Social Institutions of a Catholic State to 1620*. Cambridge, MA.: Harvard University Press, 1971.

Rollo-Koster, Joëlle. 'From Prostitutes to Brides of Christ: The Avignonese *Repenties* in the late Middle Ages' *Journal of Medieval and Early Modern Studies* 32:1 (2002): 109-144.

Rostinio, Pietro. *Trattato del mal francese*. Venice: Lodovico Avanzi, 1559.

Sansovino, Francesco. *Venetia cittá nobilissima et singolare*. Venice: I. Sansovino, 1581.

Sanuto, Marin. *I diarii*. Venice: G. Berchet, 1879-1881.

Schleiner, Winfried. 'Infection and Cure through Women: Renaissance Constructions of the French Disease' *Journal of Medieval and Renaissance Studies* 24:3 (1994): 499–517.

Schleiner, Winfried. 'Moral Attitudes toward Syphilis and Its Prevention in the Renaissance' *Bulletin of the History of Medicine* 68 (1994): 389-410.

Shilts, Randy. *And the Band Played On: People, Politics, and the AIDS Epidemic*. New York: St. Martin's Press, 1987.

Siena, Kevin. *Venereal Disease, Hospitals, and the Urban Poor: London's 'Foul Wards' 1600-1800*. Rochester: University of Rochester Press, 2004.

Steele, Brian. 'In the Flower of Their Youth: "Portraits" of Venetian Beauties ca. 1500' *Sixteenth Century Journal* 28:2 (1997): 481-502.

Sudhoff, Karl. *The Earliest Printed Literature on Syphilis*. Florence: R. Lier, 1925.

Treichler, Paula A. 'AIDS, Gender, and Biomedical Discourse: Current Contests for Meaning' pp. 190-206 in *AIDS: The Burdens of History*, eds. Elizabeth Fee and Daniel M. Fox. Berkeley: University of California Press, 1988.

Yavneh, Naomi. 'The Ambiguity of Beauty in Tasso and Petrarch' pp. 133-157 in *Sexuality and Gender in Early Modern Europe: Institutions, Texts, Images,* ed. James Grantham Turner. Cambridge: Cambridge University Press, 1993.

The French Connection: Syphilis and Sodomy in Late-Renaissance Lucca

Mary Hewlett

The venereal disease known to us as syphilis first appeared in Italy in the 1490s during the French campaign to claim Naples. The Neapolitans, and subsequently other Italians, described this new disease as the *mal francese* or 'French Disease,' thereby blaming the army of King Charles VIII for introducing the nasty scourge into Italy. The French on the other hand, named the disease the 'Neapolitan Pox' claiming Neapolitan prostitutes had infected French soldiers. Thus, as the disease rapidly spread throughout Europe, the pattern was set in place for blaming the disease on various forms of the 'other:' be they 'foreigners' (especially enemy foreigners[1]) and social or sexual deviants.

This article looks at one aspect of this process by examining (what I have termed) the 'French Connection,' that is, the connection made by the government of the Italian city-state of Lucca between the *mal francese* and the practice of sodomy. Lucca was a city-state republic ruled by a narrow oligarchy, made up of families whose roots went back several centuries.[2] In order to maintain their power base, these families controlled the political, social, moral, and religious lives of Lucchese citizens. Those who behaved in an unorthodox manner or disregarded the laws of the city ran the risk of prosecution. As in other cities, the government assumed there was a connection between physical and moral corruption. Just as the appearance of the Black Death had led moralists to speculate on the reasons why sufferers were being punished with the affliction, so this new contagious ailment provoked a similar response. When the disease took hold all over Europe, many perceived it as a form of divine punishment inflicted on an erring society. Those seeking scapegoats readily found them. In various ways

---

[1]In Lucca, as in other cities in Italy, foreigners were those from other cities and regions as well as from other countries.

[2]For more on the background history of Lucca and the formation of principal families, see Meek, *Lucca 1369–1400*; Bratchel, *Lucca 1430–1495*; Bertini, *Le grandi famiglie*.

moralists could view the morally lax, those living on the margins, or outsiders as deviant, thereby conveniently branding them as culprits. It was argued that the horrible symptoms of the new plague were signs of a parallel moral depravity in the sufferer. The external sores on the body of the syphilitic were seen as evidence of the victim's inward corruption. In this climate of moral castigation, it is no wonder that even the victims of the new scourge themselves feared it as a punishment for their sexual sins.

Fear of Sodomy

Some Italian moralists saw the foreign invasions and destructive wars of the peninsula as a punishment for the sins of the people, and especially for the crime of sodomy, which they described as a crime against nature. A Bull issued by Pope Pius V in 1566 declared that the Italian wars of the late-fifteen and early sixteenth century were God's punishment for the sins of the Italian people, specifically mentioning the arch-sin of sodomy. Nicholas Davidson explores this connection in his work on sodomy in Venice.[3] In particular, he examines the diary of a Venetian patrician named Girolamo Priuli, who made the observation that Venetian men were becoming more effeminate in their dress and manners, thereby luring each other into sodomy.[4] In Lucca, those who practiced 'the nefarious vice of sodomy' were also seen as corrupting the city, both physically and morally. For these reasons sodomites became one of the government's prime targets for moral reform.

Sodomy had been a concern for the Lucchese from the mid-fourteenth century when, like many other cities searching for culprits, Lucca feared that by tacitly allowing the vice of sodomy it had provoked divine punishment in the form of the Black Death. This concern was aggravated by fear of further population depletion in the wake of the plague, which had already reduced the city's population by a third. As a non-procreative form of sexual intercourse sodomy threatened the numerical strength of Lucca just at a time when more citizens were desperately needed to compensate for recent losses and labour deficiencies. As a result, sodomy, whether between same-sex partners or opposite-sex partners, was deemed to be a crime.

---

[3]Davidson, 'Sodomy in Early Modern Venice,' p. 67. See also Ruggiero, *Boundaries of Eros*. For fifteenth-century Florence, see Rocke, *Forbidden Friendships*. For attitudes to sodomy in northern Renaissance cities, see Boes, 'On Trial for Sodomy in Early Modern Europe,'(for a discussion of Strasbourg) and Naphy, 'Sodomy in Early Modern Geneva'; Puff, *Sodomy in Reformation Germany and Switzerland*.

[4]Davidson, 'Sodomy in Early Modern Venice,' p. 67.

Matters came to a head in 1369 during a state visit to Lucca by the Holy Roman Emperor Charles IV and his consort. The urgency of this problem was graphically and embarrassingly brought to the attention of the authorities when the royal party and other dignitaries standing on the balcony of the municipal palace witnessed a man sodomizing a boy in the courtyard below. The government acted swiftly and brutally: despite being a member of the patrician class, the man was burnt alive; the boy narrowly escaped the same fate thanks to the intervention of a high-ranking official.[5]

In 1448 the government institutionalized the drive to eradicate sodomy when it set up a special court known as the *Offizio sopra l'Onestà* or Office of Decency, specifically to hear and try cases of sodomy.[6] The General Council elected three magistrates from among citizens who had a right to vote and hold office in the Commune.[7] In the mid-1500s, the General Council revamped the office as part of a policy of moral policing designed to maximize patrician control over the city.[8] The government revised legislation concerning sodomy and sent orders to the Office of Decency urging the court to escalate what was frequently described in the documents as the 'war on sodomy.'[9] These magistrates served for a term of one year and met on a regular basis – by the sixteenth century at least once a week. The law stipulated that they had to be selected from among men of the highest calibre. In 1533 a revision of the laws stated that one of the three citizens chosen must hold a doctorate in law and all must be over the age of forty.[10] Since this was deemed to be an onerous office, after their one-year term magistrates did not have to serve again for another three years.

The government continued to view sodomy as a serious concern throughout sixteenth and into the mid-seventeenth century.[11] Government

---

[5]Bongi, *Bandi lucchesi del secolo decimoquarto*, pp. 377–388.

[6]Unfortunately, the records of the *Offizio sopra l' Onestà* from 1448–1547 are lost.

[7]ASL, *Serie Statuti del Comune di Lucca 1308–1549*, fol. 343.

[8]*Decreti penali*, p. 121 (1533).

[9]*Decreti penali*, p. 121. For more information on the threats faced by the Lucchese government in the sixteenth century, see Berengo, *Nobili e mercanti* especially pp. 83–334; Adorni-Braccesi, *'Una città infetta,'* pp. 53–143; Seghieri, '1554: un anno difficile per Lucca,' pp. 3–12; Hewlett, 'A Republic in Jeopardy,' pp. 9–22.

[10]*Decreti penali,* p. 120 (1533).

[11]Over this period Lucca built a massive wall that surrounded the city and kept a large military contingent in response to supposed outside threats, mainly from Florence. This policy in itself brought problems, because the soldiers often appear in the criminal records, including records of the *Onestà* and the *Protettori delle meretrici*. They were also undoubtedly a factor in the spread of the *mal francese*.

records contain dispatches strongly urging the Office to be more diligent in tracking down sodomites, whom it saw as threats to the well-being and right order of the city. Fears of divine punishment mingled again with anxiety that sodomy might stunt the future population growth of Lucca. The connection between moral and physical disease was further cemented by yet more visitations of pestilence. Apart from the syphilis epidemic, Lucca was also hit by sporadic plague epidemics, two of which were particularly serious. One occurred in 1575–1577 and the other in 1630–1631. It is interesting that 1630–1631, which saw the last major outbreak of plague decimate the Lucchese population, also marks a start to the decline in the number of sodomy trials.[12]

Work done on other cities shows that sodomy was prosecuted in other European cities to varying degrees. Michael Rocke's ground-breaking work on Florence in the fifteenth century shows that sodomy was part of the natural cultural development of Florentine males, who in their pre-pubescent youth acted as *patiente* or passive partner, progressing as they aged to becoming the active partner with younger boys, before usually ceasing sex with other males when they married. The Florentine Office of the Night prosecuted sodomites in large numbers, but failed to stamp out sodomy, and prosecutions declined in the sixteenth century.[13] Recent work by Nicholas Davidson builds and expands on Guido Ruggiero's classic study of sex in Renaissance Venice. Davidson found that, despite its harsh laws against sodomy, Venice seemed increasingly reluctant to prosecute the crime by the mid-sixteenth century when, as in Florence, the number of prosecutions declines. Davidson concludes that the reluctance of people to denounce sodomites indicates a tacit acceptance of sodomy in society. This reluctance may have been due to a more secular outlook, though Davidson also suggests that socio-economic factors such as the tendency of Venetians to later and less frequent marriages meant that there was less opposition to non-procreative sex; thus sodomy became less of a threat to the city.[14]

While there are also indications that the population of Lucca, like that of Venice, may not have agreed altogether with the strict policy of the oligarchy, Lucca's situation was more perilous than that of Venice. Lucca

---

[12]For more information on the plague in Italy, and the response of the city governments, see Cipolla, *Public Health and the Medical Profession*; Carmichael, *Plague and the Poor in Renaissance Florence*.

[13]See Rocke, *Forbidden Friendships*, pp. 43–84 for a description of the Office of the Night. The peak of the prosecutions was late 1495 to early 1496. The office was disbanded in 1502. See Rocke, *Forbidden Friendships*, pp. 232–235.

[14]Davidson, *Sodomy in Early Modern Venice*, pp. 89–90.

was a city in fear of being swallowed up by its predatory neighbour, Florence. The narrow oligarchy was determined to make sure that there was no excuse for Florence, or another external power such as the papacy, to intervene in its internal affairs; therefore, control of the political, social, religious, and moral lives of its citizens was imperative. These practical considerations combined with the very real fear of divine punishment drove the government's opposition to sodomy.

The Lucchese authorities defined sodomy as anal sex, either between two males or between a male and a female. Despite the fact that the term 'sodomy' could be interpreted as any sexual activity not permitted by the Church and depended on the legislation in a particular location, it is important to stress that in Lucca only anal sex was prosecuted. Although other forbidden acts such as *fellatio* were mentioned in passing, they never warranted prosecution in the trials of consenting adults. In cases of pedophilia however, the authorities included acts leading to anal sex in their definition of sodomy, although cases in which no penetration occurred were judged more leniently. While oral sex and masturbation were frowned upon, these practices did not in themselves merit prosecution by the State.

Between 1551 and 1647, the Office of Decency tried 260 cases involving men, women, and children.[15] Male same-sex sodomy and molestation of boys made up the bulk of the cases, accounting for 202 (77.6%) of the trials appearing before the magistrates. This number represents the actual cases that came to trial, as recorded in the first five books of the *Onestà*. Each could and often did involve several accused. The sixth book of the *Onestà* shows extensive lists of those described as the *prevenuti*, the repeat offenders. There were 1,839 preliminary prosecutions between the years 1539 and 1580 indicating that only a fraction of those accused were actually brought to trial. It also shows that prosecutions for sodomy were a lucrative process for the Lucchese government.[16]

Trials that involved multiple young men and adolescent boys caused the greatest anxiety, as the authorities feared they were fighting a losing battle. One case from 1581 dragged on for a year because many of the accused admitted having sexual relations with several others within an increasingly expanding group that eventually involved twenty-one men and teenage boys.[17] In order to find out the extent of suspected 'nests of

---

[15] ASL, *Offizio sopra l'Onestà* 1–5 (1551–1647).

[16] These documents are the only remaining lists of *prevenuti* or repeat offenders, but the large numbers recorded in these forty years indicate the enormous number of denunciations resolved out of court. ASL, *Offizio sopra l'Onestà* 6, (1539–1580).

[17] ASL, *Offizio sopra l'Onestà* 3, fols. 2^r–16^r (16 July 1581). This case involved males

sodomites,' the *Onestà* routinely tortured the majority of the accused and often some of the witnesses as well. The laws meticulously set out the various categories of punishment, ranging from public whipping and a spell in the stocks for young offenders, to death for those considered to be irredeemable sodomites. Repeat offenders over the age of fifty were seen as a serious risk to younger men and boys, and considered too old to change their ways through chastisement; for them, death was the only solution.[18] In the rare cases where executions took place, the condemned was first decapitated and then his body was burned to remove all trace of him. The magistrates were also particularly severe with adults seen to be corrupting the youth of the city, and especially adults in positions of authority over the young, such as priests abusing alter boys and teachers molesting pupils. In these cases the authorities went to great lengths to seek out and round up all those involved; those repeatedly abusing their position of trust could be sentenced to death even as young as thirty.[19]

THE FRENCH CONNECTION: THE *MAL FRANCESE* AND SODOMY

The rapid spread of the *mal francese* in Italy added fuel to these fears of sodomitical practices. As Jon Arrizabalaga's contribution to this volume shows, the sexual nature of the disease was quickly recognized and connected to 'sins of the flesh.'[20] Because for the Lucchese government the most serious of these sins of the flesh was sodomy, the pox and sodomy became closely linked in the minds of those whose task it was to police morals. Thus, the advent of syphilis played into the hands of the authorities attempting to stamp out sodomy, for the social disease of sodomy and the sexual disease of syphilis seemed to feed off each other and constitute a double-headed menace. Not surprisingly, the Lucchese authorities escalated the war on sodomy by treating the *mal francese* as a disease specifically spread by anal intercourse. Those suspected of carrying the *mal francese* were thus automatically investigated as sodomy suspects. The trial records of the *Onestà* provide ample evidence of this connection and reveal the measures the city took to combat both sodomy and the *mal francese*.

---

ranging from 14 to 50 years of age and represented a cross section of the community. It is the trial that comes closest to providing evidence of a homosexual sub-culture in Lucca.

[18]*Decreti penali*, p. 123 (1533).

[19]*Decreti penali*, p. 123 (1533). Despite the harsh wording of the law, only nine men were executed for sodomy in the period 1551–1647.

[20]For more on the spread of the disease through Europe, see Arrizabalaga, Henderson and French, *The Great Pox*.

Apart from the magistrates themselves, two important court officials contributed to the investigations. First, the court agent known as the *gattaiuola* acted as a detective or spy, going underground into taverns, barracks, and public baths to pick up gossip and information. Armed with names of suspected sodomites, he would collect evidence from various sources in order to build a solid case against them. One particularly diligent *gattaiuola* trapped several unsuspecting offenders. On one occasion he pretended to be seeking a partner for anal intercourse and thus incriminated a female prostitute willing to offer him erotic sodomy.[21] The records show another *gattaiuola* seeking out a young female rape victim who was in the *Ospedale degli Incurabili* being treated for *mal francese,* which he assumed she had contracted by being sodomized. He persuaded her that it was in her best interest to denounce and press charges against her sodomizer.[22] The *gattaiuola* was well paid for his services. He provided continuity and expertise in the *Onestà*, as he was employed year after year, whereas the magistrates rotated annually. [23]

The *Onestà* also relied heavily on medical authorities to add insight and bring the weight of medical knowledge to bear on their inquests. As an official, the medical consultant was called upon to examine both perpetrators and victims of anal rape for injuries or signs of the *mal francese*. It was on his evidence that the court frequently based its verdicts. When medical testimony pointed to violent anal rape, venereal disease, or enlargement of the sphincter due to habitual anal intercourse, the accused was likely to be found guilty. The presence (or absence) of the *mal francese* thus played a key role in Lucchese sodomy trials. With the escalation of cases involving the *mal francese*, medical witnesses became increasingly important to the magistrates.

Who were these witnesses? The records show all kinds of medical practitioners. It was not uncommon to find Latinate university-trained physicians, the most prestigious of the day, giving testimony. More frequently it was the more common barber surgeons who stood as medical experts. This is not surprising given that more people could afford their services.[24] A more surprising discovery was that women, too, offered

---

21ASL, *Offizio sopra l'Onestà* 3, fol. 36^{v} (21 November 1592).

22ASL, *Offizio sopra l'Onestà* 3, unpag. (20 June 1589).

23It appears that this office was a family business, which was handed down from one generation to another for several generations.

24An excellent description of the categories of healers can be found in Siraisi, *Medieval and Early Renaissance Medicine,* pp. 17–77 and 153–186; Lindemann, *Medicine and Society,* pp. 103–119 and 193–230. For a discussion of the range of healers treating the pox in Italy see David Gentilcore's contribution to this volume.

medical testimony. While excluded from formal education or guild membership that would allow them to become physicians, surgeons, or apothecaries, female healers were permitted to treat other women, often in matters relating to childbirth or ailments associated with the female reproductive organs. Regardless of the limitations put on their practices, female healers had a considerable clientele, as some women turned for help more readily to their midwives or female popular healers than to male doctors. Because they generally charged less for their services than other healers, female healers may also have provided an alternative for poorer women as well as for those hoping to keep their condition a secret.[25] The fact that women so often consulted these female healers meant that the magistrates also called female practitioners as medical witnesses in sodomy trials involving women. What is interesting for this particular study is that these women tended to know far more about the various venereal diseases of their female patients than did their male colleagues. Despite the clear hierarchy within medicine, the sodomy inquests demonstrate that these socially insignificant female healers could in fact command weighty medical authority.

Given the wide range of healers called to testify in sodomy trials it is not surprising to find conflicting interpretations of the *mal francese*. The disease was notoriously hard to diagnose. As a result, interpretations of its wide ranging symptoms held crucial importance for those contesting sodomy in the courts. This is illustrated by a case from 1597 in which it was the testimony of a female healer, Mattea di Federico da Encoli, that swung the opinion of the magistrates in favour of Lucretia, a prostitute denounced for offering erotic sodomy. The *gattaiuola* had brought the denunciation, claiming that Lucretia had been treated for the *creste*, that is sores indicating infection by *mal francese*. Three male medical witnesses gave conflicting testimony before the court called Mattea. She readily admitted she had treated Lucretia with an ointment, but specified that it was not for *creste,* but for *morice*. When the authorities cross-examined her about her knowledge in such matters, Mattea confidently explained to them the difference between *creste* and *morice*. *Creste* were like a cock's comb and *morice* were more like granules in varnish.[26] This case not only indicates the respect given

---

[25]For a discussion of this in London, see Siena, 'The "Foul Disease" and Privacy,' pp. 214–223.

[26]ASL, *Offizio sopra l'Onestà* 4, fols. 63^{v}–67^{r} (7 July 1597). 'Creste' refers to *condyloma accumata spegalososis*. The *Oxford English Dictionary* describes them as 'wart-like tumours of skin near the genital area or anus, generally associated with syphilis'. The term *morice* also surfaces in other cases. It is more difficult to define, because it does not seem to have consistent symptoms. The symptoms indicate it could have been one of several complaints, including gonorrhea.

this female healer's professional opinion, it demonstrates how the presence, or in this case the absence, of the disease played a pivotal role in sodomy prosecution. Moreover, it also demonstrates how attempts to establish infection as a medico-legal 'fact' in sodomy trials could be highly contested.

On a number of similar occasions conflicting medical opinions resulted in hurt pride and professional rivalry. Such tension played itself out in the courtroom in front of the judges, as one case from 1629 vividly illustrates.[27] On this occasion a father, Bastiano, brought a complaint against his own son-in law Michele, whom he accused of sodomizing and infecting his daughter with *mal francese*. Bastiano revealed under questioning that Michele had married his daughter, Leonora, without his consent. He claimed he had been reluctantly prepared to accept the marriage to avoid a scandal, until he found that his daughter was sick.

The barber surgeon Flamminio was the first witness called for the prosecution. He testified that he had examined Leonora and found that she had been sodomized and was now suffering greatly from a severe case of *mal francese*.[28] He also told the court that Leonora had confessed to him that her husband had infected her. When it was Leonora's turn to testify, she indignantly protested that she had never confided in Flamminio. She flatly denied that Michele had ever sodomized her or that she was suffering from the *mal francese*. She did, however, admit that her husband had 'taken her from behind,' but in the 'natural part.'[29]

She then requested that the magistrates call her own midwife as a witness. This woman's evidence conflicted with the barber surgeon's. The midwife testified that although there was some evidence of disease there was no reason to believe that just because it had invaded the anal area that the couple had been practicing sodomy. She stated that Leonora was suffering from *morice* and not *mal francese*. The midwife went on to say that she had considerable experience in treating women; therefore, she knew what she was talking about. She volunteered details about how it was possible to tell if anal sex had taken place. She claimed that Leonora did not exhibit any of these symptoms. Thus, she could safely say that the girl had not been sodomized.[30] Although the midwife did not go into detail as to how she diagnosed sodomy, information from other cases reveals that

---

27 ASL, *Offizio sopra l'Onestà* 5, fols. 1^r–10^v (4 September–13 October 1629).

28 ASL, *Offizio sopra l'Onestà* 5, fol. 1^v (5 September 1629).

29 ASL, *Offizio sopra l'Onestà* 5, fol. 3^r (7 September 1629).

30 ASL, *Offizio sopra l'Onestà* 5, fol. 3^v (7 September 1629). In this case Leonora's *morice* sounds like gonorrhea. She complained of extreme pain on urination, one of the symptoms typical of gonorrhea.

enlargement and inflammation of the rectal sphincter was frequently offered as evidence of anal sex.

The case became further complicated when more witnesses gave evidence, including another midwife who Bastiano called to support Flamminio's testimony. Another factor confusing the case was whether or not Leonora was in the early stages of pregnancy, which she herself claimed. Pregnancy would indicate to the authorities that the couple had practiced at least some procreative sex. The main concern with conjugal sodomy was that it was practiced as a way of preventing procreation.

Faced with cases in which medical witnesses provided conflicting evidence, the magistrates had to fathom out the various biases that might affect testimony, especially when the parties divided into camps, each with their own loyal witnesses. On this occasion, it appears they chose to believe Leonora and her husband Michele, who claimed that Leonora's father had bribed both of his medical witnesses, namely Flamminio the surgeon and the second midwife. Leonora also accused her father of trying to break up the marriage and attempting to destroy Michele's reputation. She insisted that she did not have the *mal francese,* that she was pregnant, and that her disease was one that she had suffered from sporadically since her childhood.[31] Again we see how the disease impacted these proceedings, not only in the attempts to prove or deny that sodomy had occurred, but also in attempts to establish reputation – the father insisting that his caddish son-in-law had infected his daughter, and Leonora flatly denying it.

The Commune's response to *mal francese* also meant that the city lent considerable support to private charitable institutions dealing with the disease, such as the *Spedale di san Luca* and the *Spedale degli Incurabili,* that is the Hospital for the incurably ill.[32] Arrizabalaga, Henderson, and French have illustrated that these hospitals for the incurable treated patients with the French Disease in many communities throughout Italy.[33] The extant records of these institutions provide another source of information to explore the intersection of sodomy and syphilis in Lucca. The *Spedale degli Incurabili* opened in 1537 to accept and treat patients with chronic and

---

[31]ASL, *Offizio sopra l'Onestà* 5, fol. 9^{v} (3 October 1629). The suspicion seems to have been that Leonora may have been pregnant and then lost the baby.

[32]Although it is apparent that all over Italy private citizens initiated the funding of charitable organizations, this can be misleading. The prominent families who ran the oligarchy in Lucca were also the leaders in social and religious life; therefore, it was often the same citizens who sat on the General Council, the committee of a confraternity, and on the magistracies concerned with moral policing.

[33]Arrizabalaga, Henderson, and French, *The Great Pox,* pp. 145–233.

incurable diseases including syphilis, but excluding plague victims and lepers who were treated elsewhere.

Disappointingly, very few records of the actual activities and treatment methods of the *Incurabili* remain in Lucca. Most of what survives deals with the administration of the confraternity that ran the hospital and not with the patient records. Nevertheless, some information can be gleaned from the scanty remnants. A brief list of patients admitted for treatment between 1650 and 1663 gives a glimpse of some aspects of the daily running of the *Incurabili*. There are dates of admission and discharge, as well as lists of clothing and belongings that patients had in their possession when they entered the institution. Unfortunately, the records provide no detail of the actual method of treatment. The patient lists show that in 1663 only two women were admitted that year out of thirty-six patients.[34] However, this seems an anomaly, because in 1664 thirty women and only twenty men were admitted for treatment.[35] A notice for 22 April 1663 records that out of sixty patients admitted that year, thirty-seven had left the establishment cured.[36] The records for 1664 and 1665 show a very similar ratio of admissions and discharges. The evidence of patients 'cured' demonstrates that by the second half of the seventeenth century the *mal francese* was no longer considered an 'incurable' disease.[37] It is interesting to note that the *Incurabili* summarily expelled difficult patients such as Domenicho di Francesco, a baker, who was insolent and therefore discharged without further treatment.[38]

The *Onestà* saw the *Incurabili* as an opportunity to expand its campaign of sexual surveillance by turning medical institutions into a forum for moral investigation. To this end, wanting to kill two birds with one stone, it sent frequent notices to doctors in the city to be on the lookout for evidence of both sodomy and the *mal francese* in their patients, and to report all such cases to the Commune. By doing so the civic authorities attempted to expand their network of informants beyond the official spy, the *gattaiuola*, hoping to draw on privileged information gleaned through the medical gaze. Physicians, barber-surgeons, and midwives worked for the Commune of

---

34 ASL, *Lo Spedale degli Incurabili*, 16, fol. 3^{v} (22 April 1663).

35 ASL, *Lo Spedale degli Incurabili,* 16, fol. 4^{v} (April 1664).

36 ASL, *Lo Spedale degli Incurabili*, 16, fol. 3^{r} (April 1663).

37 ASL, *Lo Spedale degli Incurabili*, 16, fols.. 30–31^{v}, 53^{r}, 58–59^{v} (April 1664 & April 1665). Although it is well-documented that syphilis goes through an asymptomatic dormant stage, it seems that certain treatments did appear to help. The records document several 'complete' cures. Claude Quétel discusses apparently successful cures for syphilis in *History of Syphilis,* pp. 58–66.

38 ASL, *Lo Spedale degli Incurabili*, 16, fol. 3^{r} (13 February 1663).

Lucca and in various charitable organizations such as the *Spedale degli Incurabili*, the Misericordia and the orphanages.[39] From the point of view of the Commune, when it came to matters of health, it was vitally important for the government to keep a finger on the pulse of the city. Potentially, this had the added benefit of providing the *Onestà* with additional leads to investigate both syphilis and sodomy. All doctors were required to keep a logbook, to see if there were repeated problems with any patients that the government should investigate. The surgeons' logs reveal no cases of treatment of syphilis or sodomy, but this lacuna could be interpreted in several ways: perhaps such patients avoided going to the government-paid doctors and sought help elsewhere to evade surveillance. Or perhaps doctors themselves were reluctant to make denunciations. This brings into question the effectiveness of using government-paid healers as forced spies for the *Onestà*. Certainly, there are no cases in which healers came forward willingly to denounce patients. In fact, evidence points to the opposite – healers may have tried to protect patients.[40]

Despite the zealousness of the court, in some cases the doctors or popular healers purposely did not diagnose the patient with *mal francese*. As we have seen they might diagnose some other infection. This transpired in the long case of the notorious 'Maria from the mountains of Genoa,' a prostitute accused of infecting several men with syphilis transmitted through erotic sodomy. It seems to have been a fellow prostitute and rival named Juditta, and not Maria's surgeon, who reported Maria's *mal francese* to the authorities. Juditta testified that she had held the lamp for the surgeon when he treated her colleague.[41] However, the barber surgeon denied that he had treated Maria for *mal francese*.[42] Likewise, some doctors examining victims of the *mal francese* told the court that they could not be certain if or when sodomy had occurred, in which case the accused was less likely to be found guilty. In 1568 a woman named Pellegrina accused Febo, a tailor who lived in her building, of cornering her and sodomizing her. The examining barber surgeon refused to be browbeaten by the court, saying that he could not tell if Pellegrina had been sodomized, but he did say that she certainly had the *mal francese* and had contracted it earlier. Despite considerable pressure

---

39 ASL, *Raccolte Speciali*.

40 There were a large number of anonymous secret denunciations, but often certain witnesses appear at the trials who seem likely to have brought that particular denunciation. In no case was this found to be a healer.

41 ASL, *Offizio sopra l'Onestà* fol. 3, 98^{r} (30 November 1595).

42 ASL, *Offizio sopra l'Onestà* 3, fols. 98^{r}–142^{r} & *Offizio sopra l'Onestà* 4, fols. 1^{r}–78^{r} (30 November–31 December 1595).

to make a firm diagnosis, the doctor could not attest to her having being taken by force. The magistrates repeatedly demanded that the surgeon give a more definitive diagnosis regarding the sexual act, but all he would do was diagnose the longstanding *mal francese* and refrain judgment on the possibility of sodomy. His testimony seems to have been vital. The court acquitted the accused rapist, because the surgeon's claim that Pellegrina had suffered from the disease for a long time tarnished her *fama* or reputation and somehow excused her alleged assailant.[43]

Because the city legally required that healers denounce patients and give evidence, treating patients for *mal francese* could be a risky business for doctors. Giving evidence could also pose a problem, because loyalty to their city and loyalty to the patients could conflict. In the 1597 case of the prostitute Lucretia discussed above, her barber surgeon Allexio Belensario was himself in trouble with the *Onestà*. A secret denunciation claimed that Lucretia had been sodomized and that 'Allexio had medicated her in the back part and had cut away the crests.'[44] This meant that he was now liable for prosecution for not having reported that he had treated her for venereal disease. In this particular case, it appears that Allexio was somewhat enamoured of Lucretia, who was described as very beautiful. Healers needed to keep the trust of their patients, who would be unlikely to consult them again if they denounced them to the authorities. In a closely knit society such as Lucca, word spread rapidly; not keeping faith with a patient could seriously jeopardize a doctor's reputation and severely reduce his clientele. It is also possible that some patients with *mal francese* may have preferred to consult folk healers who might not feel the same governmental pressures to report them.

Not only did the *Onestà* order the staff of the *Spedale* to report suspected victims of the *mal francese* and suspected victims of sodomy, but on at least one occasion they sent magistrates from the court directly into the *Spedale degli Incurabili*. The *gattaiuola* was also a frequent visitor, hoping to glean evidence. In 1641 the authorities became aware that a larger number of patients than usual, mostly male but also some female, were turning to the *Incurabili* for treatment of the *mal francese*. The *Onestà* elected for that year was particularly zealous and requested permission from the government to take more active measures.[45] With such permission in hand, the *Onestà*, together with the *podestà*, sent a number of deputies to the *Incurabili* to question patients under oath. The deputies had instructions to ask patients

---

43 ASL, *Offizio sopra l'Onestà* 1, fol. 46^{r} (30 October 1568).

44 ASL, *Offizio sopra l'Onestà* 4, fol. 63^{r} (7 July 1597).

45 ASL, *Offizio sopra l'Onestà* 5, fol. 597 (9 May 1641).

how, where, and from whom they had contracted the *mal francese*, and whether they could have infected anyone else. This investigation proved fruitful, as it produced a number of leads that the court followed up in subsequent months, eventually resulting in several prosecutions for sodomy. Lorenzo di Nicolai Castagnoni, for one, testified he had caught the *mal francese* through sexual relations with Jacopino Fiorentino (Florentine), who was married and had two young children.[46] Further investigation implicated another man, Ruggiero, and two prostitutes.[47] In another case, fourteen year-old Francesco claimed to have caught the disease from another boy in his workshop, and yet another youth described as 'giovanetto disonesto' (dishonest youngster) implicated three others.[48] Such action by the *Onestà* shows that the magistrates clearly linked syphilis to sodomy. The investigation also revealed to the authorities an alarming level of promiscuous sodomy involving both men and women. Evidence that so many patients afflicted with the *mal francese* had multiple partners exacerbated the alarm over networks of sodomites. Despite the fact that these were patients at the *Incurabili*, there is no evidence that it was the doctors working in the hospital who leaked information about their patients on this occasion. It is more likely that the *gattaiuola* was the source, as he had been the informant on several other occasions.

In dealing with sodomy trials in which rape had occurred, the *Onestà* recognized that infection with *mal francese* compounded the crime. The court viewed with particular seriousness the trials that involved the rape of children. In response to this concern, a document from 1592 proclaimed that sodomy with brutality resulting in serious injury and/or infection with *mal francese* was to be punished more harshly.[49] In 1614, the grandmother of a twelve-year-old boy denounced Giovannino Locci for sodomizing her grandson Filippo so brutally that he had severely damaged the boy's 'back part.'[50] When the surgeon examined Filippo on behalf of the court, he found that the boy had not only suffered severe tearing of the anal area but that he had also been infected with the *mal francese* as a result of the rape. The boy's description of his attacker included the fact that he had no nose, which may well indicate either that the accused Giovannino was in the advanced stages of syphilis or that he had been mutilated as punishment for some previous offence.[51]

---

[46]ASL, *Offizio sopra l'Onestà* 5, fols. 597–600 (9 May 1641).
[47]ASL, *Offizio sopra l'Onestà* 5, fol. 604 (9 May 1641).
[48]ASL, *Offizio sopra l'Onestà* 5, fol. 606 (31 May 1641).
[49]ASL, *Offizio sopra l'Onestà* 4, unpag. (1592).
[50]ASL, *Offizio sopra l'Onestà* 5, fol. 4^r (24 January 1614).
[51]ASL, *Offizio sopra l'Onestà* 5, fol. 4^r (24 January 1614).

In another case, from 1625, a widow brought a complaint against one Antonio Sosti, a carpenter who had accepted her son Ventura as an apprentice.[52] Ventura's mother, a widow, had been grateful for the opportunity this apprenticeship afforded her son, but within 15 days the boy had run back home to his mother, refusing to go back to work and lamenting that 'Antonio was not a good master.'[53] Shortly after, Ventura became very sick and needed medical attention on three separate occasions. Medical examination revealed that Ventura had been beaten, sodomized and infected with the *mal francese*. Suspicion fell on Antonio, who, tipped off when an angry neighbour confronted him, managed to elude the guards and escape from Lucca.[54] Although the *Onestà* condemned Antonio to death *in absentia*, this was of no help to Ventura's mother, who now despaired that she would not be able to pay for her son's treatment.[55] Normally in such cases the magistrates would inflict a heavy fine on the guilty party, part of which would go to the victim of the rape; in this case, however, Antonio's escape had precluded such financial aid. In 1641 Maria di Cesare di Paolino, who had been infected with the *mal francese* by her rapist was slightly luckier; the court ordered her attacker to pay fifty scudi to the family for this 'malissimo di sanità.'[56]

Although there were some cases of rape or seduction of apprentices by masters, it was far more common for older apprentices to abuse the younger boys. Many such cases indicate a desire for sexual experimentation on the part of the perpetrator.[57] This meant that the abuse might continue for an extended period of time. In his research on Florentine sodomy, Michael Rocke discovered that often the younger partner was afraid or reluctant to denounce his attacker because of shame, fear of reprisals, or fear of losing his job.[58] Frequently, it was the revelation that the child had been infected with *mal francese* that actually brought the case to light and led the civic authorities to prosecute for sodomy.

Because families lived in such close quarters, it was difficult to hide the evidence of injuries or infection. In 1606, the concerned father of Lorenzino went to the *Onestà* because his fourteen-year-old son had contracted the

---

52ASL, *Offizio sopra l'Onestà* 5, fol. 235 (1 June 1625).

53ASL, *Offizio sopra l'Onestà* 5, fol. 237 (1 June 1625).

54This was an all too common occurrence. It was easy for fugitives to slip over the border.

55ASL, *Offizio sopra l'Onestà* 5, fol. 239 (21 June 1625).

56ASL, *Magistrato de' Segretari* 10, fol. 75v (22 February 1646).

57Evidence also suggests that older boys sodomized younger ones as part of a bullying process.

58Rocke, *Forbidden Friendships*, p. 163.

mal francese and he feared the boy had been molested.[59] In fact, further investigation into the case revealed a still more unpleasant truth for Lorenzino's father: the boy had been working as a male prostitute. He had caught the disease from a man at an inn in Pisa and then proceeded to infect all his clients. An older boy named Momo was found to be Lorenzino's pimp, introducing him to his clients, arranging payments, and taking a cut of the profits. The two boys were actually engaged in a thriving business partnership![60]

Judging by the number of sodomy cases in which the parties were infected with the *mal francese*, this was a serious problem. In a case from 1638, two teenage boys appeared before the *Onestà* charged with sodomizing each other as well as a number of other boys.[61] The fact that the youths were seriously infected with the *mal francese* made the magistrates more eager to pursue the lead from a secret denunciation and track down all the contacts. Once again, the *Onestà* relied on medical testimony. The magistrates called Vincenzo Burlingari, a surgeon from the *Incurabili*, who confirmed that Francesco Botti, one of the boys, had blisters and a ring of sores in the 'back part.' In his opinion, the boy had 'every sign of the said sickness,' which seemed to the doctor to have originated in the anal area. When the magistrates pressed the surgeon to say how he thought the boy had contracted the disease, he replied that although it could have been caught through sex with a woman, in general it was caught through being the passive partner in sodomy. The surgeon then went on to elaborate on the symptoms of the disease: 'Having caught the *mal francese*, it begins with bleeding, and then pulsating forth through the skin, the said pustules or ulcers appear.'[62]

Another doctor from the *Incurabili* reported that in treating Francesco Botti he had administered *aqua forte*, (nitric acid) one of the common treatments for the *mal francese*.[63] Finally, the *direttore* of the *Incurabili* testified that the boy had remained in treatment for only a week. The problem was that the boy had gone out at his most contagious stage and was now probably infecting others. Here again, medical testimony about the chain of syphilitic infection served to broaden the search for sodomites. As evidence from the doctors evolved, Francesco was linked to a spate of cases, including that of

---

59ASL, *Offizio sopra l'Onestà* 4, fols. 12r–24r (30 December 1605).

60ASL, *Offizio sopra l'Onestà* 4, fol. 24r (30 December 1605).

61ASL, *Offizio sopra l'Onestà* 5, fol. 508 (28 March 1638).

62ASL *Offizio sopra l'Onestà* 5, fol. 509 (28 March 1638).

63Other treatments used in Lucca included a mercury-based ointment and guaiacum, also known as *legno santo* or holy wood.

Francesco Orsetti, his co-accused, whom the doctors had also treated for *mal francese*. The round up of all those treated for the disease as a result of Francesco's 'work' included a priest, a tailor, and a silk-worker, who, incidentally, was Francesco Orsetti's brother-in-law.[64]

Considering the number of cases involving infected men raping children leads to speculation that there may also be a close link between the high instance of pedophilia and the spread of the *mal francese*. Among the many myths associated with syphilis was one that intercourse with a virgin of either sex could cure the disease.[65] At the very least, the anxieties about catching the disease meant a partner who was young and more sexually innocent would be considered a safer option. Obviously this had some serious repercussions for the child. Both Francesco Orsetti and Francesco Botti had caught the disease while in prison from their jailer, who initiated them both into the practice of sodomy.[66]

The proactive measures of the magistrates reflected a double fear: that of the spread of moral as well as physical corruption. The xenophobia of the Lucchese, snug within their walls, also meant that they had an increasingly suspicious attitude towards non-Lucchese, known locally as *forestieri*, living, working or visiting in Lucca. It is telling that many of the persons accused were from other Italian cities such as Florence, Pisa, or Siena. There is evidence to suggest that Lucca feared moral contamination from outside, especially from Florence, a traditional enemy.[67] In one of the interviews conducted at the *Incurabili*, one of the patients, a prostitute nicknamed *La Pistoia*, told magistrates that she had caught the disease in Florence, where men liked 'to do as they pleased' with prostitutes, including sodomy. She told the magistrates that Maria, her companion, had undergone the same abuse.[68] When magistrates discovered a community of monks practicing sodomy they blamed a Sienese monk of bringing in moral corruption from Siena.[69] Just as Italy as a whole saw itself to have been infected by the invading French in 1494, so too Lucca perceived itself as under threat of sexual and moral siege from neighbouring cities. Lucca

---

64ASL, *Offizio sopra l'Onestà* 5, fol. 509 (28 March 1638).

65For more on the notion of virgins having the power to cure syphilis, see Schleiner, 'Infection and Cure through Women,' pp. 506–517.

66ASL, *Offizio sopra l'Onestà* 5, fol. 508 (28 March 1638).

67For other examples of works that discuss how syphilis was linked to the 'other,' see Foa, 'The New and the Old,' and Quétel, *History of Syphilis*, pp. 9–49. For discussion on the literature of sodomy and the 'other' see Puff, *Sodomy in Reformation Germany and Switzerland*, pp. 124–166.

68ASL, *Offizio sopra l'Onestà* 5, fol. 604 (9 May 1641).

69ASL, *Magistrato de' Segretari* 9, fol. 45^r (18 September 1637).

thus provides yet more evidence of the powerful connection between the pox and xenophobia explored in several other articles in this volume.

Yet Lucca's attitude towards foreigners was somewhat ambivalent, because it went hand in hand with the policy of recruiting foreign prostitutes to combat sodomy among Lucchese males. In 1534, prostitutes were given the freedom of the city, and a special ruling was set in place to protect them.[70] This included the creation of the *Protettori delle meretrici*; an appeal court where prostitutes could bring complaints against clients who harassed or abused them. Interestingly, there seems to have been no particular suspicion that registered prostitutes were directly blamed for the spread of *mal francese*.[71] Thus the connection between prostitution and the pox was not as simple or immediate as perhaps first thought. It is possible that the open acceptance of prostitutes going about their trade legitimately allowed them the freedom to seek medical attention without fear of reprisal: provided, that is, that they had not contracted the disease through anal sex.

This did not mean, however, that prostitutes were free from accusations in the *Onestà*. Sometimes prostitutes were prosecuted for offering erotic sodomy, or at least complying with clients' demand for anal sex and thereby spreading the *mal francese*. Prostitutes bringing accusations against clients who had forced them to perform sodomy frequently found themselves counter-accused of having complied. This often complicated cases for the judges. When the court found out that these women were also repeat offenders, they were unceremoniously banished from Lucca, but only after they had revealed the names of their sodomite clients.

Just like doctors, prostitutes might be privy to valuable information, which the *Onestà* made a point of pursuing. One such woman is particularly worthy of mention. Margarita Bismantova figures in two sodomy trials a few years apart. In the first trial, which occurred when she was only twelve, she was the plaintiff. The *gattaiuola* found Margarita in the *Incurabili* and urged her to bring a complaint. She accused Agostino, a young artisan, of abduction, both vaginal and anal rape, and infecting her with the *mal francese*.[72] The case was dismissed after Margarita admitted that there had been other men. The magistrates ordered that she be flogged for mischief

---

[70]Further legislation in 1543 and 1640 reinforced the rights and privileges granted to prostitutes. *Decreti penali*, p. 265 (24 April 1543); p. 266 (27 July 1543); p. 267 (9 August 1640).

[71]The subject of the Lucchese policy on prostitution and sodomy is covered in Hewlett, 'Women, Sodomy, and Sexual Abuse in Late-Renaissance Lucca,' pp. 125–186.

[72]ASL, *Offizio sopra l'Onestà* 3, unpag. (20 June 1589).

making and sent her back to the *Incurabili* for further treatment for the *mal francese*.[73] Her uncle, who gave evidence in this trial, told the court that Margarita's whole family, including her younger siblings with whom she shared a bed, and her grandmother 'were riddled' with the disease. Margarita later told the court that her father had put her into prostitution after she had lost her virginity to one of his acquaintances. He had since deserted the family.[74] Margarita was flogged and treated for the *mal francese*; Agostino was released.

Three years later there was second trial involving Margarita, this time as a defendant. She was denounced by one of the *sbirri* or police who overheard her boasting in a tavern that she offered erotic sodomy.[75] By this time her mother was dead and Margarita was an established prostitute. On this occasion the case developed into a much longer and more complicated trial, as Margarita attempted to implicate several clients including the policeman who had denounced her. Once again, she claimed that she was the victim of anal rape, testifying that she had contracted for vaginal sex but the men had sodomized her by force against her wishes. So convincing was her testimony, that the magistrates ordered that the men involved be subjected to torture. Interrogated individually, each of the accused men protested his innocence, despite the duress of the rope-hoist. Unsure as to who was telling the truth, the court then decided to torture Margarita, as was the normal practice in such cases where the reliability of the witness was in dispute. Faced with the *zuffoli* (sharpened reeds forced under the fingernails), Margarita swiftly admitted lying about one of the clients but not the other two. This meant these two men went back to the torture chamber, but once again they refused to confess. Finally, Margarita underwent a brief session with the *zuffoli* before reluctantly admitting that she had accused all three men out of spite. With some bravado, she told the court she had targeted one so-called client because he had rejected her and refused to pay when he found she had the *mal francese*. She counter-accused the policeman because he had denounced her. The court ordered that she be banished in perpetuity.[76]

73ASL, *Offizio sopra l'Onestà* 3, unpag. (20 June 1589).

74ASL, *Offizio sopra l'Onestà* 3, fols. 36^{v}–51^{r} (21 November 1592).

75ASL, *Offizio sopra l'Onestà* 3, fol. 36^{v} (1 November 1592).

76ASL, *Offizio sopra l'Onestà* 3, fol. 51^{r} (21 November 1592).

CONCLUSION

The cases discussed here demonstrate that there was some confusion in Lucca about both syphilis and sodomy. The indication is that the prevalence of the *mal francese* tended to make it a convenient 'catch-all' disease; but at the same time, not all those who were suspected of having *mal francese* actually had the disease, and not all doctors were 'yes' men who gave the magistrates the answers they were looking for.

The evidence also reveals the strong links that the oligarchic government of Lucca assumed between the *mal francese* and the practice of sodomy. The government recruited court agents, medical personnel, and prostitutes in an attempt to stop the spread of both sodomy and syphilis. In the eyes of the authorities, sodomy was the greater evil of the two, because it was seen as directly responsible for the spread of the *mal francese* and more. It is most telling that Lucca established the *Onestà* to combat sodomy in 1448, almost fifty years before the outbreak of the *mal francese* – that is because the authorities already saw perpetrators of sodomy as bearers of moral corruption long before syphilis arrived on the scene. In a sense, however, the city authorities can also be seen as exploiting the physical disease as a way to control the moral plague of sodomy, by meting out harsher punishments in cases where syphilis was diagnosed, and by using evidence of infection and medical treatment as an opportunity to investigate and prosecute morality. Syphilitic sodomites were doubly diseased and doubly guilty, thus subject to the full force of the law. Furthermore, the magistrates pressured doctors to make the connection between the two undesirables, thereby helping them to snare a larger number of alleged miscreants in the *Onestà*'s net. The city provided government offices that controlled the spread of infection and supported the confraternities that treated patients suffering from the disease. In this context, in the renewed spirit of Counter-Reformation charity, the *mal francese* provided pious citizens – who were often the same citizens who acted as magistrates – with an opportunity to perform good works. Nevertheless, fear of the disease and increasing suspicion of outsiders, beginning in the second half of the sixteenth century, meant that those practicing sodomy, especially when they were foreigners, were convenient scapegoats for the city's woes.

University of Windsor
Windsor, Ontario

CITED WORKS

Manuscript sources

Lucca. Archivio di Stato di Lucca (ASL)
 Compagnia e Spedale dello Spirito Santo detto degli Incurabili
 Offizio sopra L'Onestà
 Magistrato de' Segretari
 Protettori delle Meretrici
 Raccolte Speciali
 Serie statuti del comune di Lucca 1308–1549

Printed Sources

Adorni-Braccesi, Simonetta. *'Una città infetta': la Repubblica di Lucca nella crisi del Cinquecento*. Firenze: Leo S. Olschki, 1994.

Arrizabalaga, Jon, John Henderson, and Roger French. *The Great Pox: The French Disease in Renaissance Europe*. New Haven: Yale University Press, 1997.

Berengo, Marino. *Nobili e mercanti nella Lucca del Cinquecento*. Torino: Giulio Einaudi, 1965.

Bertini, Elio. *Le grandi famiglie dei mercanti lucchesi*. Lucca: Maria Pacini Fazzi, 1976.

Boes, Maria R. 'On Trial for Sodomy in Early Modern Germany' pp. 27–45 in *Sodomy in Early Modern Europe*, ed. Tom Betteridge. Manchester: Manchester University Press, 2002.

Bongi, Salvatore. *Bandi lucchesi del secolo decimoquarto*. Bologna: Tipografia del Progresso, 1863.

Bratchel, M. E. *Lucca 1430–1494: The Reconstruction of a City-State*. Oxford: Oxford University Press, 1994.

Carmichael, A. G. *Plague and the Poor in Renaissance Florence*. Cambridge: Cambridge University Press, 1986.

Cipolla, Carlo. *Public Health and the Medical Profession in the Renaissance*. Cambridge: Cambridge University Press, 1976.

Davidson, Nicholas. 'Sodomy in Early Modern Venice' pp. 65–81 in *Sodomy in Early Modern Europe*, ed. Tom Betteridge. Manchester: Manchester University Press 2002.

Decreti penali fatti in diversi tempi dall' Illustrissimo e Eccellentissimo Consiglio del'Eccellentissima Repubblica di Lucca. Lucca: Baldassar del Giudice, 1640.

Foa, Anna. 'The New and the Old: The Spread of Syphilis (1494–1530)' pp. 26–45 in *Sex and Gender in Historical Perspective,* eds. Edward Muir and Guido Ruggiero. Baltimore: The Johns Hopkins University Press, 1990.

Hewlett, Mary. 'A Republic in Jeopardy: Cosimo I de' Medici and the Republic of Lucca' pp. 9–22 in *The Cultural Politics of Cosimo I de' Medici,* ed. Konrad Eisenbichler. Aldershot: Ashgate, 2001.

Hewlett, Mary. 'Women, Sodomy and Sexual Abuse in Late-Renaissance Lucca.' Ph. D. Diss. University of Toronto, 2000.

Lindemann, Mary. *Medicine and Society in Early Modern Europe*. Cambridge: Cambridge University Press, 1999.

Meek, Christine. *Lucca 1369–1400: Politics and Society in an Early Renaissance City-State*. Oxford: Oxford University Press, 1978.

Naphy, William. 'Sodomy in Early Modern Geneva: Various Definitions, Various Verdicts' pp. 94–110 in *Sodomy in Early Modern Europe,* ed. Tom Betteridge. Manchester: Manchester University Press, 2002.

Puff, Helmut. *Sodomy in Reformation Germany and Switzerland 1400–1600.* Chicago: University of Chicago Press, 2003.

Quétel, Claude. *History of Syphilis,* trans. Judith Braddock and Brian Pike. Baltimore: The Johns Hopkins University Press, 1990.

Rocke, Michael. *Forbidden Friendships: Homosexuality and Male Culture in Renaissance Florence.* Oxford: Oxford University Press, 1996.

Ruggiero, Guido. *The Boundaries of Eros: Sex, Crime and Sexuality in Renaissance Venice.* Oxford: Oxford University Press, 1985.

Schleiner, Winfried. 'Infection and Cure through Women: Renaissance Construction of Syphilis' *Journal of Medieval and Renaissance Studies,* 24:3 (1994): 499–517.

Seghieri, Mario. '1554: un anno difficile per Lucca, convolto nel conflitto tra il Duca Cosimo e i Franco-Senese di Pietro Strozzi' *Rivista di Archeologia, Storia, Costume. Sezione Lucchese,* 15:4 (1986): 3–12.

Siena, Kevin. ' The Foul Disease and Privacy: The Effects of Venereal Disease and Patient Demand on the Medical Marketplace in Early Modern London' *Bulletin of the History of Medicine,* 75:2 (2000): 199–224.

Siraisi, Nancy G. *Medieval and Early Renaissance Medicine: An Introduction to Knowledge and Practice.* Chicago: University of Chicago Press, 1990.

The Clean and the Foul: Paupers and the Pox in London Hospitals, c.1550–c.1700

Kevin Siena

Hospitals faced something of a moral dilemma when confronted with the pox, or as it was frequently termed in early modern England, the 'Foul Disease.'[1] To heal or not to heal was the fundamental question, and it was not easily resolved. Well into the eighteenth century benefactors of English hospitals could still be found debating whether the 'foul' counted as worthy objects of their charity.[2] For those who saw the disease as a just punishment from God – and there were many – the question of medical intervention was barbed. There was a fair bit of logic to the argument that treating the poxed meant intervening with God's handiwork. For Calvinists especially, this posed a problem. If human agency could not cleanse the sins of the soul, perhaps it should not attempt to wipe away the sins of the flesh either. William Clowes, Elizabethan surgeon to St. Bartholomew's Hospital and devout Calvinist, called the pox a product of 'filthy sinne,' and 'a notable testamonie of the just wrath of God.' A full century later English doctors still called the pox 'the just punishment of God upon our sins,' or the Lord's 'reward of the Sin of Fornication.'[3] We know that English doctors displayed particular reluctance to interfere when it came to providing information on prophylaxis, something Italian doctors discussed more freely, for fear that they would contribute to debauchery, helping sinners to continue their immoral ways while avoiding the just punishment represented by *lues venerea*.[4]

---

[1]Particular elements of this argument appear in expanded forms in chaps. 1 and 2 of my *Venereal Disease, Hospitals and the Urban Poor.*

[2]The debate at the Westminster Infirmary can stand as representative. A group of trustees lobbied successfully to convince the board that 'persons infected with the Venereal Disease do generally bring it upon themselves by their own lewd and vicious Habits' and were therefore 'no means proper Objects of this Charity.' *Some Reasons of a Member of the Committee... against the Admission of Venereal Patients,* pp. 1–3.

[3]Clowes, *Brief and Necessary Treatise*, p. 150. See also Shirley, *A Short Compendium of Chirurgery*, p. 114 and Blanckaert, *A New Method of Curing the French-Pox,* pp. 117–120.

[4]Schleiner, 'Moral Attitudes toward Syphilis,' pp. 390–397, 404–410; Quétel, *History of Syphilis*, p. 59

Yet English doctors did treat the pox. Clowes justified his medical intervention as a form of Christian love for his fellow man, stressing that no one should mistake that he ever meant 'to incourage...people to wallow or continue in their beastly life.'[5] In spite of providential interpretations of this disease two factors determined that pox sufferers would always find doctors willing to treat them in Tudor-Stuart London. First, there continued an underlying notion of Christian compassion to help those in need, which was never quashed by any strand of reformation thought. Regardless of their moral slip, the poxed were often suffering horribly and few doctors who came face to face with that suffering turned their backs on them. Secondly, there was significant money to be made treating this epidemic.[6] If laws of supply and demand counted for anything, the sheer demand for their services determined a continuous supply of willing doctors. Indeed, as David Gentilcore's contribution to this volume shows for Italy, the market response to the pox was significant. Similarly, London patients with money to spend had little trouble finding a doctor.[7] However, when it came to the poor, things were a bit more complex.

Attitudes towards the poor hardened as the sixteenth century wore on,[8] and the pox played its own role in this development. As Arrizabalaga, Henderson and French have shown, authorities forged connections between the pox and the disorderly urban poverty that they witnessed in the streets. These historians argue convincingly that these connections contributed significantly towards the increasing intolerance shown towards the poor in the sixteenth and seventeenth centuries.[9] Clowes certainly made it clear that he saw the poor as the main source of London's pandemic. Evaluating the city's outbreak he exclaimed

> The causes whereof, I see none so great, as the licentiousness and beastly disorder of a great number of rogues and vagabonds, the filthy life of many lewde and idle persons, men and women, about the citie of London...[10]

What to do about them?

---

[5]Clowes, *Brief and Necessary Treatise*, p. 150.

[6]On the application of a market model to explore medicine in this period see Cook, *Decline of the Old Medical Regime*, pp. 28–69. On the London trade in venereal disease see Bynum, 'Treating the Wages of Sin'; Porter, *Health for Sale*, p. 148–155;Quétel, p. 86–93.

[7]Siena, 'The "Foul Disease" and Privacy,' pp. 199–206. Stone, *Family, Sex and Marriage*, pp. 487, 600.

[8]Jütte, *Poverty and Deviance*, pp. 158–177.

[9]Arrizabalaga, Henderson and French, *The Great Pox*, p. 282.

[10]Clowes, *Brief and Necessary Treatise*, p. 149.

Some have suggested that venereal patients' condition rendered poor sufferers beyond the reach of charity's mercy and that hospitals refused them on moral grounds. As one scholar recently put it, the pox 'was a moral problem so severe that it barred even charity itself.'[11] We now know that this view cannot hold up for Italy, Germany or Spain where studies have revealed pox hospitals treating the poor in the sixteenth century.[12] It is also untrue for England where, despite some suggestions that hospital care for the pox must await the Enlightenment,[13] both of London's main medical hospitals, St. Bartholomew's and St. Thomas's, treated poxed paupers from at least the 1550s.[14]

The late-Stuart surgeon Charles Peter poignantly asked, what should society do when confronted by 'those poor unhappy wretches where the Pox and Poverty are complicated ?'[15] It was a difficult question. However, it is clear that one answer – shunning them altogether – was not an option; or at least, it was not the option that those in charge of London's royal hospitals chose in the sixteenth and seventeenth centuries.

CLEAN WARDS, FOUL WARDS

The two hospitals took slightly different approaches when responding to the foul disease. Just like continental hospitals, St. Bartholomew's and St. Thomas's were intent on segregating venereal patients from their general patient populations. However, St. Thomas's and St. Bart's segregated differently. St. Thomas's built isolated venereal wards on the main hospital grounds. In its 'sweate wards' poor men like apprentice Randell Bryton or

---

[11]Allen *The Wages of Sin*, pp. 42–42 and 57–58.

[12]On Germany see Jütte, 'Syphilis and Confinement,'; Risse, *Mending Bodies, Saving Souls*, p. 215. On Italy see Arrizabalaga, Henderson and French, *The Great Pox*, pp. 145–233. On Spain see Terrada, 'El tratamiento de la sífilis en un hospital renacentista.'

[13]Williams, *The London Lock*, pp. 8–10; Bynum, 'Treating the Wages if Sin,' p. 7; Adler, 'History of the Development of a Service for the Venereal Diseases,' pp. 124–128.

[14]It is possible that this was the case from earlier in the century as well. One piece of evidence pointing in this direction is Robert Copland's c.1530 poem, *The Highway to the Spitalhouse*, in which the narrator, a hospital porter, includes the poxed among the patients accepted in the hospital: 'That for their living can do no labour/ And have no friends to do them succour, / As old people sick and impotent, / Poor women in childbed have here easement, / Weak men sore wounded by great violence / And sore men eaten with pox and pestilence, / And honest folk fallen in great poverty / By mischance or other infirmity; / Wayfaring men and maimed soldiers / Have their relief in this poor house of ours....'. Cit. in Orme and Webster, *The English Hospitals*, pp. 151–155. See also Fabricius, *Syphilis in Shakespeare's England*, pp. 60–61.

[15]Peter, *Observations on the Venereal Disease*, pp. 35–37.

women like Eme Danyell both described in the 1550s as 'diseased with the poxe' underwent their mercury treatment.[16] St. Thomas's governors underscored the importance of their quarantine when they stipulated that 'no patient of the fowle Disease be admitted into this house till there shall be room in the fowle wards.'[17] Records show that they enforced the segregation vigilantly. There was a quite real incarceration at work, enforced mainly by threats to expel patients who broke quarantine.

> That if hereafter any happen to be admitted into this house that have the Foul Disease they shall not goe out of their ward nor come into the house to fetch any thing nor within the chappell nor sitt upon the seats in the court yards upon pain of expulsion.[18]

Such threats begin to demonstrate the flip-side to the charitable hand. Hospitals offered mercy, but they could just as quickly rescind it for those who disobeyed.

St. Bartholomew's took a different approach. That hospital transformed former leper hospitals into 'outhouses' for the poxed poor. In a word, they treated their foul patients off-site. Margaret Pelling has noted the continued use of lazarettos to segregate particular classes of patients elsewhere in sixteenth-century England.[19] Bart's outhouses bring English practice somewhat more in line with continental examples of the *Blatternhaus* in Germany and the *Incurabili* hospitals in Italy, where the poxed were similarly segregated in institutions apart from the general hospitals. The use of institutions once meant for lepers indicates yet another way in which the pox is indebted to the cultural memory of leprosy, and one more instance in which we see Europeans scrambling to retrofit essentially medieval ideas, or in this case institutions, as they responded to the new disease.

Bart's lazarettos absorbed their new clientele rather easily. This may have been the case because the pox bore the stamp of its medieval ancestor in so many ways. As Foa and Harris have suggested, early representations of the pox drew heavily on the iconographic and discursive presentations of leprosy, the medieval venereal disease *par excellence*.[20] Indeed, many who

---

[16]LMA, HT/ST/A4/1, fol.7; Parsons, *History of St. Thomas's Hospital*, 1:191–192; SBH, HA 1/1, fols. 23–29.

[17]LMA, H1/ST/A4/5, fol. 44

[18]LMA, H1/ST/A4/6, fols. 73–75.

[19]Pelling, *The Common Lot*, pp. 90–100.

[20]Foa, 'The New and the Old,' pp. 37–42; See also Harris, '(Po)X Marks the Spot,' above pp. 121–122. On links between leprosy and sexuality see especially Williams,

argued against the newness of the disease to Europe claimed that the pox was merely a medieval wolf in renaissance sheep's clothing; the pox was not a new disease, but just a new name for an old one, leprosy. This was a minority view, but others formed imaginative links between the two ailments, claiming that leprosy had evolved into the new scourge. The pox was not leprosy itself, but its deadly offspring.[21] Such connections meant that situating the poxed in lazarettos demanded no great stretch of the imagination.

In the sixteenth century Bart's had six lazarettos at its disposal, the Lock south of the river in Southwark, the Highgate and the Kingsland (near Hackney) both to the north, the Hammersmith and the Knightsbridge each to the west, and the Mile End in the east.[22] The City of London transferred them to the hospital in 1549.[23] The need for space to care for poxed patients may have driven municipal officials to give Bart's these houses because financial evidence from the previous year demonstrates a significant number of poxed patients in the hospital.[24] One advantage of sending the foul to former lazarettos was that it ensured not just a segregation of the hospital grounds but a wider municipal quarantine as well. As the list above indicates Bart's lazarettos were situated on the outskirts of town, isolating pox sufferers well away from the city centre, quite like the Venetian institutions explored by McGough above.

By the early seventeenth century Bart's consolidated its operations, closing all but two of the outhouses; all poxed men were now shipped to the Lock Hospital in Southwark and all poxed women went north to the Kingsland. The presence of these institutions may well have enhanced the already dubious reputations of particular neighbourhoods. For example, the presence of both the Lock outhouse and St. Thomas's Hospital in

---

'Venereal Associations of Leprosy,' as well as Brody, *Disease of the Soul*, pp. 12–13; and Ell, 'Blood and Sexuality in Medieval Leprosy,' p. 158.

[21]Quétel, *History of Syphilis*, p. 33; Brody, *Disease of the Soul*, pp. 56–57. In 1596 surgeon Peter Lowe suggested that if untreated the pox would 'degenerate into leprosie.' *Easie, Certaine, and Perfect Method*. chap. 4. Plater, Cole, and Culpeper put both diseases in the same category, the principle diseases 'of Defoedation or Defilement.' 'Of these there are two kinds principally, the one is old, called *Lues Elephantica* or Leprosie, the other new called *Lues Venerea* or French Pox.' *Golden Practice of Physick*, pp. 580–598.

[22]Honeybourne, 'Leper Hospitals of the London Area,' p. 6; Orme and Webster, *The English Hospitals*, pp. 41–48.

[23]Honeybourne, 'Leper Hospitals of the London Area,' p. 9.

[24]Margaret Pelling, was the first to comment on the significant number of venereal patients recorded 'cured' by Bart's surgeons in the fiscal year 1547/8, 'Appearance and Reality: Barber-Surgeons, the Body and Disease,' p. 97.

Southwark meant that the majority of London's foul paupers were now shipped south of the river, where the presence of such institutions as the medieval stews and theatres already gave that neighbourhood a dubious reputation.[25] It may well be that Londoners were more comfortable sending the foul to a part of the city already renowned as a centre of vice. In other words a kind of moral and sexual geography can be discerned in Elizabethan and early Stuart London and this may well have influenced decisions on where to situate these hospitals.

Considering that the disease was so morally stained we still face the question of why London institutions decided to turn hospital resources to treating the impoverished foul. Numbers may tell the story.[26] After Bart's consolidated its operations in the Lock and Kingsland in 1622, its ledgers begin listing the monies paid each month to feed patients in the two outhouses. The hospital reimbursed the outhouse surgeons on a per capita basis: four pence per patient per day. This expenditure immediately reveals that poverty and the pox represented a major social problem in early Stuart London. Hospital ledgers also list the diet expenditure for patients in the main hospital (also four pence per patient per day) making it possible to relate the population in the outhouses to the total hospital population. In 1622, the first year for which figures are available, almost one out of every four of Bart's patients (23.1%) entered its venereal wards. Unfortunately, Bart's did not list the expenditure at the (male) Lock and (female) Kingsland separately, so a gender breakdown is not possible – though the available evidence suggests that they tended to treat more men than women.[27] Moreover, a precise calculation of the number of patients is similarly obscured. The numbers give us a relative sense of the scope of these operations rather than an exact calculation. The figures represent the number of beds that were kept full throughout the year, not the number of *different* patients who filled those beds. The hospital would have had the same expenditure were the outhouses filled with the same forty patients

[25]Browner, 'Wrong Side of the River,' pp. 34–71; Fabricius, *Syphilis in Shakespeare's England*, pp. 60–62, 126; Daly, 'Hospitals of London,' pp. 244–250.

[26]The figures in this discussion are based upon analysis of St. Bartholomew's Hospital's Annual Ledgers, 1622–1696. SBH, HB 1/4–1/10. More extensive analysis of the data including graphs can be found in Siena, *Venereal Disease, Hospitals and the Urban Poor*, pp. 69–73.

[27]In 1655 administrative records state that 'the [male] Lock hath recepcon for a third part more than Kingsland,' and in 1690 the board recorded that while the Kingsland had a capacity of twenty patients, the Lock could receive thirty. SBH, HA 1/5, fol. 137; HA 1/8, f. 19.

all year long as if a new group of forty patients replaced the old ones each month or each week.

Regardless, the figures demonstrate beyond a doubt that treating the pox represented one of the primary services that St. Bartholomew's Hospital provided to early modern London, devoting nearly a quarter of its resources to a single disease. 1622 was not an anomaly. The figures from the first decade show that on average foul patients represented 20.7% of the hospital's clientele. Indeed in certain years, as in 1643, they represented almost 30%.[28] Similar data does not survive for St. Thomas's, but its records suggest that Bart's was not alone. An evaluation of the ward space, based on the number of beds in each ward, shows that by the mid seventeenth century St. Thomas's similarly devoted almost one out of every five beds (18.7%) to the venereal wards.[29]

Far from refusing poxed patients, London's Royal Hospitals made treating them one of their most important duties. These figures begin to point towards a sense of civic obligation radiating from these hospitals. Unlike the later voluntary hospitals established by private initiative, which were much more discerning about whom they designated worthy objects of charity – and which indeed frequently excluded venereal patients altogether[30] – Bart's and St. Thomas's had something of a more public obligation. Both had been medieval hospitals that the Tudor state appropriated in the dissolution of the monasteries. The crown granted them to the city to care for its sick poor and endowed each institution with significant property, the rental income of which provided their main operating budgets.[31] The crown endowed them with a civic mission to serve the poor and the resources to do so. While the city fathers and elite men who served as hospital governors undoubtedly had great latitude in how they chose to steer these institutions, it is not clear that they could have entirely refused venereal patients as historians have long suggested.

[28]SBH, 1/4–1/10.

[29]This figure emerges from an analysis of an admission register for St. Thomas's covering 1679–1683, which indicates the number of beds in each ward. LMA, H1/ST/B2/1.

[30]Consider the Westminster Infirmary, above, note 2. Other such hospitals included St. George's Hospital and The Middlesex Infirmary.

[31]Daly, 'Hospitals of London,' pp. 187–188; Parsons, *History of St. Thomas's* vol. 1:128–129, 207–226; Moore, *History of St. Bartholomew's,* pp. 149–165; Honeybourne, 'Leper Hospitals of the London Area,' p. 9; On St. Thomas's activities as a landlord see Boulton, *Neighbourhood and Society,* pp. 196–198 and 203–205. On the Reformation and English hospitals see Orme and Webster, *The English Hospital,* pp. 155–166 and Daly, 'The Hospitals of London,' chap. 3.

The figures from Bart's suggest to the contrary that the poxed poor represented a major segment of the needy sick in early modern London. Whatever moral indignation one might feel towards paupers who contracted this disease, the hospital figures point towards the presence of a widespread social problem that was simply too big to ignore.

Some historians have also suggested that in this period the pox was largely confined to the wealthy.[32] Hospital records deny this picture; in Tudor-Stuart London the pox was rampant among the urban poor. The issues attending retrospective diagnosis outlined in the Introduction prevent us from using the hospital data to suggest rates of infection for syphilis. The figures merely indicate the propensity of doctors (and patients) to render the diagnosis 'venereal.' Whatever the case, that propensity was great. What is important is that sixteenth- and seventeenth-century Londoners would have seen what they termed 'the pox' all around them. When a fifth to a quarter of a city's hospital population suffers from one disease, that city faces an epidemic. London's hospitals could hardly have ignored it.

Sex, Lies and Hospital Admission

What about these patients ? While we are forced to rely on institutional records, and thus access plebeian patients' experiences through the screen of documents created by their social betters, the records are nonetheless revealing.[33] For starters, we have strong evidence that class was no barrier to the impact of the pox on one's reputation.

It is clear that English patients of means went to considerable lengths to guard their reputations and avoid public scrutiny when they became infected. English medical treaties abounded with discussions of shame. Historians should read them both as descriptive of contemporary attitudes and simultaneously productive of those very attitudes. Private physicians and surgeons, as well as quacks and empirics, stood to gain from a clientele willing to pay for discreet treatment. Doctors certainly did their part to foster patients' anxiety by highlighting the odious and shameful nature of

---

[32]Randolph Trumbach has proposed that only after 1690 did the 'gentlemen's disease became the common disease of the London poor.' *Sex and the Gender Revolution*, pp. 196–199. Trumbach here builds on the picture first drawn by Edward Shorter, who similarly suggested that venereal disease 'remained at the margins of the population' before 1850, only slowly increasing among the general populace at the end of the eighteenth century. *Women's Bodies*, pp. 263–267.

[33]On the realities of patient life in these hospitals see Daly, 'Hospitals of London,' pp. 182–190, 200–203, 258–263, 275–282, and 289–296.

the disease in their treatises and advertisements.[34] As Roy Porter described, some London pox-doctors were indeed 'trading in fear.'[35] The need for greater comparative work on the history of sexually transmitted diseases is borne out by the relative lack of this response that David Gentilcore has charted in Italy. However, elite Englishmen clearly feared the ramifications of public exposure.

Consider Samuel Pepys. The diarist enjoyed poking fun at others who contracted the pox.[36] However, like the commentators described by both Domenico Zanrè and Darin Hayton elsewhere in this volume, his tone changed dramatically when the pox hit closer to home. When his brother Thomas lay on his deathbed in 1664, Pepys shuddered at the gossip then spreading that he might be dying of the pox. 'The shame of this very thing, I confess, troubles me as much as anything.'[37] Pepys expressed relief that his family would be saved from 'that reproach which was spread against him' when the surgeon declared that Thomas was free of the disease. Yet the doctor's words were not relief enough. Pepys insisted on inspecting his brother's genitals as he lay delirious and dying, insisting on verifying for himself that Thomas was 'as clear as ever he was born.' Even this was did not quiet him, for he threatened the doctor with revenge if he dared to breathe a word about Thomas's false pox.[38] It was this sort of anxiety that drove Londoners of means to seek out medical treatment as discreetly as possible.

So too did the poor. Their room for manoeuvre, however, was significantly limited. Those who could not take advantage of the discretion provided by private practitioners in the medical marketplace had to rely on hospitals like Bart's or St. Thomas's. Their care was a much more public affair. In order to access these medical resources, prospective patients had to line up at the hospital gates on Monday mornings to be inspected by the admissions committee, which consisted of governors, members of the medical staff, and other hospital personnel. The admissions procedure demanded that patients be evaluated on multiple levels. Were they truly needy ? Was their ailment one that the hospital could treat ? Were they too contagious to admit to the main wards ? And, importantly, were they 'clean' or were they 'foul' ? Those suffering the pox had to accept this

---

34Siena, 'The "Foul Disease" and Privacy,' pp. 206–214.

35Porter, *Health For Sale*, p. 151; Davenport-Hines, *Sex, Death and Punishment,* p. 49.

36Anselment, *Realms of Apollo*, pp. 143–144.

37Pepys, *Diary,* vol. 5:84. (14 March, 1664).

38Pepys, *Diary,* vol. 5:86. (15 March, 1664); Anselment, 'Seventeenth-Century Pox,' p. 202.

identification if they had any hope of getting a hospital bed. Evidence that humble patients resisted this labeling emerges from the most common strategy employed by venereal patients at both hospitals throughout the period. Patients dutifully assembled at the hospital gates on Monday mornings and lied.

Both hospitals' governing boards continuously bemoaned the practice. As they saw it, foul patients tried to fib their way into the clean wards. In 1642 St. Thomas's yet again emphasized the importance of the quarantine that separated clean from foul. On this occasion, however, they stressed their anxiety that foul patients conspired to conceal their ailment in order to avoid the stigma of the foul wards.

> It is ordered that any patient come to this house for cure of the Pox and there be then noe roome in the sweatwards, yf they shall thereupon feyne some other disease and after it be found to be the Pox, the said patients are then to be held incapable of cure within this house.[39]

The story was the same across the river at Bart's, where hospital administrators complained about the same nagging problem throughout the century. They, too, issued orders to cast out such patients upon discovery. For example, in June 1687 they passed the following resolution.

> Patients that have the French Pox to discover it: Ordered that all patients that have the French Pox and do not discover the same att their admittance into this hosp[ital] & obtaine admittance upon the p[re]tence of some other distemper shall be forthwith discharged and shall not be sent from this hospitall to either of the outhouses.[40]

Both sets of governors read these encounters the same way; patients were trying to enter the hospital under false pretences. Both hospitals vowed to punish such patients, not by removing them to the stigmatized foul wards, but by excluding them from care altogether. Again, the hand that offered mercy could just as quickly revoke it. As for the patients, it seems to have made little difference whether they stood to enter segregated wards within the hospital (at St. Thomas's) or former lazarettos off-site (at Bart's). Wherever they might be situated, entering a venereal ward meant accepting the identity 'foul' and all that came with it. The identical strategies by patients at both hospitals to refuse that identification begin to indicate that that concern about the stigma that haunted this disease was

---

[39]LMA, H1/ST/A4/5, fol.74; Parsons, *History of St. Thomas's,* vol. 2:42.
[40]SBH, HA 1/7, fol. 199.

not exclusive to the well-heeled. Elite Londoners like Samuel Pepys had no monopoly on reputation.[41]

However, scholars need to handle this evidence carefully. It must be read in at least two ways. On the one hand, it is entirely likely that in many instances the governors' assessment of the situation was correct. Patients who had already diagnosed themselves with the pox hoped to access hospital care without disclosing the nature of their ailment publicly. We have evidence of graft in the mid-seventeenth century indicating that some patients may have even resorted to bribes.[42] Perhaps once inside they might find a way to negotiate with the surgeon, plead with them if need be, to treat them discreetly. The problem of patients lying seems so common that we must assume that many prospective patients went to the hospital gates with a story rehearsed ready to explain away their symptoms as something other than the foul disease.

However, in other cases these negotiations likely involved different dynamics altogether. Scholars must assume that many patients whom the admitting surgeon identified as poxed legitimately contested the diagnosis because they simply disagreed. In a word, some patients were not lying but arguing. Here both the muddy nature of this diagnosis as well as the unique features of early modern diagnosis itself came into play. First, so wide ranging were the symptoms that fell under the blanket diagnosis 'foul,' which included not only genito-urinary symptoms but also a host of dermatological disorders and internal pains, that a vast variety of different ailments were probably diagnosed as the pox. Indeed, this is one of the main problems that scholars have found with attempts to diagnose the pox retroactively as syphilis or any other single condition.[43] Thus it must have been entirely common for patients who did not believe themselves to be poxed to argue at the hospital gates when the surgeon so labeled them. There was a great deal more at stake in this diagnosis than mere material or medical resources. More than a diagnosis, it was a personal labeling. It is hardly surprising that many patients contested it.

There would have been opportunity to do so thanks to the nature of medical diagnosis in this period. Before the age of the 'birth of the clinic'

[41]One study that has tried to read issues of reputation and privacy further down the social scale in late-Stuart England is Lawrence Klein, 'Politeness for Plebes.' Laura Gowing has also demonstrated that issues of sexual reputation were particularly crucial for poor women. 'Secret Births and Infanticide in Seventeenth-Century England,' p. 58.

[42]In 1662 the nurse in St. Thomas's men's venereal ward was fired for taking money from several patients to get them admitted, indicating that competition for beds was high and that such patients were vulnerable to usury. LMA H1/ST/A6/1, p. 59.

[43]Arrizabalaga, Henderson and French, *The Great Pox,* pp. 16–19.

at the end of the eighteenth century, when the medical exchange came increasingly to involve the physical exam, the early modern medical exchange relied much more heavily on discussion between doctor and patient.[44] The patient's 'history' – the narrative in a patient's own words describing the symptoms and circumstances of their ailment – was all-important. Medical historians have well established that in this period diagnosis was a much more active, participatory, and discursive process than it would later become. The prevailing medical culture was one in which patients and doctors agreed that patients had an active role to play in determining their own diagnosis.[45] So it would not have been out of place for patients to disagree with the initial conclusion that a surgeon offered.

Indeed, Clowes relates the tale of such an exchange from his private practice in which a man flatly denied that he could be poxed when the surgeon suggested it. However, in this case there were important issues of class and privacy at work. This private, fee-paying patient contested his diagnosis within the confines of a private consultation, possibly in his own home. Moreover the 'patronage' aspect of the early modern doctor-patient relationship meant that doctors had to show considerable respect for the medical opinions of their well-to-do patients.[46] Clowes eventually convinced the man that his case was venereal, but his care remained a private affair.[47]

By contrast, the diagnoses that Clowes rendered at the gates of St. Bartholomew's Hospital on the people he continuously referred to as 'idle rogues and vagabonds' were hardly as discreet; nor were they likely as courteous. Importantly, the attitudes that Clowes and the hospital governors held towards pauper patients become evident and these seem to have made a difference. Accusations that hospital patients were 'feigning' some other disease indicate significant tension, stemming from underlying assumptions that hospital authorities made about pauper patients' honesty. Because they came to see patient-deception as such an ongoing dilemma, governors came to doubt the integrity of any patient whose own diagnosis differed from that of their surgeons. Here the period's increasing intolerance

---

[44]Foucault, *The Birth of the Clinic*; Porter, 'Rise of the Physical Exam'; Fissell, 'The Disappearance of the Patient's Narrative.'

[45]This well established aspect of the early modern medical exchange has been described variously. For example, see Porter and Porter, *Patient's Progress*, pp. 78–79; Lindemann, *Medicine and Society*, pp. 195–199. On lay self-diagnosis see Wear, *Knowledge and Practice in English Medicine*, pp. 105–116. A fresh look at the active patient can be found in Pelling, *Medical Conflicts*, pp. 225–274.

[46]The work on active patients owes a great deal to Jewson's 'Medical Knowledge and the Patronage System.'

[47]Clowes, *Brief and Necessary Treatise*, pp. 195–196.

towards the poor and the influence of the pox on that attitude played an important role.[48]

Such speculation about foul patients' characters held tangible ramifications. For example, both hospitals' governors assumed the worst about patients who applied for admission a second time. Since contemporaries believed strongly in a cure, hospital authorities assumed that any patient that returned to the foul wards a second time must have re-infected themselves by returning to a life of vice. For this reason both hospitals made it a standing rule to refuse readmission to foul patients. They were given one chance; notably, this rule that did not apply to clean (i.e. non-venereal) patients.[49] At Bart's some returning patients tried to avoid detection by circumventing the admissions committee and applying directly at the outhouses. However, the hospital ordered the outhouse surgeons to report all such patients. To prevent what they considered recidivism, the governors threatened to fine the outhouse surgeons if they readmitted any foul patients covertly.[50]

Such policies unique to the foul wards begin to highlight that there were two classes of patients in these hospitals, the clean and the foul. There can be no doubt that there existed a hierarchy of care and that the foul were at its bottom. One instance conveys the point especially well. Both hospitals suffered serious financial crises following the Great Fire of London when each lost many of their rental properties in the blaze.[51] In a telling development, both hospitals, independently, cut back on their provision for venereal patients. Bart's met just a few days after the fire and closed down the outhouses virtually as its first cost cutting measure.[52] Not long after, St. Thomas's struck its 'Committee on Burnt Houses' charged with reducing costs. It quickly closed half of St. Thomas's foul wards.[53] The actions of both hospitals immediately indicate where venereal patients stood within the larger schemes of care at both institutions. These hospitals considered it a duty to extend care to the venereal poor. However, when push came to shove they compromised that obligation in order to continue providing care for the 'clean.'

48Arrizabalaga, Henderson and French, *The Great Pox,* p. 282.

49LMA H1/ST/A2, p. 81; H1/ST/A4/5, fol. 160. Parsons, *History of St. Thomas's,* vol. 2:104.

50SBH, HA 1/7, fol. 147, SBH, HA 1/8, fol. 19.

51Moore, *History of St. Bartholomew's,* pp. 328–329, 505; Parsons, *History of St. Thomas's,* vol. 2:100–101.

52SBH, HA 1/6, fol. 26.

53LMA, H1/ST/A4/5, fol. 160.

The period of tight finances that followed the Great Fire also affected therapeutics. Prior to the fire the hospitals utilized guaiac for some patients. Hailed as a wonder drug that treated the pox gently, it was believed to save patients from the famous tortures of mercury.[54] However, when resources became scarce the expensive drug went on the chopping block. After the fire, St. Thomas's declared the drug too expensive and halted its use.[55] Owsei Temkin once suggested that a therapeutic class divide existed with elite patients utilizing the gentle guaiac while the poor suffered through mercury. Indeed, Temkin offered the insightful suggestion that mercurial salivation, by all accounts a dreadful process, may have served an alternative purpose as a form of harsh discipline upon the unruly poor.[56] Hospital records indicate that up to the 1660s at least some London paupers were saved mercury's torments, receiving the more gentle treatment in the royal hospitals.[57] However, as money became tight this option faded and the divide that Temkin suggests came further into focus.

These financial crises had another significant impact on the foul wards. When Bart's reopened the outhouses its governors made it incumbent on patients to pay a portion of the costs of their care.[58] Venereal patients became the first hospital patients in England required to pay admission fees. There was now no doubting that two classes of patients existed, for the fee structure at both hospitals institutionalized it. Now patients in the clean wards continued to receive care that was truly charitable (i.e. free) while patients in the foul wards had to pay to get a bed. This undoubtedly impacted the accessibility of hospital care for the London poor and likely gave patients added incentive to challenge their diagnosis at the hospital gates. Now being labeled foul by the admitting surgeon not only had possible repercussions for one's reputation, but might mean that hospital care was simply beyond one's reach. Increasingly, the very poor who

---

[54]Quétel, *History of Syphilis,* pp. 29–32; Cunningham and Grell, *Four Horsemen of the Apocalypse,* pp. 258–260; Arrizabalaga, Henderson and French, *The Great Pox,* pp. 100–102.

[55]LMA, H1/ST/A4/5, fol. 158; On the price of the guaiac cure see also Flood and Shaw, 'The Price of the Pox.'

[56]Temkin, 'On the History of "Morality and Syphilis",' pp. 474–477. On the use of mercury see Arrizabalaga, Henderson and French, *The Great Pox*, pp. 139–144; Quétel, *History of Syphilis,* pp. 83–86.

[57]On the provision of guaiac to the poor in Italian hospitals see Arrizabalaga, Henderson and French, *The Great Pox,* pp. 189–190, 199–201, 207–209 and 230–232.

[58]In 1667 Bart's demanded that foul patients pay an unnamed fee to the outhouse surgeons, and in 1668 the governors reserved some outhouse beds for private patients who paid their costs entirely. SBH, HA 1/6, fols. 40 and 76.

aspired to get a hospital bed would have to go to their parish and hope that their churchwardens might pay for their hospitalization. Even if such patients succeeded, it meant that they had to negotiate a second, entirely separate, level of bureaucracy and face public exposure twice.[59] Bart's tried to roll back the fees in 1679 when its finances improved.[60] However, another fire decimated the hospitals' rental properties in 1696 with the same financial effect. Bart's renewed its fees, and this time they became permanent.[61] St. Thomas's soon followed suit.[62] Moreover, even when the hospitals brought in fees for clean patients in the eighteenth century the fee schedule at both hospitals always determined that costs in the foul wards were considerably more expensive.[63]

Admission fees were not the only policies unique to the foul wards. Other rules related to discipline and reform. Recent studies on health care and poor relief in Protestant and Catholic Europe have made the point that a key difference in manifestations of charity was a greater tendency by Catholic benefactors to continue the medieval tradition of balancing physical healing with spiritual healing. Whereas Protestant forms of public health care tended to move away from overt attempts to save patients' souls, Catholic institutions continued to make this an important goal.[64] If saving a body *and* a soul formed the heart of their dual charitable mission, who posed a better target for Catholic care than the poxed?[65] Their disease might kill them and their lifestyle might condemn them. The desire to heal tapped into renewed Catholic vigour for *caritas* in the Counter-Reformation. If the doctrine of good works meant anything, it meant helping those who needed it the most, and few among the needy could match the pathos of those afflicted with this new crippling disease. While on the one hand the links between the *mal francese* and leprosy helped craft the poxed as people who needed to be segregated, on the other hand it also meant that

---

59On medical care at the parish level see Wear, 'Caring for the Sick Poor'; Pelling, *Common Lot,* pp. 63–102; and Siena, *Venereal Disease, Hospitals and the Urban Poor,* pp. 135–180.

60SBH, HA 1/7, fols. 78, 123.

61SBH, HA 1/8, fol. 127

62LMA, H1/ST/A4/6, fol. 172.

63For example, by 1730 venereal patients' fees were double the fees demanded of other patients; by 1771 they were triple. Siena, *Venereal Disease, Hospitals and the Urban Poor,* pp. 102–106.

64See the parallel discussions in *Health Care and Poor Relief in Protestant Europe* and *Health Care and Poor Relief in Counter-Reformation Europe.*

65Henderson, 'Charity and Welfare in Early Modern Tuscany,' p. 71; Palmer, 'Ad Una Sancta Perfettione,' p. 88.

the poxed took up the place vacated by the disappearance of lepers as one of the most poignant recipients of Catholic charity.

Indeed, Arrizabalaga, Henderson and French's exploration of Italian pox hospitals and Laura McGough's contribution to this book have borne this out. They demonstrate that Italian authorities balanced moral reformation programs alongside traditional therapeutics as significant components of the *Incurabili* hospitals' regimens of care, indicating links between these hospitals and such classic Counter-Reformation institutions as the fallen women's asylums that sought to reform prostitutes and wayward girls.[66] The picture of a subtle but important confessional divide drawn by Grell, Cunnigham and Arrizabalaga seems apt when we contrast the English and Italian hospitals that treated the pox in the sixteenth century. We do not find Bart's or St. Thomas's using the foul wards to initiate similar moral reform programs or otherwise 'save' foul patients beyond providing basic Anglican service, something they did for all patients.[67] Indeed, it would take two more centuries before English pox hospitals began establishing the sorts of fallen women's asylums similar to the Italian institutions described by McGough, a difference that again underscores the need for further comparative research. However, at the dawn of the seventeenth century we begin to see, if not attempts to reform patients, serious attempts to discipline them. Claude Quétel has suggested that the seventeenth century witnessed 'a change in the moral landscape' regarding the disease, as the pox came to be viewed with increasing contempt.[68] Looking at London hospital care, it is hard to disagree.

Beginning in 1599, St. Thomas's initiated the practice of publicly whipping its venereal patients. In July the administration stated

> forasmuch as it is credibly informed to this court by some of the almoners that very many of the poor people that are taken in to be cured in this hospitall are visited with the French Disease and that it is very likely that many of them do get the same by lewd and incontinent life. Therefore it is ordered that from henceforth such of the same people as shall be noted and known as notorious and lewde livers shall, after they be cured, have some punishment inflicted upon them at the cross before they be suffered to be pass away. That by the terror thereof others may be admonished from falling into the like vice.[69]

[66]Arrizabalaga, Henderson and French, *The Great Pox,* pp. 173–176.
[67]SBH, HA 1/5, fol. 319; HA 1/7, fols. 107 and 171.
[68]Quétel, *History of Syphilis,* pp. 73–75.
[69]Cit. in Parsons, *History of St. Thomas's,* vol. 1:240–241.

The order gave patients frightening new incentive to conceal their illness at the hospital gates and contest any surgeon who tried to declare them foul. The policy also indicates, yet again, that assumptions about patients' character made by hospital administrators counted for quite a lot. The assumption that many patients led a 'lewd and incontinent life' clearly drove the administration to implement this policy. It is significant that the order does not stipulate that every foul patient must be flogged, only those deemed to be 'lewde.' However, there is no evidence to indicate how or by whom that decision was reached. Presumably, married people and known wet nurses might stand a chance of avoiding the punishment by blaming their infection on an unfaithful spouse or infected infant. Given the non-sexual forms of contagion that physicians still believed,[70] we are probably safe in assuming that many patients did everything they could to convince hospital authorities that they caught their pox from a someone's cup, bed-linen, or dirty shirt. Unfortunately, we must also assume that the majority of those who failed in their attempts to convince suffered the flogging.

This punishment was not just intended to make patients see the errors of their ways. It was intended to send a message to others; the whipping was purposely public. It stands to reason that this beating served the same purpose as other public punishments and shaming rituals central to social policing efforts in the period. Historians have made the period renowned for rough music, the ducking stool, the stocks, and the pillory.[71] St. Thomas's public whipping mirrors other contemporary rituals of rough shaming that aimed to preserve the social order by tarnishing transgressors publicly while teaching them a painful physical lesson. When exploring the social meanings of violence, Susan Dwyer Amussen has stressed that 'spectacle was central' to corporeal punishment in early modern England, noting that rituals that combined violence and shaming, such as public whipping, were most often connected with moral offences.[72] St. Thomas's punishment of 'lewde' foul patients falls right in line with her description.

70Clowes, *Short and Profitable Treatise,* fol. 5; Lowe, *An Easie, Certaine, and Perfect Method,* chap. 3; Peter, *Description of the Venereal Disease,* p. 6; Fabricius, *Syphilis in Shakespeare's England,* p. 20

71On charivaris see Davis, 'The Reasons of Misrule,' reprinted in her *Society and Culture,* pp. 97–123. For an overview of corporeal punishment see Ruff, *Violence in Early Modern Europe,* pp. 96–100.

72Amussen, 'Punishment, Discipline, and Power,' p. 11; Dabhoiwala, 'Sex, Social Relations and the Law,' pp. 85–101; See also the work on scolds. Amussen, *An Ordered Society,* pp. 117–133; Underdown, 'The Taming of the Scold.'

Later reference to corporeal punishment indicates that the practice continued at least until the middle of the century. In 1649, the hospital reiterated that foul patients, once cured, were not to be re-admitted. In January of that year the hospital amended the rule. Instead of refusing to re-admit venereal patients altogether, the governors ordered that they be whipped: 'that henceforward none of the Fowle Disease once p[er]fectly cured and put out be after received in for the same disease except hee or shee first receive the punishment of this house for the same if by the opinion of the surgeons or credible report the same be received by ill courses.'[73] This order put the surgeons in a powerful, yet possibly compromising position. On the one hand, they could vouch for a returning patient and save them the pain and embarrassment of public whipping. However, to do so was to make a public claim to their employers that their original work was faulty. In other words, for a surgeon to save a patient from being whipped he had to claim that his original treatment had failed, and therefore the patient's symptoms represented an old pox, not one newly acquired through 'ill courses.' Considering the contemporary confidence that the disease could be cured, the importance of doctors' reputations to their livelihoods, and the assumptions made about foul patients' integrity and propensity to deceive, it becomes difficult to imagine that this happened in the majority of cases.

Conclusion: Mercy, Scorn, and Need

> I do speak it with griefe of mind, that in the Hospitall of Saint Bartholomew in London, there hath beene cured of this disease by me and three others, within five years, to the number of one thousand and more. I speake nothing of Saint Thomas Hospitall, and other houses about the citie, wherein an infinite multitude are dailey cured. The Masters of the foresaid Hospitalls, being moved with devotion, and a christianlike care towards these wicked and sinful creatures, are daily inforced to take in a number of these diseased people.[74]
>
> –William Clowes, 1596

The evidence from hospitals reveals enormous tension surrounding the issues of poverty and the pox in early modern London. With the exception of a very brief period following the Great Fire, Bart's and St. Thomas's

---

73LMA, H1/ST/A6/1, p. 81.

74Clowes, *Brief and Necessary Treatise,* p. 150.

treated venereal patients consistently – *en masse* – for a century and a half. The pox did not bar charity, despite all the cultural baggage that accompanied this disease in early modern England. The sheer numbers alone speak volumes. Clowes claimed that of every twenty patients admitted by Bart's ten had the pox.[75] It was an exaggeration. However, it was not as great as some may have thought. Half of Bart's clientele did not enter the foul wards, but almost a quarter did.

Clowes is one of the most frequently cited Elizabethan authorities on venereal disease. Of course, this is partially because his publications are some of the earliest English treatises that we have on the disease; they went into multiple editions long after his death. However, I also suspect that scholars frequently cite Clowes because he had a knack for saying a great deal in a relatively short space. Consider all that he packs into the sentence that ends the passage above: 'The Masters of the foresaid Hospitalls, being moved with devotion, and a christianlike care towards these wicked and sinful creatures, are daily inforced to take in a number of these diseased people.' In a sense all the key elements of the story of hospital care for the pox are captured in this single sentence. These elements are mercy, scorn and need.

Who can doubt that those in charge of the royal hospitals were moved by 'devotion and christianlike care?' Despite the providential interpretations of this disease, the widespread assumptions that the infected deserved it, the increasingly harsh attitudes towards the poor, the drift toward puritanism in the era of the religious wars, or the 'change in the moral landscape' regarding the pox after 1600, the royal hospitals never shunned these patients. To the contrary, they each devoted a major portion of their overall resources towards treating them. It is likely that the governors, just like Clowes himself, saw themselves as offering mercy to the needy in the name of Christ.

However, Clowes immediately describes the recipients of his Christian mercy as 'wicked and sinful.' The foul would never be ordinary hospital clients. Both St. Thomas's and St. Bartholomew's set them off as a unique class of patient. Obviously the policy of segregation made this quickly apparent. As Robert Jütte has shown, the practice of institutional isolation was itself a way of stigmatizing particular segments of the underclass.[76] However, the policies unique to the foul, which went well beyond quarantine, were informed by a set of assumptions derived from the unique

[75]Clowes, *Brief and Necessary Treatise,* p. 150.

[76]Jütte, *Poverty and Deviance*, pp. 165–167.

nature of this ailment. The hospitals offered mercy, but it was a one-time deal. Returning patients were routinely assumed to have returned to their bawdy ways and were now left to suffer the consequences, cut off from the Christian hand of charity. Moreover, while the foul were ultimately deemed worthy of care, they were the first to feel budgetary cuts when resources became scarce. If it came down to choosing between caring for a clean patient or a foul one, that choice was clear. Indeed the 'charitable' nature of care itself became malleable as both hospitals brought in admission fees, shifting some of the financial burden for treatment onto the shoulders of these 'wicked and sinful' patients. At a time when hospital fees were still unheard of in England, no one raised opposition to the proposal to make the foul pay. After all, they were fortunate to get any care at all. Further, as the seventeenth century dawned and England began to witness increased attempts to crack down on such things as alehouses, adultery, gambling, and popular religion, hospitals contributed to the cause of moral policing, rendering the divide between the clean and the foul starker than ever. Forcing the foul to face the lash, hospital authorities punished patients' bodies in a public ritual that made a statement about moral probity.

So these hospitals' 'christianlike care' for the 'wicked' demonstrated equal parts mercy and scorn. But these alone do not tell the tale. Clowes' poignant statement concluded that hospitals were 'daily *inforced* to take in...these diseased people.' [my emphasis] There was an element of obligation here. Certainly, at the individual level hospital administrators had great latitude to refuse patients, especially those who had been in the hospital before or those they deemed to be liars. However, it is not clear that they could refuse the poxed *en masse*. Clowes' general description of London's situation – its streets teeming with infected people who crowded the hospital gates week after week – seems accurate. The sheer scope of the twin problems of poverty and the pox in early modern London indicates that, as on the Continent, authorities could not simply turn their backs with a shrug of moral indignation. Lurking beneath the surface of these hospitals lies a constant triangulated conflict between that indignation, a Christian drive for mercy, and a civic obligation to address a public health crisis.

Finally, none of this was lost on the patients themselves who give every sign that they tried to negotiate their hospitalization on their own terms as best they could. Mercy. Scorn. Need. Patients undoubtedly had their own take on these factors, seeking to tap into available mercy while mitigating public scorn, all the while driven by quite considerable need.

Trent University
Peterborough, Canada

CITED WORKS

Manuscript Sources

London. London Metropolitan Archives (LMA)
St. Thomas's Hospital, General Court of Governors Minutes, 1556–1735. HT/ST/A4/1–7.
St. Thomas's Hospital, Grand Committee Minutes, 1634–1690, H1/ST/A6/1–2.
London. St. Bartholomew's Hospital Archive, (SBH)
St. Bartholomew's Hospital, Journal of Governors Minutes, 1549–1708, HA 1/1–8.
St. Bartholomew's Hospital, Annual Ledgers, 1622–1696, HB 1/4–1/10.

Published Sources

Adler, M. W. 'History of the Development of a Service for the Venereal Diseases' *Journal of the Royal Society of Medicine,* 75 (1982): 124–128.

Allen, Peter Lewis, *The Wages of Sin: Sex and Disease, Past and Present.* Chicago: University of Chicago Press, 2000.

Amussen, Susan Dwyer. *An Ordered Society: Gender and Class in Early Modern England.* New York: Basil Blackwell, 1988.

Amussen, Susan Dwyer. 'Punishment, Discipline, and Power: The Social Meanings of Violence in Early Modern England' *Journal of British Studies,* 34:1 (1995): 1 34.

Anonymous, *Some Reasons of a Member of the Committee, &c. of the Trustees of the Infirmary in James Street Westminster, near St. James Park, for his dividing against the Admission of Venereal Patients.* London, 1738.

Anselment, Raymond. 'Seventeenth-Century Pox: The Medical and Literary Realities of Venereal Disease' *Seventeenth Century,* 4 (1989): 189–211.

Anselment, Raymond. *The Realms of Apollo: Literature and Healing in Seventeenth-Century England.* Newark: University of Delaware Press, 1995

Arrizabalaga, Jon, John Henderson, and Roger French. *The Great Pox: The French Disease in Renaissance Europe.* New Haven: Yale University Press, 1997.

Blanckaert, Steven. *A New Method of Curing the French-Pox.* Amsterdam: John Taylor and Thomas Newborough, 1690.

Boulton, Jeremy. *Neighbourhood and Society: A London Suburb in the Seventeenth Century.* Cambridge: Cambridge University Press, 1987.

Brody, Saul N. *The Disease of the Soul: Leprosy in Medieval Literature.* Ithaca: Cornell University Press, 1974.

Browner, Jessica A. 'Wrong Side of the River: London's Disreputable South Bank in the Sixteenth and Seventeenth Century' *Essays in History,* 36 (1994): 34–71.

Bynum, W.F. 'Treating the Wages of Sin: Venereal Disease and Specialism in Eighteenth-Century Britain' pp. 7–47 in *Medical Fringe and Medical Orthodoxy, 1750–1850,* eds. W. F. Bynum and Roy Porter. London: Croom Helm, 1987.

Clowes, William. *A Short and Profitable Treatise Touching on the Cure of a Disease now called Morbus Gallicus*. London, I. Daye, 1579.

Clowes, William. *A Brief and Necessary Treatise, Touching on the Cure of the Disease now called Lues Venerea, by Unctions and Other Approved Waies of Curing: Newly Corrected and Augmented in the Yeare of our Lord 1596*. London, Edm. Bollifant, 1596.

Cook, Harold. *The Decline of the Old Medical Regime in Late Stuart London*. Ithaca: Cornell University Press, 1986.

Cunningham, Andrew and Ole Peter Grell. *The Four Horsemen of the Apocalypse: Religion, War, Famine and Death in Reformation Europe*. Cambridge: Cambridge University Press, 2000.

Daly, Christopher, 'The Hospitals of London: Administration, Refoundation, and Benefaction, c. 1500–1572.' D.Phil. Diss. Oxford University, 1993.

Davenport-Hines, Richard. *Sex, Death and Punishment: Attitudes to Sex and Sexuality in Britain Since the Renaissance*. London: Collins, 1990.

Davis, N. Z. *Society and Culture in Early Modern France*. Stanford, CA: Stanford University Press, 1975.

Dabhoiwala, Faramerz. 'Sex, Social Relations and the Law in Seventeenth- and Eighteenth-Century London' pp. 85–101 in *Negotiating Power in Early Modern Society: Order, Hierarchy and Subordination in Britain and Ireland,* eds. Michael J. Braddick and John Walter. Cambridge: Cambridge University Press, 2001.

Ell, Stephan R. 'Blood and Sexuality in Medieval Leprosy' *Janus,* 71 (1984): 153–164.

Fabricius, Johannes. *Syphilis in Shakespeare's England*. London, Kingsley Publishers, 1994.

Fissell, Mary. 'The Disappearance of the Patient's Narrative and the Invention of Hospital Medicine' pp. 92–109 in *British Medicine in an Age of Reform*, eds. Roger French and Andrew Wear. London: Routledge, 1991.

Flood, John L. and David J. Shaw, 'The Price of the Pox in 1527: Johannes Sinapius and the Guaiac Cure' *Bibliothèque d'Humanisme et Renaissance,* 54:3 (1992): 691–707.

Foa Anna. 'The New and the Old: The Spread of Syphilis (1494–1530)' pp. 26–45 in *Sex and Gender in Historical Perspective,* eds. Edward Muir and Guido Ruggiero. Baltimore: The Johns Hopkins University Press, 1990.

Foucault, Michel. *The Birth of the Clinic: An Archaeology of Medical Perception,* trans. Alan Sheridan. New York: Pantheon, 1973.

Gowing, Laura. 'Secret Births and Infanticide in Seventeenth-Century England' *Past and Present,* 156 (1997): 87–115.

Health Care and Poor Relief in Counter-Reformation Europe. eds. Ole Peter Grell, Andrew Cunningham and Jon Arrizabalaga, London Routledge, 1999.

Health Care and Poor Relief in Protestant Europe, 1500–1700. eds. Ole Peter Grell, and Andrew Cunningham, London: Routledge, 1997.

Henderson, John. 'Charity and Welfare in Early Modern Tuscany' pp. 56–86 in *Health Care and Poor Relief in Counter-Reformation Europe*, eds. Ole Peter Grell, Andrew Cunningham and Jon Arrizabalaga. London: Routledge, 1999.

Honeybourne, Marjorie B. 'The Leper Hospitals of the London Area' *Transactions of the London and Middlesex Archaeological Society,* 21 (1963): 1–61.

Jewson, Nicholas. 'Medical Knowledge and the Patronage System in Eighteenth-Century England' *Sociology*, 8 (1974): 369–385.

Jütte, Robert. *Poverty and Deviance in Early Modern Europe*. Cambridge: Cambridge University Press, 1994.

Jütte, Robert. 'Syphilis and Confinement: Hospitals in Early Modern Germany' pp. 97–115 in *Institutions of Confinement: Hospitals, Asylums, and Prisons in Western Europe and North America, 1500–1950,* eds. Norbert Finzsch and Robert Jütte. Cambridge: Cambridge University Press, 1996.

Klein, Lawrence E. 'Politeness for Plebes: Consumption and Social Identity in early eighteenth-century England' pp. 362–382 in *The Consumption of Culture 1660–1800: Image, Object, Text,* eds. Ann Bermingham and John Brewer. London: Routledge, 1995.

López Terrada, María Luz, 'El tratamiento de la sífilis en un hospital renacentista: la sala del mal de siment del Hospital General de Valencia' *Asclepio*, 41:2 (1989): 19–50.

Lowe, Peter. *An Easie, Certaine, and Perfect Method, to Cure and Prevent the Spanish Sicknes*. London: James Roberts, 1596.

Orme, Nicholas, and Margaret Webster, *The English Hospital, 1070–1570*. New Haven: Yale University Press, 1995.

Palmer, Richard. '"Ad Una Sancta Perfettione:" Health Care and Poor Relief in the Republic of Venice in the Era of the Counter Reformation' pp. 87–101 in *Health Care and Poor Relief in Counter-Reformation Europe*, eds. Ole Peter Grell, Andrew Cunningham and Jon Arrizabalaga. London: Routledge, 1999.

Parsons, Frederick Gymer. *The History of St. Thomas's Hospital.* 3 vols. London: Methuen, 1932.

Pelling Margaret. 'Appearance and Reality: Barber-Surgeons, the Body and Disease' pp. 82–112 in *London 1500–1700: The Making of the Metropolis,* eds. A. L. Beier and Roger Finlay. London: Longman, 1986.

Pelling Margaret. *The Common Lot: Sickness, Medical Occupations and the Urban Poor in Early Modern England*. London: Longman, 1998.

Pelling Margaret. *Medical Conflicts in Early Modern London: Patronage, Physicians and Irregular Practitioners 1550–1640*. Oxford: Oxford University Press, 2003.

Pepys, Samuel. *The Diary of Samuel Pepys,* eds. Robert Latham and William Matthews. 11 vols. Berkeley: University of California Press, 1970.

Peter, Charles. *Description of the Venereal Disease, Declaring the Causes, Signs, Effects, and Cure thereof.* London: Printed for the Author, 1678.

Peter, Charles. *Observations on the Venereal Disease, with the True Way of Curing the Same*. London: S.D. and D.N., 1693.

Plater, Felix, Abdiah Cole, and Nicholas Culpeper. *A Golden Practice of Physick in Five Books and Three Tomes* London: Peter Cole, 1662.

Porter, Dorothy, and Roy Porter. *Patient's Progress: Doctors and Doctoring in Eighteenth-Century England*. Oxford: Polity Press, 1989.

Porter, Roy. *Health For Sale: Quackery in England 1660–1850*. Manchester: Manchester University Press, 1989.

Porter, Roy. 'The Rise of the Physical Exam' pp. 179–197 in *Medicine and the Five Senses,* eds. W. F. Bynum and Roy Porter. Cambridge: Cambridge University Press, 1993

Quétel, Claude. *The History of Syphilis,* trans. Judith Braddock and Brian Pike. Baltimore: The Johns Hopkins University Press, 1990.

Risse, Guenter. *Mending Bodies, Saving Souls: A History of Hospitals.* Oxford: Oxford University Press, 1999.

Julius R. Ruff. *Violence in Early Modern Europe.* Cambridge: Cambridge University Press, 2001.

Schleiner, Winfried. 'Moral Attitudes Towards Syphilis and its Prevention in the Renaissance' *Bulletin of the History of Medicine,* 68 (1994): 389–410.

Shirley, John. *A Short Compendium of Chirurgery... With the Several Methods of Treating the French Pox.* London: W.G. and Charles Blount, 1678.

Shorter, Edward. *Women's Bodies: A Social History of Women's Encounter with Health, Ill-Health, and Medicine.* New Brunswick, N.J.: Transactions Publications, 1991.

Siena, Kevin P. 'The "Foul Disease" and Privacy: The Effects of Venereal Disease and Patient Demand on the Medical Marketplace in Early Modern London' *Bulletin of the History of Medicine,* 75:2 (2001):199–224.

Siena, Kevin P. *Venereal Disease, Hospitals and the Urban Poor: London's "Foul Wards" 1600–1800.* Rochester: University of Rochester Press, 2004.

Stone, Lawrence. *The Family, Sex and Marriage in England, 1500–1800.* London: Weidenfeld and Nicolson, 1977.

Temkin, Owsei. 'On the History of "Morality and Syphilis"' pp. 472–484 in his *The Double Face of Janus and Other Essays in the History of Medicine.* Baltimore: The Johns Hopkins University Press, 1977.

Trumbach, Randolph. *Sex and the Gender Revolution, vol. 1: Heterosexuality and the Third Gender in Enlightenment London.* Chicago: University of Chicago Press, 1998.

Wear, Andrew. *Knowledge and Practice in English Medicine, 1550–1680.* Cambridge: Cambridge University Press, 2001.

Wear, Andrew. 'Caring for the Sick Poor in the Parish of St. Bartholomew Exchange, 1580–1679' pp. 41–60 in *Living and Dying in London,* eds. W. F. Bynum and Roy Porter. London: Wellcome Institute for the History of Medicine, 1991.

Williams, David Innes. *The London Lock: A Charitable Hospital for Venereal Disease 1746–1952.* London, Royal Society of Medicine Press, 1996.

Williams, Gordon. 'Venereal Associations of Leprosy' *Trivium,* 11 (1976): 64–77.

Underdown, David. 'The Taming of the Scold: The Enforcement of Patriarchal Authority in Early Modern England' pp. 116–136 in *Order and Disorder in Early Modern England,* eds. Anthony Fletcher and John Stephenson. Cambridge: Cambridge University Press, 1985.

Notes on Contributors

Jon Arrizabalaga is the Head of the Department of History of Science at the Consejo Superior de Investigaciones Científicas - Institució Milà i Fontanals, Barcelona. He currently works on the history of medicine, health and disease in late medieval and early modern Europe. He has co-authored (with John Henderson and Roger French) *The Great Pox: The French Disease in Renaissance Europe* (New Haven: Yale University Press, 1997).

Diane Cady is Assistant Professor in English at Mills College where she teaches late medieval and early modern literature and gender studies. She is currently completing a monograph titled *Damaged Goods: Gender and Commerce in the Canterbury Tales.*

David Gentilcore is Reader in History at the University of Leicester. He is the author of two monographs, *From Bishop to Witch: the System of the Sacred in Early Modern Terra d'Otranto* and *Healers and Healing in Early Modern Italy*, and is currently completing *Mixing Medicine and Buffoonery: Charlatans and Charlatanism in Early Modern Italy*. In 2001-2002 he was Hannah Visiting Professor at McMaster University, where his contribution to this volume was written.

Jonathan Gil Harris is Professor of English at George Washington University. He is the author of *Foreign Bodies and the Body Politic: Discourses of Social Pathology in Early Modern England* (1998) and *Sick Economies: Drama, Mercantilism and Disease in Shakespeare's England* (2004), and co-editor of *Staged Properties in Early Modern English Drama* (2002). His current book project is entitled *Untimely Matter: Reworking Material Culture in Shakespeare's England.*

Darin Hayton is Assistant Professor of history of science at Haverford College. His research focuses on the interplay between science and politics in the late medieval and early renaissance period, especially in the Germanies and the Holy Roman Empire. He also works on the transmission of scientific knowledge from Byzantium into the Latin west.

Roze Hentschell teaches courses in British literature and culture of the sixteenth and seventeenth centuries at Colorado State University. Her research interests include popular literature and material culture of the Renaissance and issues of nationalism. She is specifically interested in cultural representations of the textile industry in the early modern period and is at work on a full-length study, *The Culture of Cloth in Early Modern England.*

Mary Hewlett is Assistant Professor at the University of Windsor. She has published an article on the political implications for Lucca of Cosimo I de' Medici's foreign policy and is currently working on domestic violence in Late Renaissance Lucca.

Laura McGough is finishing postdoctoral work at Johns Hopkins University and the Center for Disease Control on an Association of Teachers of Preventive Medicine fellowship. With a Ph.D. in history from North- western University, she has taught at several universities, including the University of Ghana. She plans to work in international health.

Kevin Siena is Assistant Professor of History at Trent University. He has authored articles on the history of sex and disease in early modern Europe and most recently the monograph, *Venereal Disease, Hospitals and the Urban Poor: London's 'Foul Wards' 1600-1800* (2004). He is now at work on a study of the illness strategies of the urban poor in early modern London.

Dr. Domenico Zanrè is a Lecturer in Italian at the University of Glasgow in Scotland. His main research interests focus on the area of cultural production in Cinquecento Italy, and he has worked extensively on the sixteenth-century Florentine duchy of Cosimo I de' Medici. His latest book, *Cultural Non-Conformity in Early Modern Florence*, was published by Ashgate in 2004.

Index

Publications of the Centre for Reformation and Renaissance Studies

ISBN information is for paperback edition unless otherwise specified

Barnabe Riche Society Publications

Lodge, Thomas. *A Margarite of America*. Ed. by Henry Janzen and intro. by Don Beecher (2005), pp. 205. ISBN 0-7727-2027-4

Essays and Studies

Zirpolo, Lilian. *Ave Papa, Ave Papabile: The Sacchetti Family, Their Art Patronage, and Political Aspirations*. (2005), pp. 252. ISBN 0-7727-2028-2

Fantasies of Troy: Classical Tales and the Social Imaginary in Medieval and Early Modern Europe. Ed. by Alan Shepard and Stephen D. Powell (2004), pp. 306. ISBN 0-7727-2025-8

Shell Games: Studies in Scams, Frauds, and Deceits (1300–1650) Ed. by Mark Crane, Richard Raiswell and Margaret Reeves (2004), pp. 334. ISBN 0-7727-2023-1

A Renaissance of Conflicts: Visions and Revisions of Law and Society in Italy and Spain. Ed. by John Marino and Thomas Kuehn (2004), pp. 456. ISBN 0-7727-2022-3

The Renaissance in the Nineteenth Century / Le XIXe siècle renaissant. Ed. by Yannick Portebois and Nicolas Terpstra (2003), pp. 302. ISBN 0-7727-2019-3

The Premodern Teenager: Youth in Society 1150–1650. Ed. by Konrad Eisenbichler (2002), pp. 349. ISBN 0-7727-2018-5

Occasional Publications

Estes, James M. *The First Forty Years: A Brief History of the Centre for Reformation and Renaissance Studies*. (2004), pp. 106. ISBN 0-7727-2026-6

Annotated Catalogue of Editions of Erasmus at the Centre for Reformation and Renaissance Studies, Toronto. Comp. by Jacqueline Glomski and Erika Rummel (1994), pp. 153. ISBN 0-9697512-1-4

Register of Sermons Preached at St. Paul's Cross (1534–1642). Comp. by Millar MacLure and revised by Peter Pauls and Jackson Campbell Boswell (1989), pp. 152. ISBN 0-919473-48-2

Language and Literature. Early Printed Books at the CRRS. Comp. by Willian R. Bowen and Konrad Eisenbichler (1986), pp. 112. ISBN 0-7727-2009-6

Published Books (1499–1700) on Science, Medicine and Natural History at the CRRS Comp. by William R. Bowen and Konrad Eisenbichler (1986), pp. 37. ISBN 0-7727-2005-3

Bibles, Theological Treatises and Other Religious Literature, 1492–1700, at the CRRS. Comp. by Konrad Eisenbichler, Gay MacDonald and Robert Sweetman (1981), pp. 94. ISBN 0-7727-2002-9

Humanist Editions of Statutes and Histories at the CRRS. Comp. by Konrad Eisenbichler, Gay MacDonald and C. Turner (1980), pp. 63. ISBN 0-7727-2001-0

Humanist Editions of the Classics at the CRRS. Comp. N.L. Anderson, Kenneth R. Bartlett, Konrad Eisenbichler, and Janis Svilpis (1979), pp. 71. ISBN 0-7727-2000-2

Renaissance and Reformation Texts in Translation

Du Bellay, Ronsard, Sébillet. *Poetry and Language in 16th-Century France*. Trans. and intro. by Laura Willett (2004), pp.116. ISBN 0-7727-2021-5

Girolamo Savonarola. *A Guide to Righteous Living and Other Works*. Trans. and intro. by Konrad Eisenbichler (2003), pp. 243. ISBN 0-7727-2020-7

Godly Magistrates and Church Order: Johannes Brenz and the Establishment of the Lutheran Territorial Church in Germany, 1524–1559. Trans. and ed. by James M. Estes (2001), pp. 219. ISBN 0-7727-2017-7

Giovanni Della Casa. *Galateo: A Renaissance Treatise on Manners*. Trans. by Konrad Eisenbichler and Kenneth R. Bartlett. 3rd ed. (2001), pp. 98. ISBN 0-9697512-2-2

Romeo and Juliet Before Shakespeare: Four Stories of Star-Crossed Love. Trans. by Nicole Prunster (2000), pp. 127. ISBN 0-7727-2015-0

Jean Bodin. *On the Demon-Mania of Witches*. Abridged, trans. and ed. Randy A. Scott and Jonathan L. Pearl (1995), pp. 219. ISBN 0-9697512-5-7

Whether Secular Government Has the Right to Wield the Sword in Matters of Faith: A Controversy in Nürnberg in 1530. Trans. and ed. by James M. Estes (1994), pp. 118. ISBN 0-9697512-4-9

Lorenzo Valla. *'The Profession of the Religious' and Selections from 'The Falsely-Believed and Forged Donation of Constantine'*. Trans. and ed. Olga Z. Pugliese. 2nd ed. (1994), pp. 114. ISBN 0-9697512-3-0

A. Karlstadt, H. Emser, J. Eck. *A Reformation Debate: Karlstadt, Emser and Eck on Sacred Images*. Trans. and ed. Brian Mangrum and Giuseppe Scavizzi. 2nd edition (1991), pp. 112. ISBN 0-9697512-7-3

Nicholas of Cusa. *The Layman on Wisdom and the Mind*. Trans. Mark L. Feuhrer (1989), pp. 112. ISBN 0-919473-56-3

Bernardino Ochino. *Seven Dialogues*. Trans. and ed. Rita Belladonna (1988), pp. 96. ISBN 0-919473-63-6

Tudor and Stuart Texts

The Queen's Majesty's Passage and Related Documents. Ed. and intro by Germaine Warkentin. (2004), pp. 158. ISBN 0-7727-2024-X

Early Stuart Pastoral: 'The Shepherd's Pipe' by William Browne and others, and *'The Shepherd's Hunting' by George Wither.* Ed. and intro by James Doelman (1999), pp. 196. ISBN 0-9697512-9-X

The Trial of Nicholas Throckmorton. Ed. and intro by Annabel Patterson (1998), pp. 108. ISBN 0-9697512-8-1

James I. *The True Law of Free Monarchies* and *Basilikon Doron.* Ed. and intro by Daniel Fischlin and Mark Fortier (1996), pp. 181. ISBN 0-9697512-6-5

To order books, and for additional information, contact:
CRRS Publications, Victoria University
71 Queen's Park, Toronto ON, M5S 1K7, CANADA
tel: (416) 585-4465 / fax: (416) 585-4430
e-mail: <crrs.publications@utoronto.ca> / web: <www.crrs.ca>

MEMBER OF SCABRINI GROUP
Québec, Canada
2005